WITHDRAWN FROM LIBRARY

D1558941

Geriatric Home-Based Medical Care

Jennifer L. Hayashi • Bruce Leff
Editors

Linda DeCherrie • Theresa A. Soriano
Associate Editors

Geriatric Home-Based Medical Care

Principles and Practice

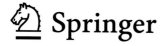

Editors
Jennifer L. Hayashi
Division of Geriatric Medicine and
    Gerontology
Johns Hopkins Bayview Medical Center
Baltimore, MD, USA

Bruce Leff
Division of Geriatric Medicine and
    Gerontology
Johns Hopkins Bayview Medical Center
Baltimore, MD, USA

ISBN 978-3-319-23364-2   ISBN 978-3-319-23365-9   (eBook)
DOI 10.1007/978-3-319-23365-9

Library of Congress Control Number: 2015956333

Springer Cham Heidelberg New York Dordrecht London
© Springer International Publishing Switzerland 2016
This work is subject to copyright. All rights are reserved by the Publisher, whether the whole or part of the material is concerned, specifically the rights of translation, reprinting, reuse of illustrations, recitation, broadcasting, reproduction on microfilms or in any other physical way, and transmission or information storage and retrieval, electronic adaptation, computer software, or by similar or dissimilar methodology now known or hereafter developed.
The use of general descriptive names, registered names, trademarks, service marks, etc. in this publication does not imply, even in the absence of a specific statement, that such names are exempt from the relevant protective laws and regulations and therefore free for general use.
The publisher, the authors and the editors are safe to assume that the advice and information in this book are believed to be true and accurate at the date of publication. Neither the publisher nor the authors or the editors give a warranty, express or implied, with respect to the material contained herein or for any errors or omissions that may have been made.

Printed on acid-free paper

Springer International Publishing AG Switzerland is part of Springer Science+Business Media
(www.springer.com)

Foreword

This is a timely and valuable book as home-based medical care or "house call medicine" is making an important and vital resurgence in American Medicine. While always a valuable and noble part of medical practice, house calls diminished dramatically over the last 50–60 years as medical specialization and sub-specialization came to dominate American health care. This specialty domination came also with increasing technical capabilities in diagnosis and treatment, predominantly available in hospitals, enabling these institutions to dominate health care in power, financing, and medical education.

Wide-ranging change in America's health care delivery system is emerging now, motivated by high health care costs and increasing concerns about patient safety and satisfaction often concerning hospital care. Because of these concerns, there is resurgence in home-based medicine among many venues. Academic medical centers, health care systems, community hospitals, health insurance companies, and community-based care delivery programs are now trying to expand or initiate programs in house calls.

Six generic trends are fueling the increasing interest in home-based medical care.

1. Changes in Patient Population: The population of seniors, especially those over 80 years of age, has increased greatly the number of individuals who are homebound with chronic disease and associated disability. Also now many younger individuals with chronic disease and disability are living in the community. The care of such individuals is very difficult and greatly burdensome for them without their being able to receive high-quality and comprehensive primary care in the home. Without high-quality home-based primary care programs such patients may require more frequent hospitalizations, visits to an emergency room, and institutionalization.

2. Health Care Delivery Innovation: Health care leaders recognize the value home-based medical care as a way to prevent recurrent hospitalizations and allow safe, early discharge of patients from hospitals and even, for selected patients, a substitute for admission to an acute care facility. These forms of hospital-linked home-based medical care have proven to be high-quality, cost-effective health care with high patient satisfaction. Even long-term care placement may be delayed or avoided with organized home-based medicine. Programs play important roles in improving care quality, patient satisfaction, and overall cost in the

management of many chronic illnesses such as heart failure, chronic pulmonary disease, and others that have been typically associated with frequent hospitalizations.

3. Ideal Care for Patients: Home visits are greatly appreciated by patients and their families. It is an altruistic pattern of care delivery and deeply rewarding for the health professional. House calls are invariably memorable and allow a clinician to know quickly a patient much more fully than possible when seen in the office or hospital. Such in-depth knowledge of a patient typically leads the health care provider to more thoughtful clinical judgments in advising ill patients and their caregivers. Visiting a patient at home builds a level of trust between patient, family, and health professional that is vital in providing the highest quality of care.

4. Team Care in Medicine: Medicine is increasingly team and multi-professionally based. Home-based medicine in recent decades has served as an exemplary model of such care. It is an ideal arena to develop and nurture effective team care and to teach trainees about the importance of and strategies for excellent interdisciplinary care. Team care is complex and requires the effective and efficient partnership of a variety of professionals. High-quality team care requires training and retraining. It demands skills not typically taught in depth in schools. Communications among professionals on a team must be punctual, focused, collaborative, respectful, pithy, wise, nurturing, patient-focused, and efficient. Team care when delivered well is superior to care provided by an individual. The patient benefits from the input of a variety of different professionals and the professionals benefit by sharing advice and insights from others.

5. Value in Medical Education: Home-based medical care in many training programs has become an important and valuable component of the education of students and postgraduate trainees. House calls require a clinician to hone his or her clinical skills in history taking and physical examination. The typical easy and immediate access to diagnostic testing in clinics, emergency rooms, or hospitals is not readily available in the patient's home and the clinician must think carefully and thoughtfully before ordering a test or procedure. This process requires that the clinician have a sensitive conversation with a patient before initiating a request for testing or treatment. Such communications are vital to high-quality care delivered in any venue but so often lost or not emphasized in hospital or clinic training venues. Being a guest as a clinician in a patient's home is a privilege that is at once informative, insightful, and humbling. All of these qualities are characteristic of clinical excellence. Scholars describing medical education in the United States over the last five or so decades suggest that we have lost the public trust by not always keeping the needs of our patients in focus. In any venue of health care delivery, the patient should always be the focus of attention and in charge of their own health care. House calls provide a poignant venue for such teaching.

6. Advances in Technology Available in the Home: The modern house call is quite different than that provided in the last century. No longer is a house call an isolated visit by a clinician. Now it is a system of care, typically team based and increasingly technologically sophisticated. Monitoring of patients, the transmission of

data and images, and the performance of sophisticated treatments are all possible at home. Technological advances do not diminish the need for the presence in the home of fine clinicians. If anything, they increase the need.

This book is edited by lifelong champions of home-based medical care. They have selected authors who are all experts and are deeply knowledgeable about the field. Most have created innovative programs. This book is a rich resource for professionals, students, trainees, and administrators who are committed to providing high-quality care for seniors.

The reader will gain useful information about home-based medical care and knowledge of the scientific work that supports their value. For society, this portends house calls as a promising and vital component of health care delivery systems. American medicine needs to regain the trust of the public in delivering appropriate, high-quality, satisfying, and cost-effective medical care that is truly patient centered. House call medicine is a vital component in regaining this public trust.

Baltimore, MD, USA   John R. Burton, M.D.

Preface

The health care system in the United States is changing. The physician house call, once the primary mode of health care delivery, was gradually relegated over the latter half of the twentieth century to a nostalgic footnote in textbooks of the history of medicine. However, tremendous growth in the population of older adults with chronic disease and disability, coupled with advances in medical technology over the past decade, has created both a need and an opportunity for a new model: medical house calls as part of a *system* of home-based medical care.

The larger health care system has been slow to adapt to this opportunity because of the economics of medical care, misconceptions about the safety and quality of home-based medical care, and a continuing bias in favor of facility-based medical care over care provided in the community setting. Comprehensive experiential education in home-based medical care is still rare in most physician, nurse practitioner (NP), and physician assistant (PA) training programs. This book is intended for clinicians who recognize the need for specialized knowledge, skills, and attitudes in providing care in the home setting, whether they are considering making their first medical house call or are already regularly caring for patients within an established home-based medical care program.

Experts in home-based medical care from highly respected programs and institutions across the country have collaborated to create this practical reference based on decades of shared experience and solid scientific evidence. We anticipate that the evidence base will continue to grow as this system of care expands and succeeds, along with meaningful quality assessments and outcome measures. We hope that this book serves both as a useful compendium of hands-on clinical advice and as a foundation for future development of the field of home-based medical care.

Baltimore, MD, USA

Jennifer Hayashi, M.D.
Bruce Leff, M.D.

Contents

Contributors

Sonica Bhatia Department of Geriatrics and Palliative Medicine and Department of Medicine, The Mount Sinai Hospital, New York, NY, USA

Peter A. Boling Virginia Commonwealth University, Richmond, VA, USA

John R. Burton Johns Hopkins Bayview Medical Center, Baltimore, MD, USA

Silvia Chavez The Mount Sinai Health System, New York, NY, USA

Jessica L. Colburn Division of Geriatric Medicine and Gerontology, Johns Hopkins University School of Medicine, Baltimore, MD, USA

Thomas Cornwell Home Centered Care Institute, Northwestern Medicine Hospital, Wheaton, IL, USA

Ericka L. Crouse Virginia Commonwealth University, Richmond, VA, USA

Linda DeCherrie Department of Geriatrics and Palliative Medicine, Icahn School of Medicine at Mount Sinai, New York, NY, USA

Christian Escobar Department of Medicine, The Mount Sinai Hospital, New York, NY, USA

Thomas Finucane Department of Geriatric Medicine and Gerontolgoy, Johns Hopkins Bayview Medical Center, Baltimore, MD, USA

Peter M. Gliatto Departments of Medicine and Medical Education, Geriatrics and Palliative Medicine, Icahn School of Medicine at Mount Sinai, New York, NY, USA

Lyons T. Hardy Virginia Commonwealth University, Richmond, VA, USA

Jennifer L. Hayashi Division of Geriatric Medicine and Gerontology, Johns Hopkins University School of Medicine, Baltimore, MD, USA

Cameron R. Hernandez The Mount Sinai Health System, New York, NY, USA

Elizabeth M. Jones Visiting Doctors Program, Mount Sinai Hospital, New York, NY, USA

K. Eric De Jonge MedStar Washington Hospital Center, Washington, DC, USA

Department of Geriatrics, Medstar Washington Hospital Center, Washington, DC, USA

Helen Kao Department of Geriatrics, Internal Medicine, University of California San Francisco, San Francisco, CA, USA

Fred C. Ko Brookdale Department of Geriatrics and Palliative Medicine, Icahn School of Medicine at Mount Sinai, New York, NY, USA

M. Victoria M. Kopke The Mount Sinai Health System, New York, NY, USA

Claire K. Larson Department of Medicine, Division of Geriatrics, University of California-San Francisco, San Francisco, CA, USA

Bruce Leff Division of Geriatric Medicine, Johns Hopkins University School of Medicine, Baltimore, MD, USA

Yasmin S. Meah Medical Education, Medicine and Geriatrics and Palliative Care, Icahn School of Medicine at Mount Sinai, New York, NY, USA

Kara R. Murphy DuPage Health Coalition, Carol Stream, IL, USA

Ritesh A. Ramdhani Movement Disorders Division, Department of Neurology and Neurosurgery, Icahn School of Medicine at Mount Sinai, New York, NY, USA

Jonathan A. Ripp Departments of Medicine, Geriatrics and Palliative Medicine, and Medical Education, Mount Sinai Hospital, New York, NY, USA

Christine Ritchie Division of Geriatrics, Department of Medicine, University of California San Francisco, San Francisco, CA, USA

David Skovran Department of Medicine, Icahn School of Medicine at Mount Sinai, New York, NY, USA

Theresa A. Soriano Department of Geriatrics and Palliative Medicine, Icahn School of Medicine at Mount Sinai, New York, NY, USA

George A. Taler MedStar Washington Hospital Center, Washington, DC, USA

Department of Geriatrics, Medstar Washington Hospital Center, Washington, DC, USA

Martha L. Twaddle Palliative Medicine, Northwestern University Feinberg School of Medicine, Chicago, IL, USA

Ania Wajnberg Department of Medicine and Department of Geriatrics and Palliative Medicine, The Mount Sinai Hospital, New York, NY, USA

Meng Zhang Department of Medicine, Department of Geriatrics and Palliative Medicine, Icahn School of Medicine at Mount Sinai, New York, NY, USA

Part I

Fundamentals

Introducing Home-Based Medical Care

1

Jennifer L. Hayashi and Bruce Leff

Abstract

As the population ages, home-based medical care becomes increasingly important in the care of frail, functionally impaired older adults. Unfortunately, formal education in home-based medical care is limited, and misconceptions abound. This book is intended to be a practical clinical reference for health care providers who practice medicine in the home. Home-based medical care is highly relevant to the evolving health service delivery system in the USA, but terminology related to this field can be confusing. We adopt the term "home-based medical care" to emphasize the relevance of this practice model as part of the contemporary health care system.

Keywords

Home-based medical care • Medical house calls • Medical home visits • Geriatric medicine

1.1 Key Points

1. Home-based medical care is important in the care of frail, functionally impaired older adults.
2. Formal education in home-based medical care is limited, and misconceptions abound.
3. Home-based medical care is highly relevant to the evolving health service delivery system in the USA.

J.L. Hayashi, M.D. (✉) • B. Leff, M.D.
Division of Geriatric Medicine and Gerontology, Johns Hopkins University School of Medicine, 5200 Eastern Avenue- Suite 2200, Baltimore, MD 21044, USA
e-mail: jhayash1@jhmi.edu

© Springer International Publishing Switzerland 2016
J.L. Hayashi, B. Leff (eds.), *Geriatric Home-Based Medical Care*,
DOI 10.1007/978-3-319-23365-9_1

3

4. This book is intended to be a practical clinical reference for health-care providers who practice medicine in the home.
5. Terminology related to this field can be confusing. We adopt the term "home-based medical care" to emphasize the relevance of this practice model as part of the contemporary health care system, in contrast to the evocative but outdated image of the quaint country doctor making house calls in the pre-antibiotic era.

It is not uncommon for papers on house calls or home-based medical care, in both the lay and academic literature, to begin with an image of a doctor, black bag in hand (perhaps even driving a horse-drawn carriage), on her way to deliver care to a sick patient in need. Such images are usually accompanied by prose extolling the quaint and archaic nature of the house call and how it has not disappeared entirely from medical practice, in the face of a medical system that has evolved into a high-technology-focused juggernaut.

Such an image also evokes some of the best aspects of the practice of medicine. We are inspired by the dedication of a physician who cares enough about her patients to accommodate their convenience by seeing them in their homes. We visualize the sick patient comfortable at home, happy to have avoided the challenge and trauma of visiting the doctor's office, an urgent care center, or a hospital emergency department.

The clinicians making these visits know that seeing their patients at home will provide important information that may not be discernible in the office. Imagine the patient who has experienced multiple recent hospitalizations for recurrent heart failure. The house call reveals a second-floor bathroom and a kitchen stocked with sodium-rich canned and frozen foods that a friend buys for her, because she cannot go to the supermarket herself. Only when the clinician asks about her ability to climb the stairs does the patient admit that she often "can't make it in time," so she only takes her diuretic when she goes upstairs for the evening. The clinician now proposes useful solutions for this complex set of medical, functional, and social problems contributing to the patient's recurrent hospitalizations.

By taking medical care directly to the place where the patient spends the most time, home-based medical care exemplifies patient-centered care. At home, the physician easily assesses the patient's function in her own environment and helps address barriers to care and social determinants of health. Coming to see the patient at home is an unspoken endorsement of the patient's importance and helps to build a level of trust and communication that may be difficult to create in a typical office visit [1].

Unfortunately, the quaint image of the doctor in the horse-drawn carriage can trivialize the field of home-based medical care, as it undermines its other attributes that are critical to the delivery of truly modern medical care in the twenty-first century. In the wake of the Affordable Care Act, there has begun an inexorable shift from volume-based to value-based care. Special attention is now paid to the care of "high-need, high-cost" patients by government officials, health service delivery system leaders, payers, health-care providers, health advocacy and consumer organizations, and others.

In this context, home-based medical care has much to offer. Home-based medical care has been demonstrated to be a critical component for a range of health service delivery models that improve the quality of care, while reducing the costs of care. Such models include care transition models, home-based primary care, geriatric resources for assessment and care of elders (GRACE), and hospital at home [2–4]. Home-based primary care can also facilitate the discussion of goals of care that allow frail older adults to forgo burdensome and futile interventions at the end of life. Home-based medicine is a critical strategy for population health management [5]. This has been recognized by the development of important policy initiatives such as the Independence at Home Act (section 3024 of the Affordable Care Act) [6]. The business case for home-based medical care is also gaining recognition; venture capital is flowing into the field. In addition, the first accountable care organization that caters exclusively to homebound patients was recently launched.

Unfortunately, relatively few physicians, nurse practitioners, and physician assistants are engaged in providing home-based medical care. Most clinicians receive little or no training in home-based medicine, so they are unaware that this type of care is possible. Lack of training can lead to fear of the unknown and to misconceptions about the quality of home-based care and associated malpractice risks. "Fear of the unknown" may also include concern for personal safety in providing care in neighborhoods different from those they usually frequent. Finally, there may be significant concerns regarding the financial viability of providing home-based medical care.

These ideas are not supported by experience or evidence. Technological advances allow rapid, accurate point-of-care evaluation at home with equipment and services equivalent to or superior to that available in the typical ambulatory practice, if not the hospital. Medicolegal issues in home-based medical care medicine are much less common than in other sites of care, perhaps due to the enhanced therapeutic relationship described above. Although no data exist to indicate an increased threat to personal safety of clinicians who make home visits, anecdotal experiences suggest that such concerns are not justified. The only misconception that is rooted in fact is the concern for financial viability. While it is true that the volume of patients seen by a single clinician in an office setting is greater than in a typical home-based medical practice, the office requires greater financial resources to manage and maintain. Home-based medical care can generate "downstream" revenues for the medical system in the form of shorter non-emergent hospitalizations, specialist visits, and ancillary laboratory and imaging studies [7]. The emerging emphasis on the shift to value-based care means that home-based medical care will play a much greater role in the future of health care for an aging population and that models to more appropriately compensate home-based medical providers will emerge.

Despite the dearth of home-based medical providers relative to the need for their services, data suggest that the field is expanding. From 2000 to 2006, there was a 100 % increase in the number of house calls provided to Medicare beneficiaries. Approximately 1 million non-podiatry home-based medical visits were provided in 2006 and 2.49 million in 2013. Interestingly, while the number of home-based medical visits has increased rapidly, the number of providers performing those visits has decreased, suggesting that the health-care providers delivering these services are focusing their practice on home-based medical care [8].

This book, then, is intended to serve as a reference for these clinicians who seek a concise, practical guide to the principles and practice of home-based medical care. Experts actively involved in direct clinical care, research, education, and administration across the USA have condensed their vast knowledge and experience into these pages, with the goal of making home-based medicine accessible to all of the clinicians and patients who need it. Whether you are a nurse practitioner contemplating home visits for the first time, a physician assistant considering an expansion of services, a primary care physician wondering how to help your frail older adult patients achieve their health goals, or an experienced home-based medicine provider, we hope this book will help you to deliver excellent medical care at home to the patients who need it most. We hope that, over time, home-based medical care will continue to expand exponentially and that this volume will serve the needs of those who provide such care.

We will know that home-based medical care has truly come of age when papers begin not with descriptions of the doctor in a horse-drawn carriage but with descriptions of providers delivering state-of-the-art care to the neediest and most vulnerable patients.

We conclude this introduction with a note on terminology. The terms "house call" and "home visit" have commonly been used in the context of caring for patients in the clinical contexts described above. These terms are not incorrect, but these terms fail to convey the full scope of medical care in the home and may even trivialize it. When, for instance, a physician or nurse practitioner from a high-quality home-based primary care practice sees a patient at home, they are providing the patient with holistic interdisciplinary team-based care and community-based resources that address the medical, social, and functional needs of the patient and their families and caregivers. It is not simply an isolated encounter but a true system of care. Further, important stakeholders at the national level do not consistently understand the term "house call medicine" and commonly conflate it with services such as skilled home health care.

As such, we prefer the term "home-based medical care" to refer to house calls and home visits provided in the context of home-based primary care, home-based palliative care, and other home-based medical care models that are evolving in the ever-changing health care delivery system. Much of this text focuses on home-based primary care.

As care moves increasingly toward the home setting, home-based medical care will expand in scope. We look forward to watching that evolution, and hope this is the first of many editions of this book. In that spirit, please feel free to send us thoughts and ideas on topics to address in future editions via email at jhayash1@jhmi.edu or bleff@jhmi.edu.

References

1. LoFaso V. The doctor-patient relationship in the home. Clin Geriatr Med. 2000;16:83–94.
2. Counsell SR, Callahan CM, Clark DO, et al. Geriatric care management for low-income seniors: a randomized controlled trial. JAMA. 2007;298:2623–33.
3. De Jonge K, Jamshed N, Gilden D, Kubisiak J, Bruce SR, Taler G. Effects of home-based primary care on medicare costs in high-risk elders. J Am Geriatr Soc. 2014;62:1825–31.
4. Edes T, Kinosian B, Vuckovic NH, Nichols LO, Becker MM, Hossain M. Better access, quality, and cost for clinically complex veterans with home-based primary care. J Am Geriatr Soc. 2014;62:1954–61.
5. Boling PA, Leff B. Comprehensive longitudinal health care in the home for high-cost beneficiaries: a critical strategy for population health management. J Am Geriatr Soc. 2014;62:1974–6.
6. http://innovation.cms.gov/Files/fact-sheet/IAH-Fact-Sheet.pdf
7. Desai NR, Smith KL, Boal J. The positive financial contribution of home-based primary care programs: the case of the Mount Sinai Visiting Doctors. J Am Geriatr Soc. 2008;56:744–9.
8. Leff B, Carlson CM, Saliba D, Ritchie C. The invisible homebound: setting quality-of-care standards for home-based primary and palliative care. Health Aff (Millwood). 2015;34:21–9.

Part II
House Calls in the Health Care Ecosystem

Getting Started with Home-Based Medical Care

2

K. Eric De Jonge and George A. Taler

Abstract

This chapter reviews the three major issues relevant to getting started with a home-based medical service. They are (1) defining the clinical and geographic aspects of a target population, (2) how to build a practice and team structure for a defined population, and (3) what are the financial options for long-term sustainability. Building an effective and sustainable home-based medical practice depends on creating a dedicated core team to deliver comprehensive medical and social services focused on avoiding high-cost events, successful integration of community service partners, establishing a strong administrative structure, and a diversified financial model.

Keywords

Home-based medical care • Home-based primary care • House calls • Frail elders • Community services • Population health • Geographic area • Financial sustainability

2.1 Overview

When starting a home-based medical practice, a core guiding principle is to provide "the right care, for the right patient, by the right provider, at the right time, with the right tools." Home-based primary care (HBPC) is, by definition, centered on meeting patient and family needs in their place of residence.

K.E. De Jonge, M.D. (✉) • G.A. Taler, M.D.
MedStar Washington Hospital Center, 110 Irving St., NW, East Building- Room 3114, Washington, DC 20010, USA

Department of Geriatrics, Medstar Washington Hospital Center, Washington, DC, USA
e-mail: karl.e.dejonge@medstar.net

© Springer International Publishing Switzerland 2016
J.L. Hayashi, B. Leff (eds.), *Geriatric Home-Based Medical Care*,
DOI 10.1007/978-3-319-23365-9_2

When starting such a home-based medical practice, there are at least four major questions to answer in defining your practice:

• What is the main mission?
• What is the target population and geographic service area?
• What is the practice and team structure?
• What are the financial options for sustainability?

We approach these questions with a focus on building a dedicated home-based primary care (HBPC) practice to serve elders with complex medical and social needs [1–3]. We recognize that some providers make house calls as an extension of an office-based practice, on an episodic basis, to patients recently discharged from the hospital or to younger populations with permanent disabilities. We will touch on these other options but will concentrate on how to build an HBPC model for chronically ill elders. Common factors among all potential home-based medical approaches are the need for 24/7 clinical access for patients and family members and imperatives for high-value care for private insurance and governmental payers. These priorities are most achievable by taking a comprehensive and long-term approach to care.

2.1.1 What Is the Target Population and Geographic Area?

Home-based primary care is woven into the fabric of the community and thus based upon the needs of the local patient population and environment. Patient selection characteristics can include age, clinical conditions, functional status, and stage along the illness trajectory. The local environment includes the specific zip codes to be serviced, the population density, and socioeconomic and ethnic demographics. Some of the key initial steps are to decide which population to serve and what exact geographic area to cover.

2.1.1.1 Patient Population
Initially, a practice needs to select a primary target population, usually from one (or more) of four major types:

• Elders (65 and over) with severe chronic disabling disease
• Younger disabled persons affected by neurologic or mental health disorders
• Post-hospital or urgent care populations (without long-term primary care)
• Convenience populations in home, office, or hotel settings

A common target population for HBPC is older homebound patients with chronic illness and functional disability. They are usually 65 years of age and over, have chronic disabling disease, and are at high risk of hospitalization [1–3]. Most HBPC programs focus on elders who face obstacles getting to a doctor's office and for whom home-based medical care provides access to primary care and is more effective than office-based care. These patients and their families need a trusting long-term relationship with an interdisciplinary team that can offer prompt management of acute and chronic illness as well as compassionate end-of-life care.

Some home-based medical practices extend services to younger populations with neurologic disability, developmental disabilities, or severe mental illness. Other niche home-based medical care programs focus on high-intensity micropopulations such as persons with ventilator dependence, recent hospital discharges, or people with end-stage heart disease on intravenous medication pumps or ventricular assist devices. While home-based medical services can help these niche populations, they each have special needs that require specific personnel and specialty services that are different than that needed for general primary care of frail elders. Customized teams are best suited to meet the challenges of these subgroups.

A target population can also be defined by its stage along the illness trajectory or setting of care. For example, a practice may focus on the immediate post-hospital 30-day period to prevent readmissions. This may require that a practice loosen its criteria for functional disability and refer patients back to office-based practice as patients improve or when the 30 days end. Others provide episodic, urgent care as a high-end convenience service on a private-pay basis in the home, the workplace, or for travelers in local hotels. The decision on which population to serve will inform subsequent decisions about staffing and the business model.

2.1.1.2 Geographic Area

Choice of a specific geographic catchment area is a second major consideration in defining practice parameters. Neglecting to do so is a common cause of practice failure due to costs of overly long travel distances and associated greater amounts of unproductive "windshield" time. A key issue is driving radius, which determines extent of travel time from the "home-based" office. We advise that this radius be limited to a 20–25-min driving time. This limit can represent different mileage distances depending on the urban, suburban, or rural nature of the practice. A driving time limit enhances the ability to cluster visits each day in a smaller area, so individual visits can be less than 5–10 min apart on a particular day. Driving represents time in which you cannot see patients or (safely) text or use the phone and may or may not be reimbursable (see "financial considerations" about potential private-pay trip charges).

To choose a geographic area, we suggest using a detailed local map with zip code boundaries, sites of senior communities, and major thoroughfares in and out of population centers. One can then map a program's service area by matching demographic data on the location of a target patient population within the driving radius. We suggest that a catchment area minimize crossing of natural boundaries such as rivers or large parks with restricted traffic patterns. Be mindful of daytime traffic congestion due to rush hours, schools, sports arenas, or large shopping malls. It also helps a practice to define the catchment territory with specific zip codes for ease of describing a service area to the public.

Once defined, avoid "boundary creep," except for exceptional circumstances. For example, stretching the program zip code boundaries beyond a 25-min driving radius may be worthwhile for high population density opportunities, such as continuing care retirement communities, assisted living facilities, or "NORCs" (naturally occurring retirement communities).

When starting up, a practice should also assess the socioeconomic strata of patients within its territory. This is often available from US Census data tracts. Interestingly, high numbers of low-income patients can confer the benefits of traditional Medicaid or Medicaid waiver programs that offer social work and daily aide supports. What such patients may lack in financial resources can be balanced by the presence of government-funded support services for aging at home. Serving a high-income population can bring opportunities to offer private-pay services.

A practice needs to consider the availability of relevant service partners in an area. For example, when serving an elderly population, a program needs a close working relationship with a local and high-quality hospital and emergency department, to ensure continuity of care across these settings. The practice will also need a partner pharmacy that can deliver medications and supplies and social service agencies to organize daily support services.

A practice should assess the penetration of Medicare Advantage and Shared Savings programs (also known as accountable care organizations) in the area. Many local health systems have access to this data in their managed care or insurance divisions. Payers recognize that groups of high-cost patients require clinical care beyond the capacity of office-based primary care. These payers may provide payment options based on cost savings that expand revenues beyond limits of fees-for-service.

After defining a geographic area, the practice can further identify subareas within the region, to allow clustering of visits and enhance daily clinician efficiency. For example, if one team covers eight zip codes, clinicians can plan to focus visits each day on two contiguous zip codes to lessen driving time. Driving patterns for 1 day can either resemble a fishbone with nearby visits along a major residential thoroughfare or a small circle of visits along a clockwise path that brings you back to the home base.

In summary, a practice first needs to define their primary mission and then select the primary population their team aims to serve to meet the main mission of the practice. Then, the practice must define its geographic reach, demographic characteristics, and payer mix in the catchment area. Some key elements of success are to maintain a strict driving time radius, to partner with senior congregate communities, to determine availability of local service partners, and to seek payers who can offer value-based payments such as shared savings, a sizable per member per month, or partial capitation approach.

2.1.2 What Is the Practice and Team Structure?

After defining its mission, patient population, and geographic area, a home-based medical care program faces early decisions about practice and team structure. Initial structural decisions based on clinical mission and business approaches then guide the resources needed, staffing, and range of services offered. Some early decisions include:

1. Whether to build a dedicated HBPC practice or add house calls to existing office practice
2. Whether to focus on long-term primary care or short-term or episodic care
3. Whether to set up a not-for-profit or a for-profit entity
4. Whether to be part of large integrated health system or function as an independent entity in the community

Once a practice addresses these structural questions, it can proceed with creating the structure of the business model and clinical team.

2.2 Dedicated HBPC Team versus Extension of Office Practice

Given the disparate duties of operating both an office practice and a home-based medical practice, some providers choose to make a clean break and fully commit to a mobile primary care service. Building a dedicated HBPC team has the advantage of setting a clear mission, building a team focused on a single goal, and developing infrastructure for unique clinical and business aspects of home-based medical care [1, 4].

Early steps to develop a dedicated HBPC team include:

- Make your practice known in the local health-care community and neighborhoods (e.g., primary care practices, emergency rooms, home health and hospice agencies, senior housing communities).
- Determine which practice partner entities are available to serve the target population (e.g., pharmacy, durable medical equipment delivery, skilled home health agency services, home-based personal care services, subspecialty physicians, and hospital care).
- Hire core team members (physicians, nurse practitioners, and/or physician assistants, social workers, and office coordinators) with start-up funding from a sponsoring health system, philanthropy, or private investment.
- Build strong administrative infrastructure support for financial practice management and data analytics.

A more modest approach to starting a home-based medical practice is an existing office-based practice. This can start with clinicians who make visits to previous office patients that are now homebound. Patients transfer to the home-based service from the office practice when their disability impairs access to the office. In this case, practice supports are organized through the office structure for scheduling, phone triage, billing, and prescription refills. Coordination with community agencies falls to the individual provider and office staff, and after-hours coverage relies on the on-call service of the office practice.

As the home-based medical practice pulls more complex and time-consuming patients from the office practice, this can enhance office efficiency and satisfaction of the providers and staff. A medical group that extends itself to the home also improves the community reputation of the practice. Case-mix severity in the office practice may decline, and there can be little net gain financially. There is a potential financial advantage of home-based medical care, if the practice is rewarded by payers for preventing high-cost events and total cost savings.

Practices that assign house calls to a nurse practitioner or physician may find that volume-based productivity drops in order to manage the most complex patients. As patient volume grows, a house call workload can generate greater time commitment per patient and pull resources away from scheduled office duties [5]. Challenges for an office extension approach include:

1. Difficulty providing urgent visits when needed, as an office schedule limits flexibility.
2. Increased on-call demands due to greater care needs of home-based patients.
3. Practice of home-based medicine requires a distinct skill set for clinicians and administrative staff.
4. Potential differences in productivity between office and home-based medical practices.

Our experience is that building a home-based primary care service from an office-based practice can be a starting point, but the team should set specific milestones to determine when to create a subsidiary or independent HBPC team.

2.3   Long-Term Primary Care versus Short-Term or Episodic Services

Before embarking on a home-based medical practice, providers need to decide if they want to offer a comprehensive and long-term primary care approach or a more short-term and episodic approach. The long-term approach commits to coordinate medical and social services for a population of older patients across settings and over time, from the home to the hospital, to skilled nursing facilities, and to hospice. Such an HBPC team assumes responsibility for a high-cost and ill population and is accountable for clinical and cost outcomes of the population. These teams generally offer 24/7 phone access to clinical staff, urgent visits when needed, and coordination of social and medical specialty services. This type of a mobile interdisciplinary team can offer greater depth of services and potential for clinical and financial success than episodic house calls extended from an office practice.

Home-based medical care can come in many shapes and sizes. Some health systems have shown modest benefits of home visits as a short-term post-hospital intervention in heart failure patients, to prevent hospital readmissions and to lower costs [6, 7]. In this type of short-term intervention, the post-hospital service aims to help the hospital avoid hospital readmission penalties under Medicare.

Other practice types provide urgent, consultative house calls as an added service to usual office-based primary care. This arrangement occurs mostly in the context of entities that are at financial risk for health service utilization, e.g., Medicare Advantage plans and Medicare Shared Savings (accountable care organization) programs. Yet other home-based medical care providers deliver episodic visits to travelers in hotels, employees in the workplace, or people at homes on a private-pay basis to meet a demand for convenient urgent care. These practices usually eschew insurance payments, and fees are negotiated prior to delivery of the service.

2.4 Not-for-Profit Versus For-Profit Entity

Providers need to make an early decision about whether to be part of a not-for-profit or for-profit entity. There are benefits and risks to each approach and no right or wrong strategy.

The benefits of being a not-for-profit are the ability to raise start-up or ongoing funds through philanthropy and to define the practice's mission based on public service rather than purely financial performance. The risks of being a not-for-profit include a harder path to replication and financial sustainability and uncertainty of consistent funding from grants, a sponsoring entity (such as a hospital or health-care system), or government resources.

The benefit of being a for-profit entity is the clear mandate that the service needs to be financially viable. This focuses the mind of managers and clinicians and ensures close attention to efficiency, revenue cycle, and practice management methods. The risk of being a for-profit entity is a potential for tension between the clinical mission and the pressure to achieve financial results or to answer to investors whose primary goal is financial gain.

2.5 Large Integrated Health System or Independent Community-Based Practice

Another early decision for a home-based medical practice is whether to base the practice within a large integrated health system, often with a strong hospital base, or to create an independent community-based practice. There are advantages and disadvantages to each approach. Providers need to assess which environment makes the most sense for their goals and local geographic area.

Advantages of being health system-based include the presence of clinical and financial infrastructure to support the practice. This includes access to emergency, subspecialty, and hospital care, plus operational support such as human resources, information systems, billing, and legal counsel. A practice can receive start-up funds and ongoing support from health system resources if revenues do not fully cover program costs. The main risk of being part of a hospital-oriented health system is being in conflict with incentives and associated infrastructure that drive such a system. Hospitals are still often driven by goals of maximizing admissions and procedure volume, which can run counter to the home-based medical practice's mission to prevent hospital admissions and minimize risky invasive procedures. The financial infrastructure of a hospital is skilled at billing for inpatient events and less familiar with unique practice management aspects of home-based medical care (e.g., monthly home care certification, care plan oversight, or negotiating shared savings and other value-based payment methods). Ideally, a large integrated health system would value population health outcomes and embrace a move away from the volume-driven mentality. Such larger health systems are proliferating in response to payment reforms based in the 2010 Affordable Care Act (ACA).

One advantage of being a community-based practice includes being closer, both literally and figuratively, to the patients, families, and service partners in the neighborhood. Such proximity encourages close working relationships and a shared mission to keep elders at home, rather than bringing them to the emergency department or hospital. A community practice can build practice management tools that specialize in home-based medical care and support a population health mission to deliver more appropriate care in lower-cost settings. However, being community-based does remove the health system's safety net on the financial end. This means that practice survival depends on volume productivity, the results of value-based contracts, and effectiveness of the internal financial systems.

A future option may be to base an HBPC team in a skilled nursing facility (SNF) within a large integrated system. SNFs are beginning to diversify their clinical capabilities and support a value-based system. Most patients in an HBPC practice are close to being nursing home eligible, and patients discharged from subacute rehabilitation programs following a hospital stay are a good source of referrals. Although not as extensive as the hospital, the ancillary resources available at an SNF can be advantageous to prevent high-cost events. The financial resources of an SNF can rarely match that of a large hospital, and the home-based medical practice will need to be more financially self-sufficient in the SNF arena.

2.6   Home-Based Primary Care: Team and Practice Structure

This section will outline the core daily elements of an HBPC model. All such home-based medical care programs need to have certain essential service competencies in order to ensure delivery of excellent care to ill patients and their families [1, 2, 4, 8]. These capacities include:

- Skilled medical clinicians who can provide intensive management of serious chronic illness
- Continuity of care across settings (e.g., home, hospital, skilled nursing facility, or hospice)
- 24/7 access for urgent clinical triage and decisions
- Social work case management and caregiver support
- Mental health services
- Compassionate end-of-life care
- Mobile electronic health record (EHR)

An HBPC practice needs to build a core team of physicians, nurse practitioner or physician assistant staff, social workers, office coordinators, and managerial staff. The clinical disciplines provide the daily direct care and coordinate specialty services needed by an older population with chronic illness and disability. Each HBPC team within the overall practice has a small number of providers and office staff who, working as a team, can achieve familiarity and intimate knowledge of each patient and family. In our practice, panel size for a full-time individual clinician ranges from 150 to 200 patients, depending on efficiency of scheduling and degree of administrative support. We recommend that a practice develop a plan for managing growth as patient volume expands, as a team of several clinicians approaches capacity of 300–350 patients. In typical urban setting, in a geographic service area of 8–10 zip codes, programs often reach a steady-state census of 600–800 patients. Reasons for this include a focus on a relatively small subgroup of a highly targeted population and a high annual attrition rate, with annual mortality rate for the population that approaches 20–25 % percent.

In addition to the core medical and social service staff, the array of other clinical services that a team must coordinate includes:

1. Medical services
   (a) Mobile labs and radiology
   (b) Mental health
   (c) Emergency department/hospital care
   (d) Subspecialty services (e.g., podiatry, ophthalmology, other subspecialty physician care)
   (e) Medicare skilled home health agencies
   (f) Hospice care
   (g) Private ambulance and wheelchair van transport
   (h) Inpatient rehab and skilled nursing facilities (SNF)
   (i) Pharmacy/durable medical equipment delivery
2. Social support services
   (a) Family caregiver support and counseling
   (b) Legal counsel and guardianship
   (c) Coordination of home health aides
   (d) Pest extermination and minor home modifications
   (e) Food and utility resources
   (f) Housing transitions
   (g) Nursing home placement

In terms of actual operations, the initial patient care process starts with intake of new patients. There needs to be simple access for new patients, with a single phone number and engaging office staff who answer the phone, determine if the prospective patient is appropriate for the practice (has difficulty leaving home and has a reliable caregiver/contact person), and start the intake process. In our practice, we have found significant value in having an in-person orientation at the practice's administrative office for the family caregiver or power of attorney. This ensures a level of commitment from family or caregiver to participate in the program.

We recommend holding new patient orientation sessions at least once a week for new family caregivers. At these intake sessions, we collect standardized patient and family data and educate caregivers about the home-based medical practice's unique philosophy and mission and approach to scheduling, teamwork, and practice policies.

Patient visit scheduling is based on patient and family need. We recommend seeing new patients within 1–2 weeks of the intake session. In our practice, the next few medical visits are usually conducted by nurse practitioners and scheduled based on patient or family need and degree of clinical instability. The goal is to prevent medical and social crises and thereby avoid unneeded hospitalizations or nursing home stays. We recommend applying open access where unstable patients are seen urgently within 24 h. These urgent visits can displace routine visits as needed to ensure that the team sees the highest-priority patients first. Routine visits occur every 1–8 weeks to stay ahead of any instability in a patient's medical or social problems. Our office staff confirms visits only 1 day ahead of time and offers flexible 4-h time windows (AM or PM) to the patient and caregiver.

In our practice, all medical care comes from a physician/nurse practitioner dyad. The physicians perform new patient visits, see the patient every few medical visits, and also provide direct inpatient hospital care. The nurse practitioners perform a majority of the house calls for chronic and urgent visits. The patients and families need a single number for 24/7 phone access, so the team can provide phone triage, address issues promptly, and manage care in and out of hospital. Each clinician carries a "black bag," which is a rolling multi-compartment case. The black bag and the clinician's car contain a host of mobile diagnostic and therapeutic tools (see Table 2.1) that support care at a level commensurate with an urgent care center.

A home-based primary care team's success depends in large part on holding an effective and in-person weekly interdisciplinary team meeting. All team members are present to review status of new patients, hospitalized patients, unstable patients, deaths, and several other special categories of high-risk patients. The team meeting list is built by getting patient names from all staff members, and the final list is compiled by the office nurse. Other attendees at the weekly team meeting are representatives from pharmacy, mental health, and a partner skilled home health agency. See Table 2.2 for a sample template of the weekly team meeting. As reimbursement policies change to reward coordination and value, we envision this template being used to document coordination of care time and to justify billing for case management and coordination time.

A robust electronic health record (EHR) and a practice management database are essential tools. This means that all clinicians work on one mobile EHR, where they view data from other sectors of health system (e.g., hospital, home care agencies). Where possible, a practice can also link to local health-care integrated advanced information management systems to track patients across settings (e.g., Chesapeake Regional Information System for Our Patients, or CRISP).

The information technology structure needs to produce data extraction and analysis based on care coordination and outcomes, rather than just documentation for billing. The practice administrative team needs a data analytics capacity with ability to query for outcomes on patient survival, vital status, emergency department visits

Table 2.1 Supplies for portable "black bag" and car

Pulse oximeter
Blood pressure cuff with multiple sizes
Digital ear thermometer
Portable digital scale
Stethoscope
Rechargeable otoscope/ophthalmoscope
Hemoccult cards and developer
Ear curettes
Small forceps
Bandage scissors
Bionex ear irrigation kit
Toenail clippers
Water-based lubricant (K-Y jelly)
Vinyl gloves
Hand sanitizer
Finger splints
Scalpels (Nos. 10, 11, and 15)
Phlebotomy supplies—Butterfly 23G needles, vacutainer
Sharps needle box
Silver nitrate sticks
Suture kits
Syringes and needles
Skin staple remover
Wound care supplies—*saline, gauze, Kerlix, Opsite and thin hydrocolloid dressings, hydrogel ointment, triple antibiotic ointment, elastic bandage, ABD pads*
Povidone-iodine swabs
Injectables—*epinephrine, triamcinolone, lidocaine, vitamin B12, furosemide, pneumococcal and influenza vaccines, tetanus/diphtheria toxoids*
Disposable measuring tape
Urine cups
Bacterial culture swabs
Vaginal speculums
Flashlight or headlamp
Batteries
Garbage can (regular and hazard red bag)
Disposable chucks
N95 disposable masks
Hand sanitizer
Portable laptop PC
Cell phone and car charger
Hazmat suit—*masks, booties, disposable jumpsuit*
Forms box—*For do-not-resuscitate and comfort care orders, advance directives, new patient packets and brochures, patient labels, consent forms*

Table 2.2 Template for weekly interdisciplinary HBPC team meeting

Patient category	Physician name	Nurse practitioner name	Social worker name	Active issue
New patients				
Hospitalized				
Unstable patients				
New hospice or skilled home health patients				
Anticoagulation				
On hold (SNF facilities, bedbug infestation)				
Recent deaths				

and hospital admissions, patient and family experience, and financial collections. Such data creates the ability to prove both clinical effectiveness and financial viability of the practice, which are important for value-based contracts and shared savings payment models. As home-based medical practices mature, there will be opportunities or requirements for accreditation. This will require strong administrative resources to collect and present data on practice process and patient outcomes.

Some ancillary services such as laboratory or mobile radiology can be an internal part of the business, while others may require partnership with community agencies. For example, a larger diversified for-profit home-based medical care business may own their own lab and radiology services and hospice, while a not-for-profit community practice more often must find external service partners to fill these needs.

In the final section, we address strategies for home-based medical care practices to reach financial viability.

2.6.1 What Are Financial Options for Long-Term Sustainability?

As one gets started with home-based medical care, the issue of a financial viability is a central concern. A practice needs to consider all options for creating a sustainable financial model. Long-term viability depends on careful monitoring of costs and on building diverse sources of revenue. Major revenue options include:

1. Fee-for-service billing
2. Focus on high-density older populations in assisted living facilities (ALFs)
3. Income from related services (e.g., radiology, lab, hospice, home health, pharmacy, DME)
4. Shared savings or per-member per-month payments based on quality and cost reductions
5. Private-pay fees for uncovered services

A standard first source of revenue for most home-based medical practices is fee-for-service billing from a primary insurance payer, of which Medicare is the dominant entity. There are several Medicare CPT codes for home-based medical care, including evaluation and management (E and M), home health certification, care plan oversight (CPO), a new code in 2015 called chronic care management (CCM), and advance care planning (ACP) code that may be active in 2016. All these codes require detailed documentation by clinicians and a vigilant billing and coding operation to submit and track collections. Detailed recommendations for billing Medicare are beyond the scope of this chapter. This revenue stream will likely continue as a core source but will gradually become less important as value-based payment methods take hold over the next few years.

Most home-based medical practices in the USA struggle to achieve financial viability solely on fee-for-service Medicare revenues. This is due to the inefficiency of travel and the high amounts of indirect time spent on coordination of care, family communication, and counseling for very ill older persons [8]. A small number of entrepreneurial home-based medical care companies have achieved positive financial margins on largely fee-for-service revenues, with rigorous billing/collections systems, plus the addition of supplementary funds from other revenue streams. Even with highly effective billing/coding operations, entrepreneurial practices have relied on other revenue sources such as high volumes in assisted living facilities, ancillary services such as mobile laboratory and radiology, or private-pay travel fees, in order to achieve a positive margin.

Within a fee-for-service-environment, there are advantages to focusing a practice on senior congregate housing. Such places provide economies of scale with higher volumes of patients at one site, reduced travel time, and improved volume fee-for-service productivity. There are some advantages for the congregate housing management for encouraging their residents to receive their health care through a home-based medical care provider. An HBPC team can reduce the need for transporting elders to outside health-care facilities and provide 24/7 access for clinical triage to lessen unnecessary 911 calls. Our experience is that some more financially successful programs have 30–90 % of patients in assisted living facilities, depending on characteristics of their service area.

Another path to financial viability entails integrating other related health services into a larger business entity or medical services organization (MSO). This type of diversification can make both clinical and business sense, as patients need many other services, such as mobile radiology and laboratory, skilled home health, hospice, pharmacy, and durable medical equipment. A larger business entity that includes a wider array of home-based services creates a streamlined clinical operation plus new streams of revenue to supplement the fee-for-service professional fees.

The US health insurance system is moving steadily toward paying for value (outcomes/cost) rather than for the volume of procedures or visits provided. In this environment, a home-based primary care team that can demonstrate high patient and family satisfaction and prevent high-cost events is in position to receive payments based on shared savings. This requires negotiation with payers regarding the outcome metrics and the formula for calculating shared savings or a per-member per-month coordination payment. With sufficient strategic planning and resource allocation, shared savings programs can provide a significant revenue stream. Examples of this approach include an active Medicare demonstration program, Independence at Home (IAH), private sector agreements with Medicare Advantage programs, and some accountable care organizations. These options can offer a monthly coordination of care payment and/or annual shared savings payment based on results achieved. Of note, value-based purchasing for care of high-cost patients is an emerging mode of payment for special populations based on a health system receiving lump-sum payments for an episode of care for a high-risk hospitalized population.

Some home-based primary care providers have incorporated private-pay fees to supplement fee-for-service billing for professional services not covered by insurance. These include a monthly membership fee for services such as travel time, 24/7 direct access to medical providers, and coordination of care. These arrangements can require an Advance Beneficiary Notice (ABN) within Medicare, signed by the patient. In the private-pay arena, any practice needs to carefully examine Medicare rules on what constitutes "uncovered" services and clarify the payment plan with new patients and families upon enrollment. Other examples of services that are billed in the private-pay market include social work case management, private duty nursing care, companion services, and other special services, such as shopping, housekeeping, handyman, transportation, and nutritional programs.

In summary, the key principles to support financial viability for a home-based medical practice are to build a rigorous billing and collections system, to seek diverse streams of revenues from both volume- and value-based payments, and to build a data analytics system that can track financial data and patient outcomes in real time.

2.7 Legal Considerations

Legal considerations specific to home-based medical practices include malpractice, general liability, and collaboration agreements with nurse practitioner and physician assistant professionals. While difficult to obtain in past years, access to reasonable cost malpractice coverage is no longer a difficult matter for most physicians who wish to practice home-based medical care. Nurse practitioners in independent practices can still experience problems identifying carriers, so this needs to be addressed before creating this type of practice. General liability coverage, workman's compensation, and health insurance can affect decisions about creating an independent practice versus partnering with larger health system where these costs are less. Liability also plays a role in the decision about provider transportation vehicles. Other options are for cars to be provided by the practice, use of private vehicles that are subsidized for mileage reimbursement, or left to the provider to seek a deduction on their personal taxes. Collaboration agreements are needed for independent nurse practitioners and physician assistants in states that do not allow independent practice.

Such providers need to ensure that the collaborating physician is supportive, is aware of the patient complexity, and can assure timely turnaround on signatures of notes, medical necessity forms, drug authorizations, and, where applicable, narcotic prescriptions.

2.8 Conclusion

The experience of providing home-based medical care is profoundly satisfying for the clinician, patients, and families. There is no better way to understand the life and values of the patient and to then create a care plan that then promotes dignity and well-being of that person. This chapter highlights the major issues for a provider considering a home-based medical practice—defining a primary mission, choosing a highly targeted population and geographic service area, creating a skilled practice team, and building a diverse source of revenues to support longer-term sustainability.

References

1. De Jonge KE et al. Effects of home-based primary care on medicare costs. J Am Geriatr Soc. 2014;62(10):1825–31.
2. Edes T et al. Better access, quality, and cost for clinically complex veterans with home-based primary care. J Am Geriatr Soc. 2014;62(10):1954–61.
3. Boling PA, Leff B. Comprehensive longitudinal health care in the home for high-cost beneficiaries: a critical strategy for population health management. J Am Geriatr Soc. 2014;62(10):1974–6.
4. Reckrey JM et al. The team approach to home-based primary care: restructuring care to meet individual, program, and system needs. J Am Geriatr Soc. 2015;63(2):358–64.
5. Pedowitz EJ et al. Time providing care outside visits in home-based primary care. J Am Geriatr Soc. 2014;62(6):1122–6.
6. Naylor MD et al. Transitional care of older adults hospitalized with heart failure: a randomized, controlled trial. J Am Geriatr Soc. 2004;52(5):675–84.
7. Naylor M et al. Comprehensive discharge planning and home follow-up of hospitalized elders: a randomized clinical trial. JAMA. 1999;281(7):613–20.
8. Pedowitz E et al. Time providing care outside visits in a home-based primary care program. J Am Geriatr Soc. 2014;62(6):1222–6.

Part III

Clinical Approach to Caring for Patients at Home

Care Planning and Coordination of Services

3

Thomas Cornwell and Kara R. Murphy

Abstract

Patients who have limited or no ability to leave their home (home limited or homebound) usually have a constellation of physical, emotional, financial, and social problems. Most have family or other caregivers who need education and support. These complex patients and their caregivers are best served by an interdisciplinary team. This chapter describes community resources available to assist home-based medical providers to care for homebound patients. We focus on medical home health services, as well as home- and community-based resources, and describe how such assets may be used effectively by home-based medical care clinicians.

Keywords

Skilled home healthcare • Older Americans Act • Home- and community-based services • Home care services • Community resources • Home-based medical care

3.1 Introduction

Patients who have limited or no ability to leave their home (home limited or homebound) usually have a constellation of physical, emotional, financial, and social problems. Most have family or other caregivers who need education and support. These complex patients and their caregivers are best served by an interdisciplinary team.

T. Cornwell, M.D. (✉) • K.R. Murphy
Hospital: Northwestern Medicine, Home Centered Care Institute,
1800 N. Main Street, Wheaton, IL 60187, USA
e-mail: Thomas.Cornwell@CadenceHealth.org

© Springer International Publishing Switzerland 2016
J.L. Hayashi, B. Leff (eds.), *Geriatric Home-Based Medical Care*,
DOI 10.1007/978-3-319-23365-9_3

For most home-based primary care (HBPC) practices, the interdisciplinary care team is comprised of personnel from the practice, along with a host of outside home healthcare and community-based resources. HBPC providers need to exercise medical leadership and collaboration with this interdisciplinary team by performing patient-centered care planning and coordinate the services required for optimal care of patients and families. This requires clear and timely interdisciplinary team communication of assessments and diagnoses, orders, and opportunities for reevaluation and appropriate changes in the care plan. This coordinated care planning can require considerable time [1] and effort but produces improved patient outcomes and satisfaction while substantially reducing healthcare costs [2, 3].

3.2 The Care Planning Process

The term "patient-centered care plan" is used frequently, but there is no standard template or recommendations for what constitutes a care plan. An interdisciplinary team is required to provide input on the domains of care relevant to the patient's needs. In addition to the patient and the HBPC provider, other potential interdisciplinary team members include social workers, pharmacists, chaplains, home health agency (HHA) providers, mental health workers, lawyers, and family members/caregivers. Some of the team members may be employed by the HBPC practice, but more often they are a part of a HHA or other community agencies that the HBPC program partners with. The team members involved in creating the care plan will vary among home-based medical care practices, depending on practice staffing and local resources. If the patient does not have a need that requires skilled home health services and the practice does not have a social worker, the care plan will mainly be developed by the provider with support from office staff.

Patients can be referred to the local area agency on aging (AAA) case managers who can perform a financial evaluation and determination of benefits (see "Services Commonly Available in the Home" below). It is helpful to have a main contact at the social service agency that provides case management services for the AAA. Clergy can be contacted to visit patients. Packets of patient education materials on community resources, legal issues, and advance directives can be given to patients.

If a patient has a skilled need requiring home health services, a spectrum of capabilities from the HHA can add to the care plan. Social workers are of immense value in the care of the complex HBPC patients, but most programs do not employ them because of cost. For those that have their own social worker, the care plan can be populated by both the provider and the social worker.

HBPC programs that include social workers often have interdisciplinary case conferences to discuss complicated patients. Practices that share a large number of patients with a particular HHA often find it useful to have regular, interdisciplinary team conferences to discuss patients they collaborate in the care of. Case conferencing is much less common when HBPC team members are with different agencies. Some electronic medical records have community partner portals that enable community agencies to view medical records on select patients (with consent) and also send HIPAA-compliant messages to team members, dramatically improving communication and thus patient care.

Domains for comprehensive patient-centered care plans are:

- Patient goals of care (their desires and wishes for the domains below)
- Professional care team members (specialists, home health personnel, mental health providers, social services), contact information, and course of treatment (goals and frequency)
- Caregivers and contact information (family, private duty)
- Pertinent diagnoses/symptoms and plan for each
- Medications and justification (why each medicine is needed)
- Allergies
- Supplies needed and contact information for supplier (e.g., tube feeding supplies, wound care supplies)
- Durable medical equipment (DME) and supplier
- Cognitive status
- Functional status
- Activities permitted/recommended
- Nutritional requirements/recommendations
- Emotional status/mental health
- Social status (friends, visitors)
- Spiritual status (faith, spiritual needs being addressed/met)
- Financial status/determination
- Caregiver burden
- Safety measures/environmental assessment
- Abuse/neglect
- Health maintenance (immunizations, screening tests)
- Prognosis
- Advance care planning (power of attorney for healthcare, living will, advance directives)

3.3 Categories of Home Health and Community-Based Resources for Homebound Patients

Home health and community-based resources can be classified into five categories:

1. Skilled home healthcare paid for by health insurers such as Medicare or commercial insurance
2. Custodial or personal care services that may be covered under long-term care insurance (including Veterans Health Administration benefits), Medicaid, or paid for directly by patients
3. Government-funded resources and services through the Older Americans Act (OAA) managed through area agencies on aging along with state and local governmental organizations

4. Nonprofit organizations providing services through government funding or charitable donations
5. Other licensed professionals who provide services in patients' homes (audiologists, dentist, optometrist, podiatrists, mental health providers)

Table 3.1 shows the wide range of healthcare and community resources available to home-limited patients. This chapter will detail these important resources and their value to home-limited patients and their caregivers.

3.4   Home Health Defined

In the United States, the term "home health" has come to represent the home visiting services and supports provided by HHAs. Generally speaking, there are two types of HHAs:

1. Medicare-certified agencies that primarily provide "skilled" services such as nursing, physical therapy, and occupational therapy. These services are paid for by Medicare and commercial insurance companies when patients meet certification criteria.
2. Private duty agencies that primarily provide home health aide and companion services and are paid for either privately by the patient or family and by long-term care insurance or, for patients who meet eligibility criteria, through the Medicaid or Veterans Health Administration (VA) long-term care benefit.

Many home health organizations provide both skilled and private duty services and a range of other community services and supports such as hospice and palliative care, transitional care, telehealth, care coordination, social work services, and pre-natal and early childhood programming.

Throughout this chapter, we will refer to the Medicare home health regulations which cover the majority of skilled home health services in the country [5]. These regulations change frequently. Medicare-managed care organizations and commercial insurance often have preferred providers and varying benefits that need to be determined on a case-by-case basis. Home-based medical providers can contact their local HHA billing specialists for home health coverage determination for different insurance plans.

3.5   Skilled Home Health Services

The goal of home health is to maximize the patient's health and function in the home, reduce acute episodes of care, and support the caregiver. Services include nursing care, rehabilitative therapy, personal assistance (hygiene), and social work services. Quality HBPC coupled with the resources of home health services can improve the health and quality of life of home-limited patients through

Table 3.1 Home care services

Home-based medical care	Other medical services
• Diagnostic	• Audiology
• Urgent care	• Dentistry
• Hospital at home	• Podiatry
• Transitional care	• Optometry
• Chronic primary care	• Behavioral health services
• Palliative care	**Pharmacy**
Home health agency	• Medication review
• Nursing	• Pillboxes, bubble pack, delivery
– Infusion	**Medical equipment**
– Wound care	• Walker, wheelchair
– Education	• Hospital bed, commode, tub bench
– Assessment	• Hoyer lift, mattress
– Psychiatric nursing	• Oxygen, ventilators, CPAP
• Therapy	• Adaptive devices (e.g., "long arm grabber,"
– Physical	"buttonholer," large-handled utensils, etc.)
– Occupational	• Emergency response system
– Speech	**Supplies**
• Social work	• Wound care
• Home health aides	• Continence care
Hospice	• Enteral nutrition
• Medical director/hospice physician	**Diagnostics**
• Nurse	• Self-testing (glucose, INR, vitals, weight)
• Chaplain	• Mobile X-Ray
• Social worker	• Ultrasound, Doppler
• Home health aide	• Point of care lab
• Volunteer	• Facility-based lab
• Durable medical equipment	**Telemedicine**
• Hospice medications	• Telephone
• Complimentary therapies (e.g.,	• Video interface
music, pet, massage)	• Vital sign monitor
• Bereavement counseling	• Medication monitoring
Supportive care	• GPS tracker
• Personal care aide	• Email, patient portal
• Homemaker	• Emergency helpline
• Meals on Wheels	**Smart house**
• Transportation	• Adaptive technology
• Home modification	• Universal design
• Respite care	• Emergency response system
• Friendly visitor	
• Case managers	

Adapted from Medical Management of the Home Care Patient: Guidelines for Physicians 4th Ed. [4]. Used with permission from the American Academy of Home Care Medicine

comprehensive primary medical care, nursing, and rehabilitative services. It is important to note that to receive Medicare home health services, the patient must have a skilled need. Per Medicare, skilled nursing services are covered when an individualized assessment of the patient's condition demonstrates that the specialized judgment, knowledge, and skills of a registered nurse are necessary to maintain the patient's current condition or prevent or slow further deterioration. In addition, physical, speech, and occupational therapy is a skilled service if the inherent complexity of the service is such that it can be performed safely and/or effectively only by or under the general supervision of a skilled therapist. The skills of a qualified therapist must be needed to restore function, establish or design a maintenance program in order to ensure the safety of the patient and effectiveness of the program, or perform maintenance therapy.

3.6 Home Health Nursing

Nursing care provides comprehensive patient assessments and education on disease process, medications, diet, and self-management skills. Goals of care include improvement or stabilization in symptom control (e.g., pain, dyspnea), medication management and compliance, and improvement in knowledge of disease process and symptoms to report. Teaching and training activities can include self-administration of injectable medications, administration of oxygen, self-catheterization, maintenance of peripheral and central venous lines and administration of intravenous medications, bowel or bladder training, and proper body alignment and positioning to prevent pressure sores. Nursing treatments/procedures include wound and ostomy care, urinary catheter and gastrostomy tube changes, injections, and venipuncture. Some agencies also have specialized home health nursing services including certified wound and ostomy care, infusion services (intravenous hydration, parenteral nutrition, and antibiotics), and psychiatric care. Many but not all HHA provide 24/7 nursing availability, by telephone or with in-person nurse visits. Venipuncture for the purpose of obtaining a blood sample cannot be the sole reason for Medicare home health services. If the patient has a qualifying skilled need, venipuncture can be done as part of the plan of care.

3.7 Home Health Therapy

Home health therapy provides rehabilitative treatment in the home. The goals of therapy are to maximize safety in the home environment, train the patient and family in a home exercise program, optimize assistive devices, attain maximum function, and possibly progress to the appropriate next level of care (such as outpatient therapy).

The three areas of therapy are described below:

- Physical therapy: provides skilled evaluation/assessments of individuals with mechanical, physiological, and functional limitations and disabilities. Physical therapy evaluates and treats functional deficits through use of therapeutic exercises, neuromuscular reeducation, gait training, range of motion, maintenance therapy, as well as physical modalities such as heat, cold, ultrasound, shortwave, and microwave diathermy treatments. They also evaluate for proper use of medical equipment to optimize physical function.

- Occupational therapy (OT): provides skilled evaluation/assessments of individuals with mechanical, physiological, and functional limitations and disabilities with an emphasis on evaluation and treatment of deficits in ADLs (activities of daily living) and IADLs (instrumental activities of daily living). Treatment modalities include selecting and teaching task-oriented therapeutic activities (e.g., cooking); teaching compensatory techniques to improve the level of IADLs (e.g., teaching a person who lost the use of her arm due to a stroke on how to chop vegetables with one hand); designing, fabricating, and fitting orthotic and self-help devices; and vocational and prevocational assessment and training directed to restoration of function in ADLs. OTs in home care can also evaluate home safety, provide education, and recommend modifications to environment as needed. OTs are trained to administer cognitive assessments.
- Speech therapy (speech-language pathology (SLP) services): speech-language pathology therapy (SLPT) evaluates and treats disorders of communication development, speech, language, voice, or swallowing. SLPTs can also assess cognitive status and teach patient and caregiver self-management skills.

3.8 Social Work

Social workers provide intervention and consultations for social or emotional problems that are or are expected to be an impediment to the effective treatment of the patient's medical condition or rate of recovery. They can assess the relationship of the patient's medical and nursing requirements to the patient's home situation, financial resources, and availability of community resources (note: Medicare does not cover the social worker completing applications for Medicaid, as federal regulations require the state to provide this assistance). Short-term counseling can be provided to patients or caregivers when the HHA can demonstrate that a brief intervention (2–3 visits) is necessary to remove a clear and direct impediment to the effective treatment of the patient's medical condition or rate of recovery. They also assist patients in accessing community resources.

3.9 Home Health Aides

Per Medicare, to receive home health aide services, the patient must have a skilled need (e.g., nursing care) and need hands-on personal care to maintain the patient's health or to facilitate treatment of the patient's illness or injury. Personal care involves bathing, dressing, grooming, and oral hygiene needed to facilitate treatment or to prevent deterioration in health. Examples of additional services include changing bed linens, shaving, skin care, feeding, assistance with elimination including enemas, routine catheter and colostomy care (if determined safe for aide to do), assistance with ambulation, changing bed position, and assistance with transfers. Aides can also provide non-skilled wound care and reinforcement of the home therapy program.

3.10   Medicare Skilled Home Health

Skilled home health is a valuable partner to the HBPC provider. In our experience, approximately one-third to one-half of HBPC practices' patients require skilled home health services in a given year. The service is relatively ubiquitous, with over 99 % of Medicare beneficiaries in 2012 living in a zip code with at least one HHA and 84 % living in an area with five or more HHAs [6].

3.11   Who Qualifies for Medicare Skilled Home Health?

To qualify, the patient must:

1. Have a skilled home health nursing, physical therapy, or speech therapy medical need on an intermittent basis
2. Meet Medicare's homebound definition (see below)
3. Be under the care of an allopathic, osteopathic, or podiatric doctor and have a face-to-face visit 90 days before or 30 days after start of care that documents the need for skilled home care and that the patient meets the homebound definition
4. Receive home health services under a plan of care established and periodically reviewed by a physician [7]

It is important to note that patients do not need to meet Medicare's homebound definition to receive medical care at home. The home-based medical provider must document a medically necessary reason for the visit, but the patient can be fully ambulatory and not homebound. Examples include patients with mental illness, poor compliance, failure to follow up in the provider's office, or recurrent hospital admissions.

3.12   Medicare Homebound Definition

For a patient to be eligible to receive covered home health services under both Medicare Part A and Part B, the law requires that a physician certify in all cases that the patient is confined to his/her home. The following two criteria must be met:

Criterion one: The patient must either, because of illness or injury, need the aid of supportive devices such as crutches, canes, wheelchairs, and walkers; the use of special transportation; and the assistance of another person in order to leave their place of residence *or* have a condition such that leaving his or her home is medically contraindicated. If the patient meets one of the criterion one conditions, then the patient must *also* meet two additional requirements defined in criterion two below.

Criterion two: There must exist a normal inability to leave home; *and* leaving home must require a considerable and taxing effort.

The Medicare regulation states the patient may leave the home and still be considered homebound if absences are infrequent, for short duration, or are attributable to the need to receive healthcare. They go on to provide specific examples of permitted absences from the home including therapeutic, psychosocial, or medical treatment in an adult day care program licensed or certified by a state, outpatient dialysis, outpatient chemotherapy or radiation therapy, attendance at religious services, occasional trip to the barber, a walk around the block or a drive, and attendance at a family reunion, funeral, graduation, or other infrequent or unique events [8].

The final requirement to receive skilled home health services is being under the care of an allopathic, osteopathic, or podiatric doctor and have a documented face-to-face visit 90 days before or 30 days after start of care. The face-to-face note must include the visit date and document how the patient's clinical condition (including primary diagnosis and clinical findings) supports the patient's homebound status and need for skilled services. In situations when a physician orders home healthcare for the patient based on a new condition that was not evident during a visit within the 90 days prior to start of care, the certifying physician or nonphysician practitioner must see the patient again within 30 days after admission. The specific home health services being ordered need to be documented. The face-to-face encounter does not need to be done by the certifying doctor. Examples include the face-to-face visit being done by a hospitalist or post-acute care provider upon discharge or by a resident or nurse practitioner under the supervision of the certifying physician. The patient must require nursing care, physical therapy, or speech therapy as the qualifying service. Occupational therapy, social work, and aide services can also be ordered but by themselves do not constitute a basis for eligibility for Medicare reimbursement. Medicare permits HHAs to inform the certifying physician of their findings from their comprehensive assessment that supports the patient eligibility for skilled home healthcare. The certifying physician can sign the additional information and incorporate it into his/her medical record to further substantiate need for home health services. The face-to-face documentation must corroborate the HHA's findings. Below is an example of face-to-face documentation:

> John Smith seen today at home for exacerbation of congestive heart failure with hypoxemia (oxygen saturation 86 % on room air). Did not desire hospitalization and ordered increased diuretics and oxygen. He is also having increased difficulty transferring and decreased gait. Ordered home health nursing to follow response to change in medication and addition of oxygen, and to provide education regarding congestive heart failure and low salt diet. Ordered physical therapy to evaluate and treat decreased gait and transfer difficulty. Ordered occupational therapy to evaluate and treat difficulty with transfers and recommend assistive equipment to help with ADLs. The patient is homebound because of dyspnea with minimal exertion from his heart failure and inability to walk more than 20 ft.

3.13   Recertification

Home health certifications are for 60-day episodes of care. At the end of the initial 60 days, if the patient still has a skilled need, services can be recertified for subsequent 60-day episodes, with recertification required for each episode.

Medicare does not limit the number of recertifications for beneficiaries who continue to be eligible for the home health benefit. The recertification assessment must be done during the last 5 days of the previous episode and signed and dated by the physician who reviews the plan of care indicating a continued need for skilled services. The need for continued OT may be the basis for recertification even though it cannot be used for the initial certification. Medicare also requires an estimate of how much additional time the skilled services will be required. Examples of appropriate recertification include patients with chronic urinary catheters requiring monthly and "as needed" catheter changes or wounds that have not healed and require continued skilled nursing services.

3.14   Maintenance Therapy

As the result of a January 24, 2013, settlement of a class action lawsuit challenging Medicare's improvement standard, Medicare clarified its stance on paying for home health services when a skilled provider was needed to maintain functional gains [9]. The updated "Medicare Benefit Policy Manual" now clarifies that services that are required to maintain the patient's current function or to prevent or slow further deterioration that require skilled nursing care or therapy be covered. In addition, coverage of skilled nursing care or therapy to perform a maintenance program does not turn on the presence or absence of a patient's potential for improvement from the nursing care or therapy, but rather on the patient's need for skilled care. Skilled care may be necessary to improve a patient's current condition, to maintain the patient's current condition, to prevent or slow further deterioration of the patient's condition [7]."

3.15   Start of Care

According to the Medicare Conditions of Participation (CoPs) [10], the HHA is required to see the patient within 48 h of the referral if the patient allows. An initial comprehensive assessment is performed by a nurse (or physical therapist) of the patient, the home, and the availability of caregivers. The patient assessment includes a history and physical along with the completion of the Outcome and Assessment Information Set (OASIS-C1/ICD-10 version).

3.16   The Home Health Agency Care Plan

The final product from the initial comprehensive assessment performed by the HHA is the care plan which for Medicare has to include defined key elements and be signed by the physician (a nurse practitioner or physician assistant cannot sign). The CMS Form 485 (the Home Health Certification and Plan of Care) meets regulatory and national survey requirements [11]. HHAs are not required to use Form 485 and may submit any document that contains all the required data elements and is signed by the physician. The key elements for certification are listed below.

3.16.1 Key Elements for Certification

- Patient demographics, start of care, 60-day period
- Home care provider name and provider number
- Diagnoses, surgical procedures, medications, allergies
- Durable medical equipment, supplies
- Nutritional requirements, fluid needs or restrictions, parenteral or enteral nutrition
- Safety measures, functional limitations, activity level
- Mental status, prognosis
- Types of services required, measurable therapy treatment goals, frequency and duration of visits for each home health discipline

3.17   Home Healthcare During the Certification Period

During the 60-day home health episode of care, the home health personnel carry out the plan of care and make necessary changes in communication with the home-based medical provider. Goals include reaching maximizing function and self-care, healing and/or proper care of wounds, and teaching family and caregivers how to safely care for patients. Laboratory and point of care (such as finger-stick anticoagulation monitoring) tests can be done. Advance care planning including resuscitation wishes and healthcare power of attorney may be discussed.

Effective and efficient communication between home health personnel and the home-based medical provider optimizes care. Non-emergent home health communications can be called to the home-based medical provider's office or sent electronically and dealt with during non-patient care time. There should be guidelines for emergent communication that can include calling the home-based medical provider directly. Effective collaboration can reduce hospitalizations. The rate of hospital readmission within 30 days of initial discharge to home health has remained high at 28 % [12]. Home-based medical providers can work with HHAs to provide better primary care and more timely acute care in the home to reduce unnecessary readmissions [13].

3.18   How Home Health Agencies Are Paid by Medicare

Knowledge of home healthcare reimbursement can help home-based medical providers work more effectively with agencies by understanding financial limitations and incentives that can affect patient care decisions. HHAs are paid on a prospective basis. Payment is based on which of 153 home health resource groups (HHRGs) a patient falls into. Determination of HHRGs includes a clinical, functional, and service severity level based on the number of therapy visits during the certification. The degree of impairment and needs in these areas are derived from the OASIS [14]. The 2015 national standardized 60-day episode payment is about $2900 [12]. The great majority of Medicare home health is paid for by Medicare Part A, for which there is no co-pay. Rarely, patients do not have Medicare Part A, in which case Medicare Part B, if available, will cover.

Medicare requires HHAs to cover all medical supplies while the patient is under a home health plan of care. Medical supplies are bundled into the prospective payment. Medicare supplies are classified as routine and nonroutine. Routine supplies are customarily used in small supplies in the course of most home care visits, such as alcohol preps, paper tape, cotton balls and 4×4's, and infection control protection such as non-sterile gloves, masks, and gowns. Nonroutine supplies are identifiable to an individual patient, are furnished at the direction and order of the patient's physician, and are specifically identified in the plan of care. Examples of nonroutine supplies include more complex dressings, intravenous supplies, ostomy supplies, and catheters and catheter supplies. The cost of non routine supplies is also factored into the prospective payment. If supplies are still needed when the patient is discharged from a HHA, the HBPC provider needs to arrange for them, often from a Medicare Part B supplier.

Understanding that the HHA is responsible for supplies can help the medical provider order cost-effective wound care products. Dressings that require less frequent nurse visits can help reduce HHA costs. It is also important to realize the current system to determine prospective payment favors patients with high therapy needs but low nursing needs. This makes patients with high nursing needs but low therapy needs such as bedbound patients with wounds and significant supply costs more expensive to the agency. HBPC providers need to work with HHAs on these highly complex, high-nursing care patients both to make sure they are cared for in a cost-effective manner and to advocate for them to make sure they get all the care they need.

3.19 Choosing a Home Health Agency

Patients have the right to choose their HHA and must be provided with care options. However, they often look to their home-based medical provider for guidance. Home-based medical providers should exercise the same care in choosing a HHA as they would a hospital affiliation. Providers often work with several agencies to ensure geographic coverage and appropriate services for all their patients. The home-based medical provider is responsible for recommending agencies that provide high-quality care necessary to meet the needs of the homebound patient.

To evaluate the quality of a HHA, consider the following resources, questions, and strategies:

- Accreditation: Accreditation is voluntary and signifies an agency meets national standards. Examples of certifying organizations include the Joint Commission (www.jointcommission.org) and the Community Health Accreditation Program (CHAP: www.chapinc.org).

- Home Health Compare (www.medicare.gov/homehealthcompare): This web site lists all Medicare-certified home health agencies in a given zip code and provides information on the agencies. Information includes services provided, results of thirteen processes of care measures and nine outcomes of care measures from OASIS-C, and results from patient surveys (the Home Health Consumer Assessment of Healthcare Providers and Systems (HHCAHPS) instrument).
- Does the agency employ all services or use subcontractors for direct clinical care?
- Does the agency specialize or have certain niche services? Examples can include heart failure care including telehealth, certified wound/ostomy nurse, lymphedema, post-orthopedic surgery rehabilitation, psychiatric nursing, pediatrics, infusion services, nutritionist, diabetic educator, and others.
- Does the agency provide culturally sensitive and linguistically appropriate care?
- How effectively does the agency communicate care needs and updates to the medical provider? Are communications timely, effective, and efficient?
- How responsive is the agency in managing care?
- Do they provide 24/7 coverage, and what is their staffing on nights and weekends that can help prevent unnecessary emergency department visits?
- Talk to home health agencies owners and ask them the questions noted above.
- A good resource to ask about local home health agencies is an experienced hospital discharge planner. They will have made numerous home health referrals and will be aware of agencies that communicate well and see patients in a timely manner.
- Avoid working with agencies that may be engaged in fraudulent behavior. Some red flags include agencies that:
  - Directly solicit Medicare patients by phone to whom they have not provided services
  - Add on extra therapy visits to increase payments
  - Continue to recertify patients when the skilled need no longer exists
  - Offer payments for referrals

3.20 Physician Payments for Overseeing Home Health

Medicare pays physicians for reviewing and signing certifications and recertifications for home health as well as for care plan oversight (CPO) of home health medical personnel when 30 min or more is spent in a calendar month on such activities. CPO time includes discussing care with home health personnel, reviewing and signing the care plan and orders, reviewing the patient chart for issues related to home health, and completing durable medical equipment forms. All time for these activities need to be documented in the chart. Time talking to patients, family members, or non-HHA caregivers does not count toward CPO. Communication with HHA personnel that is part of a home or office visit also does not count. Table 3.2 provides the different types of payments, the codes involved, payments, and descriptor of the service.

Table 3.2 Medicare payments for overseeing home health and chronic care management

	Medicare 2015 payment[a] ($)	Description
Home health certification	53.99	Physician certification for Medicare-covered home health services under a home health plan of care
Home health recertification	41.48	Physician recertification for Medicare-covered home health services under a home health plan of care
Home healthcare plan oversight	108.34	Physician oversight of Medicare-covered services provided by a HHA of 30 min or more in a calendar month
Hospice care plan oversight	109.41	Physician oversight of Medicare hospice services of 30 min or more in a calendar month
Chronic care management services	42.91	(Home healthcare not required) 20 min or more of clinical staff care management directed by a physician or qualified healthcare professional for patients with multiple (two or more) chronic conditions

[a]Payments vary by geographic location

3.21 Private Duty Custodial Care Services

Private duty custodial care involves home health aides or companions that assist with activities of daily living (bathing, dressing, toileting, etc.) and/or homemaker services (cleaning, meal preparation, and others). Services are paid either privately, with long-term care insurance, or through government sources for those who qualify for them such as Medicaid, the Veterans Health Administration, or funds from the Older Americans Act (see below). Private duty agencies usually charge approximately $22 per hour depending on the level of care. Private pay care can be from a few hours to 24 h per day. It is important for patients and families to make sure agencies are licensed and bonded. If patients or families hire caregivers directly on their own, it is recommended to have background checks done.

3.22 Community Resources

The maze of available community resources can be both overwhelming and confusing. Well-informed home-based medical providers can direct patients and families toward resources that can support them. A home-based medical care practice's ability to develop collaborative partnerships with community resources can reduce fragmentation and duplication of efforts and ensure that the provider has all the information and support needed to provide outstanding care to the patient and caregivers. These partnerships can also serve as a key referral source for home-based medical care programs.

There is a national emphasis to redirect federal dollars from institutional care (nursing homes) to home- and community-based services (HCBS) to enable patients to remain in the community. Since Medicaid is a state-administered program, eligibility and coverage vary widely by state. Nationally, Medicaid spending for long-term services and supports (LTSS) has grown steadily over the past 15 years due both to more funding being directed to LTSS and less funding going to nursing homes. This increased emphasis on supporting patients to remain in the community increases demand for the home-based medical provider.

Our review of LTSS will highlight both government-funded and nonprofit social and community health providers, identifying resources for patients and their caregivers. Although this section will provide background on resources available nationally, the breadth of local resources available to clinicians varies widely. While they may share a common funding stream, methods and logistics will vary significantly across locales.

The most efficient manner to learn about community resources for seniors is to go to Eldercare Locator at www.eldercare.gov. The tool provides local resources for Administration on Aging (AOA)-coordinated services (www.aoa.gov) primarily funded by the Older Americans Act (OAA). Since funding began in 1965, the OAA promotes the well-being of older individuals by providing services and programs designed to help them live independently in their homes and communities.

All individuals 60 years of age and older are eligible for services under the OAA, although priority attention is given to those who are in greatest need. Patients are often unaware that many of the services provided through OAA are free of charge.

OAA funding for programs is allocated to a region (often a county) based primarily on the number of persons 60 years of age and over. National funds are therefore distributed locally, with a local area agency on aging (AAA) evaluating the unique needs of seniors in their catchment and subcontracting with local partners to fund needed services. Each region offers a range of senior supporting services, including Information and Referral Services intended to help families connect to services.

Given community-level and regional variation, HBPC providers are advised to reach out and develop a relationship with a contact at their local AAA or subgranting agency; this minor investment of time will yield valuable guidance but may also offer secondary benefits in regard to facilitated or improved referrals, timely guidance about changes in resources/eligibility, and even referrals of appropriate patients to your clinical practice.

Some of the services most typically available through AAA include:

3.23 Center-Based Programming

3.23.1 Information and Referral/Assistance (I&R/A) Information Services

This is a key resource for senior services and available as a funded program through virtually all AAA. Information specialists are available to provide assistance and linkage to available services and resources, often accessible by telephone and in person at a local site. In addition to linking seniors with all of the services on this list, they can also provide consultative assistance with options counseling for housing, helping families to make informed decisions about the best housing available to meet their needs.

3.23.2 Adult Day Care Centers

Adult day care centers offer social, recreational, and health-related services to individuals in a protective setting who cannot be left alone during the day because of healthcare and social need, confusion, or disability. Senior centers offer a variety of recreational and educational programs, seminars, events, and activities for the active and less active older adult. Another center-based program is congregate meals, detailed in "Nutrition Services" below.

3.24 Services Commonly Available in the Home

3.24.1 Caregiver Programs

Caregiver burden has been associated with increased hospitalization and mortality in community-dwelling older care recipients. Providing support and reducing caregiver burden thus not only helps caregivers but may reduce adverse health outcomes for care recipients [15]. The National Family Caregiver Support Program provides programs and services for caregivers of older adults and some limited services to grandparents raising grandchildren, at no charge to patient or caregiver. The age of the caregiver is typically not material, as the qualifying event is caregiving for a senior. These services often include support groups, counseling services (individual or family), and crisis services. Services may be provided in the home or at a local community site.

3.24.2 Case Management

Case managers under OAA work with family members and older adults to assess, arrange, and evaluate supportive efforts of seniors and their families to remain independent. These services are typically provided free of charge. Case managers can assess clients either at the request of medical providers, through patient self-identification, or caregiver referral. Case managers provide an exhaustive review of the patient's situation with a typical assessment including the following:

- Patient goals
- Assessment of patient caregiving needs, supports, and resources
- Assessment of caregiver capacity
- Physical health (reported)
- Behavioral health, including cognition evaluation

- Screening for depression, suicidality, substance abuse, and cognition
- Functional status evaluation (ADL)
- Medication assessment
- Transportation
- Environmental scan (structure, sanitation, hazards)
- Evaluation of financial resources and stability
- Benefitting assessment (linking patients with resources)
- Utility assistance
- Legal issues
- Socialization

Identified needs result in ongoing case management with reassessment frequency from weekly to biannual depending on need.

3.24.3 Elder Abuse Prevention Programs

Allegations of abuse, neglect, and exploitation of senior citizens are investigated by trained protective service specialists. Intervention is provided in instances of substantiated elder abuse, neglect, or exploitation. While referrals will result in a comprehensive assessment, individuals with decisional capacity may decline assistance despite a finding of neglect or other risks. See also Chap. 11, "Social and Ethical Issues in Home-Based Medical Care."

3.24.4 Financial Assistance

While not available in every community, some areas offer no-cost benefit counseling programs that can be accessed through the Information and Referral Assistance specialist at local AAA to help older adults to manage their finances. Some AAA and subgrantee agencies offer paid or volunteer financial counselors who can work intensively with families to improve financial stability. Some agencies may also function as representative payees for seniors who need additional assistance.

3.24.5 Home Repair and Home Modification Programs

Community partners may offer programs through vetted tradesmen or volunteers that help older people maintain the condition of their homes and provide repairs as needed. Home modification programs provide adaptations and/or renovations to the living environment intended to increase ease of use, safety, security, and independence. There are some local, state, federal, and volunteer programs that provide grants and loans to support these efforts, and programs may offer either fixed or reduced fee programs for eligible seniors.

3.24.6   Legal Assistance

More than 1,000 legal aid services provide over one million hours of senior legal advice per year with funding from AAA. Services are available to persons aged 60 and over for certain types of legal matters including government program benefits, tenant rights, and consumer problems. Legal services under Title III-B also protect older persons against direct challenges to their independence, choice, and financial security. These legal services are specifically targeted to "older individuals with economic or social needs." [16] Most communities have a designated grantee agency to which all referrals for senior legal assistance can be made, and the lawyers available have special content knowledge. Homebound patients can receive assistance telephonically, and lawyers can visit patients at home as needed. In many cases, the local legal aid provider may also be the provider of AAA services, but eldercare.gov can offer direction to the local resource.

3.24.7   Nutrition Services

Popularly known as "Meals on Wheels," this service delivers nutritious meals to the homes of seniors and persons with disabilities. Another typically accessible resource is Congregate Meals, providing the opportunity for persons aged 60 and over to enjoy a meal and socialize with other seniors in the community. Individuals desiring nutrition services are typically assessed for income, and the agency suggests a donation or fee to defray the cost of food. Although policies vary by community, Meals on Wheels providers often defray program fees for lower-income seniors with fundraising, and many participate in the food stamp program as well.

3.24.8   Personal Care/"Cash and Counseling"

Seniors identified to have functional impairments may qualify for paid caregiver assistance and receive help with bathing, dressing, toileting, walking, meal preparation, shopping, and homemaker services. Care can be provided through agencies or in some cases through caregivers identified by the senior or person with disabilities. "Cash & Counseling" programs (states may use different names) are now available in 43 states and provide cash assistance to the beneficiary with the flexibility to "consumer direct" the spending to meet their needs. This includes hiring care providers of their choice including family members. The "Counseling" involves helping the beneficiary consider a broad range of needed services, create a budget, and manage the paperwork required to pay employee wages and withhold taxes. If the client is unable to do this, further counseling can involve appointing a representative to assist. These programs are usually funded through Medicaid waivers, which vary by state but offer state-enhanced flexibility in reimbursing long-term care services and supports for select populations where provision of those services is deemed especially valuable and/or cost-effective.

Outside of Medicaid waiver-funded programs, similar resources may be available through veteran's benefits and insurance-funded programs. More information can be found at www.hcbs.org and http://tinyurl.com/kxhoevc.

3.24.9 Respite Care

Respite provides support for the caregiver. Respite programs offer limited relief or rest from the constant/continued supervision, companionship, and therapeutic and/or personal care of a person with a functional impairment. Respite programs through OAA are free of charge, but typically limited to several hours per week. Respite providers, some of whom may be volunteers, are paired with a family to offer continuity of care over time. Some states or localities include brief nursing home stays as respite for the caregiver.

3.24.10 Telephone Reassurance

Although not available in all areas, this service provides regular contact and safety checks by trained volunteers providing reassurance and support to homebound senior citizens and persons with disabilities.

3.24.11 Transportation

Some communities provide reduced or no-cost door-to-door transportation for the elderly or persons with disabilities who do not have private transportation and are unable to utilize public transportation. Most senior ride programs have specific geographic service areas.

3.25 Behavioral Health

In addition to services funded through the OAA, every community has a designated agency tasked with providing comprehensive healthcare services for seriously and chronically mentally ill patients. The agency may be the health department or a government-designated private nonprofit entity. This designated agency is typically credentialed with many governmental as well as select private payors to provide key services. Unlike traditional counseling agencies, these agencies provide comprehensive behavioral health services for seriously and chronically mentally ill patients including intensive outpatient services, 24 h crisis services, services for dually diagnosed mentally ill and substance-abusing patients, and often limited home-based services for homebound and/or seriously mentally ill clients. Many of these designated agencies have resources supporting free or reduced cost treatment for qualifying patients. There is a shortage of mental health workers in many areas

Table 3.3 Community mental health services

Organization	Description of services	Web site
Substance Abuse and Mental Health Services Administration (SAMHSA)	SAMHSA offers an outstanding array of resources targeted to both consumers and caregivers, including: • Education on mental health and substance abuse • Search engine that offers an array of treatment options and links to providers • Referral lines and phone numbers for individuals who prefer to talk to someone • Crisis resources • Recommendations regarding self-help, peer support, and consumer groups • Clinical trials • VA resources • Government resources For providers, the SAMHSA web site offers additional resources, topic-specific guidance and grants, and research on effective behavioral health interventions	https://findtreatment.samhsa.gov/locator/home http://www.samhsa.gov/
Geriatric Mental Health Foundation	Established by the American Association for Geriatric Psychiatry, the foundation offers treatment recommendations, promotes health aging strategies, and offers tools for connecting to treatment The site includes a geriatric psychiatry search engine	www.gmhfonline.org

of the country, especially those that provide home-based mental healthcare, so these services may be very difficult to access.

Patients, caregivers, and professionals seeking behavioral health treatment will find helpful information through the tools shown in Table 3.3.

3.26 Parish Nursing

Parish nursing, also known as faith community nursing or church nursing, involves more than 15,000 registered nurses around the world with most operating in the United States. Parish nurses seek to integrate the practice of faith and healing. Parish nurses are generally affiliated with and sponsored by a particular congregation. Faith-based nursing is also found in Jewish congregations, mosques, and other places of worship.

Faith Community Nurse Roles
- Health advisor
- Health education
- Home and hospital visits
- Community referral resource
- Health system navigator
- Development of support groups
- Training and coordination with volunteers
- Provision of health screenings

Ways to determine if parish nursing is available in a given community include contacting the local hospital information and referral network or the area agency on aging. The Health Ministries Association also has a partial list of parish nurse programs which can be found at http://hmassoc.org/get-connected/networks/.

3.27 Other Key Community Partners

3.27.1 Long-Term Care Ombudsman Program

Long-term care ombudsmen are advocates for residents of nursing homes, board and care homes, and assisted living facilities. Ombudsmen provide information about how to find a facility and receive quality care. They are trained to resolve problems and can assist with complaints, but will also maintain confidentiality unless given license to communicate to others. Reports can also be made anonymously. Under the OAA, every state is required to have an Ombudsman Program that addresses complaints and advocates for improvements in the long-term care system [17].

3.27.1.1 Who Can Benefit from Ombudsman's Services?
- Residents of any nursing home or board and care facility, including assisted living facilities
- A family member or friend of a nursing home resident
- A nursing home administrator or employee with a concern about a resident at their facility
- Any individual or citizen's group interested in the welfare of residents
- Individuals and families who are considering long-term care placement

Individuals wishing to speak to an ombudsman can call their local designated senior services provided or their local area agency on aging or can search for resources at the National Long-Term Care Ombudsman Resource Center at www.theconsumervoice.org, which will identify both state and local resources. The web site also offers a consumer clearinghouse with a host of patient- and family-focused resources intended to help them make decisions and advocate for their desired services.

3.27.1.2 Money Follows the Person and Balancing Incentive Program

The Money Follows the Person (MFP) Rebalancing Demonstration Grant (authorized by the Congress in the Deficit Reduction Act of 2005) [18] and Balancing Incentive Programs (BIPs, authorized by the Affordable Care Act 2010) [19] provide financial and practical supports for transitioning chronically ill and disabled patients from nursing homes back into the community. Program goals for MFP include increasing use of home- and community-based services, reducing institutional services, and eliminating barriers that restrict Medicaid funds to institutional care settings. Patients can self-refer or be referred by others for assessment. Care managers working on returning patients to community settings help them identify appropriate residential placement and address practical considerations such as furniture, rental obligations, and sources of medical care including home-based primary care.

Similar to MFP, the Balancing Incentive Program authorizes state grants to increase access to noninstitutional long-term services and supports (LTSS). The increased dollars provided to states can only be used to support new or expanded community-based LTSS.

HBPC providers connecting to local administrators or BIP and MFP services can offer a valuable resource to patients and social service partners alike. If community partners are aware of a resource to support ongoing primary care in a residential setting, it removes one potential barrier to nursing home discharge, and many ultimately extend the capacity of both patients and community partners to support ongoing community placement.

3.27.1.3 Villages

Across the country, senior communities are organizing membership-driven grassroots organizations called Villages. There are currently 150 Villages in operation in the United States and abroad, with at least 120 more in development in 2015. Villages are run by both volunteers and paid staff. They coordinate access to affordable services including transportation, enrichment activities, educational activities and trips, health and wellness programs, and home repairs. They are directed by the seniors that they serve. More information on this developing trend is available through the Village to Village Network web site at www.vtvnetwork.org.

3.27.1.4 Department of Rehabilitative Services

Although many of the services detailed in this chapter offer specific benefits to seniors, most states also have similar services available to younger patients through their Department of Rehabilitative Services or Office of Rehabilitation Services. At a federal level, the Rehabilitation Services Administration (RSA) oversees grant programs supporting individuals with disabilities to obtain employment and live more independently. Supports include medical and psychological services, counseling job training, procurement of assistive technology, and rehabilitative training programs. More information about federally funded programs is available on the RSA web site at http://www2.ed.gov/about/offices/list/osers/rsa/programs.html.

3.28 The Department of Veterans Affairs Home-Based Primary Care Program

The VA has approximately 330 HBPC programs across the country serving more than 36,000 veterans with multiple complex chronic diseases through an interdisciplinary team approach [20]. The interdisciplinary team is made up of a physician medical director, nurse practitioner or physician assistant, nurse, social worker, therapist, dietician, pharmacist, and mental health provider. Despite providing considerable resources in the home, the program produced significant overall cost saving by reducing VA nursing home days and hospitalizations [3]. The VA has a variety of other noninstitutional programs for veterans who qualify including:

- Homemaker Home Health Aide (HHHA): contracted program to provide homemaker or home health aide through a local HHA
- Respite services
- Home Telehealth: provides telehealth services for ongoing monitoring and assessment
- Adult Day Health Care (ADHC): provides health assessment, rehabilitation, and socialization to veterans in a congregate setting
- Veteran-Directed Home and Community-Based Services (VDHCBS): a program where a VA Medical Center purchases a package of consumer-directed services from an entity in the state's aging services network

Veterans and families desiring to look into VA services can contact a social worker at their nearest VA healthcare facility, which can be located through www.va.gov under "Locations."

3.29 National Foundations and Associations

Table 3.4 details a number of associations and foundations organized around support of individuals living with select diseases as well as nonprofit supporting seniors.

3.30 Other Medical Professionals Making House Calls

Other medical professionals make house calls, but communities vary greatly in available services. There are no search engines that can easily report availability on a national scale. Home health agencies, assisted living facilities, or the area agency on aging can provide more information about local resources. HBPC clinicians can also encourage other professionals to make house calls.

- **Audiology**: diagnostic hearing evaluations, hearing loss education and counseling, selection and fitting of hearing aids, hearing aide cleaning and repairs, cerumen removal

Table 3.4 National foundations and associations

Agency	Description	Web site
The ALS Association	Links to regional care and clinics Clinical trials information Printed educational material and newsletters Support groups Equipment loan programs Respite programs Caregiver resources	www.alsa.org
Alzheimer's Association	Local offices and 24-h helpline Caregiver center Online guide to helping individuals and families find the right care options; Community Resource Finder Library services Brain health quizzes and games	www.alz.org
American Cancer Society	Support programs and services Patient lodging programs Road to recovery (transportation) Reach to recovery (breast cancer support) Hair loss and mastectomy products Look Good Feel Better program: helps with appearance-related side effects of treatment Online communities and support I Can Cope (online cancer education classes) Patient Navigator Program	www.cancer.org
American Parkinson Disease Association	Web site publications Young onset information guide Links to veteran services Tool to search for local services and support Research updates	www.apdaparkinson. org
BenefitsCheckUp	Large easily navigated resource tool supported by National Council on Aging Helps consumers find benefit programs for prescription drugs, healthcare, rent, utilities, and other needs Includes information from more than 1650 public and private benefit programs National network, local referrals, and resources	www.benefitscheckup. org
Brain Injury Association of America	Information about and living with traumatic brain injury (TBI) Treatment and rehabilitation Family and caregiver information Support group resources Webinars TBI prevention Legal issues Local state chapters	www.biausa.org

(continued)

Table 3.4 (continued)

Agency	Description	Web site
Easter Seals	Easter Seals provides many services across the spectrum. Senior services include: Mature workers Adult day programs In-home and center-based services Services for caregivers Medical rehabilitation National Center for Senior Transportation Military and veterans Employment and training Camping and recreation Brain health	www.easterseals.com
Muscular Dystrophy Association (MDA)	MDA clinics Support groups Equipment assistance Support for caregivers Educational resources Tips for success kit Emergency resources for MDA families	www.mda.org
National Academy of Elder Law Attorneys—Consumer Resources	Elder Law Attorney finder Elder Law and Special Needs Law education Government resources State and community resources Law topics	www.naela.org Select About/ consumers
National Association of Professional Geriatric Care Managers	"Find a Care Manager" tool Description of typical services and benefits Standards of practice Position papers Education tools	www.caremanager.org
National Multiple Sclerosis Society	Extensive educational publications for clinicians and laypersons Family services, insurance, and financial info Tool to search for local services and support Treatment information Current research (clinician and patient focused)	www.nationalmssociety.org
National Parkinson Foundation (NPF)	Helpline for patients Search engine for local resources including providers, centers of care, local chapters, and support groups Discussion groups Clinical trials Patient education library NPF white papers Practical tools including Parkinson's ID Bracelet, Medical Alert Card, and hospital action plan booklet Publications, online learning, webinars, and tools Multipronged training for professionals	www.parkinson.org

- **Dentistry**: routine dental X-rays, exams and cleaning, treat cavities, fillings, tooth extraction, dentures
- **Optometry**: refraction; tonometry; retinal exams; dispensing, fitting, and adjustment of glasses
- **Podiatry**: routine care of foot and ankle; debridement of nails, corns, and calluses; ulcer care including diabetic ulcers; ingrown toenails; orthotics; diabetic shoes

References

1. Pedowitz E, Ornstein K, Farber J, DeCherrie L. Time providing care outside visits in a home-based primary care program. J Am Geriatr Soc. 2014;62(6):1122–6.
2. De Jonge KE, Jamshed N, Gilden D, Kubisiak J, Bruce S, Taler G. Effects of home-based primary care on Medicare costs in high-risk elders. J Am Geriatr Soc. 2014;62(10):1825–31.
3. Edes T, Kinosian B, Vuckovic N, Olivia Nichols L, Mary Becker M, Hossain M. Better access, quality, and cost for clinically complex veterans with home-based primary care. J Am Geriatr Soc. 2014;62(10):1954–61.
4. American Academy of Home Care Physicians. Medical management of the home care patient: guidelines for physicians. 4th ed. Chicago, IL.
5. http://www.cms.gov/Regulations-and-Guidance/Guidance/Manuals/index.html. Accessed 25 July 2015.
6. Medicare Payment Advisory Commission. Report to congress: Medicare payment policy. Washington, DC; 2014.
7. Centers for Medicare & Medicaid Services. Medicare benefit policy manual: chapter 7 - home health services [Internet]. 2015 [cited 10 Feb 2015]. Available from: http://www.cms.gov/Regulations-and-Guidance/Guidance/Manuals/downloads/bp102c07.pdf
8. Department of Health and Human Services Centers for Medicare & Medicaid Services. Medicare learning network (MLN) matters [Internet]. 2013 [cited 10 Feb 2015]. Available from: http://www.cms.gov/Outreach-and-Education/Medicare-Learning-Network-MLN/MLNMattersArticles/Downloads/SE1436.pdf
9. Medicareadvocacy.org. Jimmo v. Sebelius, the Improvement Standard Case FAQ [Internet] 2013 [cited 10 Feb 2015]. Available from: http://www.medicareadvocacy.org/jimmo-v-sebelius-the-improvement-standard-case-faqs/
10. Department of Health and Human Services Centers for Medicare & Medicaid Services. Medicare and Medicaid program: conditions of participation for home health agencies [Internet]. Washington, DC: Department of Health and Human Services Centers for Medicare & Medicaid Services; 2014. Available from: http://www.gpo.gov/fdsys/pkg/FR-2014-10-09/pdf/2014-23895.pdf
11. Department of Health & Human Services Centers for Medicare & Medicaid Services. Medicare program integrity manual [Internet]. 2002 [cited 10 Feb 2015]. Available from: http://www.cms.gov/Regulations-and-Guidance/Guidance/Transmittals/downloads/R23PIM.pdf
12. Medicare Payment Advisory Commission: Report to Congress. Impact of home health payment rebasing on beneficiary access to and quality of care [Internet]. Washington, DC: Medicare Payment Advisory Commission; 2014. Available from: http://www.medpac.gov/documents/reports/dec14_homehealth_rebasing_report.pdf?sfvrsn=0
13. Eric De Jonge K, Jamshed N, Gilden D, Kubisiak J, Bruce S, Taler G. Effects of home-based primary care on Medicare costs in high-risk elders. J Am Geriatr Soc. 2014;62(10):1825–31.
14. CMS.gov. OASIS user manuals - centers for Medicare & Medicaid services [Internet]. 2015 [cited 10 Feb 2015]. Available from: http://www.cms.gov/Medicare/Quality-Initiatives-Patient-Assessment-Instruments/HomeHealthQualityInits/HHQIOASISUserManual.html

15. Kuzuya Me. Impact of caregiver burden on adverse health outcomes in community-... - PubMed - NCBI [Internet]. National Center for Biotechnology Information, U.S. National Libraru PubMed.gov. 2011 [cited 10 Feb 2015]. Available from: http://www.ncbi.nlm.nih.gov/pubmed/20808120

16. Aoa.acl.gov. Administration on aging (AoA) legal assistance - title III-B providers [Internet]. 2014 [cited 10 Feb 2015]. Available from: http://www.aoa.acl.gov/AoA_Programs/Elder_Rights/Legal/title_providers.aspx

17. Ltcombudsman.org. NORC - National long-term care ombudsman resource center: about Ombudsmen [Internet]. 2015 [cited 10 Feb 2015]. Available from: http://www.ltcombudsman.org/about-ombudsmen

18. Medicaid.gov. Money Follows the Person (MFP) | Medicaid.gov [Internet]. 2015 [cited 10 Feb 2015]. Available from: http://www.medicaid.gov/medicaid-chip-program-information/by-topics/long-term-services-and-supports/balancing/money-follows-the-person.html

19. Medicaid.gov. Balancing Incentive Program | Medicaid.gov [Internet]. 2015 [cited 10 Feb 2015]. Available from: http://www.medicaid.gov/Medicaid-CHIP-Program-Information/By-Topics/Long-Term-Services-and-Supports/Balancing/Balancing-Incentive-Program.html

20. Va.gov. Home based primary care - geriatrics and extended care [Internet]. 2015 [cited 10 Feb 2015]. Available from: http://www.va.gov/geriatrics/guide/longtermcare/home_based_primary_care.asp

How to Perform a House Call

4

Jennifer L. Hayashi, Jonathan Ripp, and Jessica L. Colburn

Abstract

This chapter addresses the general approach to conducting a home-based medical encounter, clinical factors that are especially important to focus on in providing care for patients who cannot routinely leave their homes for office visits, and the basic equipment needed for home-based medical care. The medical equipment used in home-based medical care is essentially the same as that used in a typical office visit, and many ancillary services ordered in an office visit can also be performed in a patient's home. Home-based medical care provides unique opportunities for the clinician to perform a comprehensive assessment of the patient, understand social determinants of health that impact the patient's care, and integrate these factors into highly patient-centered care plans. This approach balances evidence-based medicine with patient prognosis, preferences, and ability to travel to a medical center for specialized testing or treatment. Similarly, preventive screening and health maintenance in the homebound population require an individualized approach that includes an understanding of prognosis, as well as disease and screening-test characteristics.

Keywords

Medical home visits • House calls • Home-based medical care

J.L. Hayashi, M.D. (✉) • J.L. Colburn, M.D.
Division of Geriatric Medicine and Gerontology, Johns Hopkins University School of Medicine, 5200 Eastern Avenue, Suite 2200, Baltimore, MD 21224, USA
e-mail: jhayash1@jhmi.edu; jcolbur1@jhmi.edu

J. Ripp, M.D., M.P.H.
Departments of Medicine, Geriatrics and Palliative Medicine, and Medical Education, Mount Sinai Hospital, 1 Gustave L Levy Place, 1216, New York, NY 10029, USA
e-mail: jonathan.ripp@mountsinai.org

© Springer International Publishing Switzerland 2016
J.L. Hayashi, B. Leff (eds.), *Geriatric Home-Based Medical Care*,
DOI 10.1007/978-3-319-23365-9_4

Medical house calls, or visits to patients' homes for the purpose of providing medical care, are a critical element in the delivery of health services to frail homebound older adults. The previous chapters have outlined important considerations for structuring a home-based medical practice and identifying community resources for homebound patients in your geographic area. The next step is to gather the tools you need to provide home-based medical care. These tools include not only medical equipment and access to ancillary services but also a comprehensive approach to assessment and screening that incorporates all of the social and functional information that is uniquely available to a home-based medical care provider, as well as the prognosis and preferences of the individual patient.

4.1 Home-Based Medical Care Tools

To start, think about the sequence of events that occurs in a typical office visit. The patient arrives, registers with the receptionist, takes a seat, and completes a health questionnaire or other forms while waiting to be seen by a provider. A medical assistant or nurse takes the patient to the clinical area to measure vital signs and enter the reason for the visit into the medical record. Then the clinician obtains a history, performs a physical exam, and discusses the findings and plan with the patient. Prescriptions, imaging, labs, or consultations may be ordered as part of the plan, and the patient leaves with instructions on following up these studies.

The events that occur in home-based medical care are essentially the same as outlined above, except that the clinician is often the person to perform all of the tasks, not just the medical evaluation and management. The equipment for home-based medical care, then, is basically the same equipment that can be found in any

Table 4.1 Common minor procedures and equipment

General supplies	Alcohol swabs
	Local anesthetic with syringes and needles
	Topical antiseptic (chlorhexidine or iodine)
	Sterile and nonsterile gauze pads
	Sterile and nonsterile gloves
	Surgical tape
	Hemostats
	Sutures
	Suture and staple removal kits
	Sharps container
Toenail removal	Iris scissors
	Nail splitter/lifter
Wound care and debridement	Scalpels
Skin biopsy	Flexible shave blades
	Punch biopsy devices
	Fixative solution

office, as described in Chap. 2 (Table 2.1). One notable difference is the possible need for a mobile device that can securely access the electronic medical record if the clinician is providing longitudinal primary care in the patient's home, or a HIPAA-compliant paper chart with key clinical information for the clinician who is making occasional home visits to supplement office-based care.

In addition, many minor primary care procedures can be performed safely in the home, avoiding the burden of requiring the patient to travel to an office solely for these procedures. Table 4.1 lists common procedures that can be performed in the home and useful equipment for a home-based medical visit.

Although portable ultrasound and x-ray equipment for plain films might be cost-prohibitive for a clinician who is adding occasional house calls to an existing office practice, many communities have mobile imaging companies who provide these services, which are often covered by insurance.

4.2 Comprehensive Home-Based Assessment

Once the clinician has assembled the basic equipment needed for a house call, the next step is to plan the visit to take full advantage of the array of information available to the clinician by virtue of seeing the patient at home. Comprehensive assessment identifies key challenges, barriers, and facilitators to patient care that may not be easily identifiable in an office visit. The comprehensive assessment framework can help the clinician understand factors that may contribute to one patient's refractory hypertension or to troubleshoot another patient's persistent medication nonadherence.

The approach to conducting a comprehensive assessment must be applied judiciously, taking into account individual patient preferences: for instance, if looking into medicine cabinets or cupboards seems important to the goals of the visit, the clinician must first ensure that the patient accepts this level of scrutiny and does not consider it an invasion of privacy.

Table 4.2 lists key considerations in a comprehensive home-based assessment. The INHOMESSS mnemonic [1] can promote recall of many of these specific considerations, but it is also useful to think about comprehensive assessment within three major domains: medical, functional, and psychosocial. Medication reconciliation, immobility, and home safety are issues in each of these domains that warrant special attention in the home-based comprehensive assessment, because these problems are prevalent, have potentially catastrophic consequences, and are especially well-suited to accurate evaluation in the home setting.

Medication reconciliation (medical domain): Medication reconciliation in the home can be very different from that in the office or hospital, because the clinician can review all of the actual medication bottles in the house, not just the ones the patient remembers or chooses to bring to these other settings. Importantly, the list that many patients bring to ambulatory settings can be reviewed and updated in the home by direct comparison with the pill bottles. Dates and prescriber information on the prescription labels can provide clues to adherence. Similarly, asking open-ended questions about medication administration ("how do you take this one?"

Table 4.2 Home-based assessment [1]

Mnemonic: INHOMESSS	
Immobility/impairment	• Activities of daily living (ADLs) • Instrumental ADLs (IADLs) • Health literacy • Balance and gait problems • Sensory impairments • Cognitive impairment • Pain • Depression • Severe mental illness – Schizophrenia – Bipolar disorder – Obsessive-compulsive disorder – Agoraphobia
Nutrition	• Availability of food • Variety and quality of foods – Pantry – Refrigerator – Freezer • Nutritional status – Obesity – Malnutrition – Medical diet restrictions • Alcohol presence/use
Housing	• Neighborhood • Exterior of home – Maintenance – Safety • Interior of home – Crowding – Housekeeping – Privacy – Pests – Pets – Memorabilia
Other people	• Social supports • Caregiver burden • Neighbors • Advance directives • Financial resources • Visitors
Medications	• Prescription medications • Nonprescription medications – Interactions – Topical treatments – Dietary supplements • Medication organization/administration • Medication adherence • Treatment burden • Diversion risk

(continued)

Table 4.2 (continued)

Mnemonic: INHOMESSS	

Examination	• Vital signs
	• General physical examination
	• Gait/balance observation
	• Functional assessment
	• Ancillary services
	   – Laboratory testing
	   – Radiology
	   – EKG

Safety	• General household risks
	   – Personal emergency response system (direct link to EMS)
	   – Carpets/rugs
	   – Lighting
	   – Electrical cords
	   – Stairs
	   – Furniture
	   – Fire, smoke, CO detectors
	   – Fire extinguishers
	   – Evacuation route
	   – Hot water heater
	   – Heating and air conditioning
	   – Water source
	• Bathroom
	   – Grab bars
	   – Slippery surfaces
	   – Tub chair
	• Kitchen
	   – Gas/electric range
	   – Cooking-related fire hazards
	   – Fire extinguishers
	   – Food safety
	   – Household poisons

Spiritual health	• Religious services and activities • Lay visitors • Pastoral visits • Patient attitudes, beliefs, and health goals

Services	• Medicare/Medicaid home health
	• Private-pay agencies
	• Community resources
	   – Agency on aging
	   – Senior centers
	   – Day care

instead of "do you take this one three times a day?") can reveal problems with understanding or memory that may prompt changes in management, including negotiation with the patient or informal caregivers for more assistance.

Immobility (functional domain): "Immobility" in Table 4.2 captures general functional impairment. Activities of daily living (ADLs) include feeding, toileting, dressing, bathing, transferring, and managing continence. ADLs are the basic tasks required for minimally independent function. The home-based medical provider can usually quickly identify problems with ADLs just by noticing features of the patient's environment that may not be apparent in an office visit: the presence or degree of involvement of a caregiver, visible stains or odor of urine in the home, or a refrigerator that is empty or filled with trays from "Meals on Wheels" can all be indicators of ADL impairment. Patients with ADL deficits require hands-on personal assistance to function in the home, and the absence of a caregiver who can help with these basic needs may mean that the patient cannot remain in the community but must transition to a care facility. Instrumental activities of daily living (IADLs), in contrast, are tasks necessary to continue living in the community but do not necessarily require direct physical contact with the patient. They include meal preparation, housekeeping, medication management, money management, telephone use, and transportation. Patients with deficits in IADLs can often remain safely at home if they have a caregiver who can prepare meals and medications a few days in advance and visit or call a few times a week to check for any additional needs. A key advantage of assessing functional status in the home is the ability to ask patients to demonstrate their actual ability to complete a task, rather than having them simply report on their ability to perform activities.

Home safety (psychosocial domain): Basic home safety is easily assessed by asking the patient or caregiver to give a tour of the home, in which the clinician looks for potentially remediable fall risks (loose rugs, poor lighting, low contrast), hand rails, smoke alarms, carbon monoxide detectors, bathroom grab bars, and the layout of furniture and equipment. Evidence of cognitive impairment may also become apparent, in the form of reminders posted around the living space, safety measures such as child-proof door locks or missing stove knobs, or unusual placement of everyday objects that might signal simple misplacement by the patient (television remote control in the refrigerator) or serve as behavior prompts to maintain function (television remote control inside a box with daily medications).

Another important safety consideration that may not be as obvious on inspection is the accessibility of firearms, which can have serious implications for patients with cognitive impairment, depression, and suicide risk or for those with young children living in the home or visiting. Additionally, the safety of the home-based medical care provider may be at risk if a patient with cognitive impairment or psychiatric illness has access to a gun and misconstrues the provider as an intruder. Our practice is to ask patients "Do you feel safe at home?" which may encompass abuse, neglect, or neighborhood crime issues and then to follow up with "Are there any guns in the home?" If the answer is affirmative, then additional questions about children, ammunition, and safeguards to prevent accidental shootings may be warranted. Very rarely, a patient or caregiver may become defensive about this topic and require reassurance that the question is intended only to optimize the safety of the patient, provider, caregiver, and any associated children, not for any reporting purposes.

Figure 4.1 illustrates key clinical data that we have found useful to keep in an easily visible and accessible section of the physical or electronic medical record ("face sheet").

Figure 4.2 provides a template for home-based medical providers to perform a comprehensive assessment on an initial visit.

HOME-BASED MEDICAL CARE FACE SHEET TEMPLATE

Patient Name:_____
Medical Record #: _____
SSN_____**DOB:** _____
Address: _____
_____
Patient's Phone #: _____
Pharmacy & Phone #: _____
_____
Caregiver name: _____
    Phone:_____
    Relationship:_____
    Availability: _____
    Date of Entry to Program: _____

ALLERGIES:_____

PROBLEM	DATE OF ONSET	ICD-9
_____	_____	_____
_____	_____	_____
_____	_____	_____
_____	_____	_____
_____	_____	_____
_____	_____	_____
_____	_____	_____
_____	_____	_____
_____	_____	_____
_____	_____	_____
_____	_____	_____

MEDICAL EQUIPMENT:
Type   Vendor/phone number
_____
_____
_____

FUNCTIONAL STATUS
(*Independent, Assist, Dependent*)

Continence	__	Medications	__
Toileting	__	Telephone	__
Transfers	__	Meal Prep	__
Bathing	__	Finances	__
Dressing	__	Laundry	__
Feeding	__	Housework	__
		Shopping	__
		Driving	__

ADVANCE DIRECTIVES
Health Care Agent: _____
Relationship: _____ Phone #: _____
Advance Directive Y/N Living Will Y/N

CODE STATUS
Refer to progress note(s) dated _____
A: Full
B: DNR, DNI, Hospitalize
C: DNR, DNI, Do Not Hospitalize
D: DNR, DNI, DNH, Comfort measures only

HOMEBOUND DUE TO: _____

HOME ENVIRONMENT
Home type:
    Single Family
    Apartment
    Senior Apartment
    Group Home/ALF
Set-up:
    Single-floor: Y / N
    Number of stairs
    Into home: Front ____Back ____
    Inside Home ____
Living Situation__Alone ___ w/Family ___ w/Non-Family
HIPAA
    Notice of Privacy Practices _____
    Acknowledgment of Receipt _____

Other important information :
Weapons in home Y   N
Pets in home   Y   N
    Type:
    Need for sequestration:
Other people in home:
_____
_____

© Bruce Leff and Jennifer Hayashi

Fig. 4.1 Face sheet template (©Bruce Leff and Jennifer Hayashi)

4.3 Additional Considerations

There are some additional considerations specific to home-based medical care that are particularly relevant to clinicians who plan to provide longitudinal primary care to patients at home. These include the time required to visit functionally impaired,

Home-Based Medical Care
Initial Visit Template

Patient: **DOB:**
Date of visit:
Primary language: English Other _____   □ Interpreter present
Present at visit:
    □ Informal caregiver   Hearing impairment   Y   N
    □ Paid caregiver   Hearing aids   Y   N
    □ Other informant   Visual impairment   Y   N
    □ Fellow   Visual aids   Y   N
    □ Resident
    □ Student
    □ Other learner

Reason for referral to home-based medical care:

History
History of Present Illness

Medical History   Surgical history

Recent hospitalizations (within 1 year): diagnosis and hospital

© Linda DeCherrie, Jennifer Hayashi, Bruce Leff, Theresa Soriano

Fig. 4.2 Home-based medical care initial visit template (©Linda DeCherrie, Jennifer Hayashi, Bruce Leff, and Theresa Soriano)

sometimes socially isolated patients at home, the additional challenges of dealing with caregivers suffering from burden or burnout, the logistics of "no-shows," connectivity of the electronic medical record, and patient access to specialty services and consultation. For a more detailed discussion of these factors, please refer to Chap. 2, "Getting Started."

Medications (review for polypharmacy)   Allergies/medication reactions

Socioeconomic conditions
Education level: Amount   Duration
Literacy   Y   N   EtOH use
Former employment: Tobacco use
Unpaid caregiver   Other substances
    Name _____
    Relation _____   Spiritual community   Y   N
    Availability _____   Type:
Other people in home_____

Medicare HHA care: RN   PT   OT   PC   Guns in home?   Y   N
    Certification ends: _____
Social services
    Meals on Wheels
    Personal care aide
    Respite   Is the patient safe at home? Y   N
    Other: _____
Pharmacy _____
    Phone: _____
    Fax: _____

Family history □ Noncontributory

Cognitive/mental health
Memory complaints
    Patient   Y   N
    Caregiver   Y   N

© Linda DeCherrie, Jennifer Hayashi, Bruce Leff, Theresa Soriano

Fig. 4.2   (continued)

One additional important clinical service that can be particularly challenging to coordinate in a home-based medical practice is anticoagulation management. The traditional method of drawing a tube of blood, sending it to the lab, and calling the patient or caregiver with the results and instructions for dose adjustments is labor-intensive, time-consuming, and potentially dangerous for clinicians who are

Functional ability

ADLs (circle one):

Activity	Independent	Needs some assist	Needs full assist
Feeding	3	2	1
Transfers	3	2	1
Bathing	3	2	1
Dressing	3	2	1
Toileting	3	2	1
Continence	3	2	1
Ambulation	3	2	1

IADLs (circle one):

Activity	Independent	Needs some assist	Needs full assist
Telephone use	3	2	1
Medication mgmt.	3	2	1
Food preparation	3	2	1
Housekeeping	3	2	1
Laundry	3	2	1
Transportation	3	2	1
Finance mgmt	3	2	1

Environment/safety   Falls in last 6 months (number)
   Stairs   Syncopal
      Into home   Mechanical
         Front ____   Continence-related Y   N

         Back ____
      Inside ____

   Single-story set-up Y   N
   Smoke detector   Y   N
   CO detector   Y   N

   Fall risks   Assistive devices: Prescribed   Used
      Lighting   Cane
      Rugs   Walker
      Cords   Wheelchair
      Clutter   Reacher
                                        Hospital bed

   Home modification
      Stair rails
      Ramps
      Grab bars
      Shower chair
         Tub rail
         Bedside commode
     Other:

© Linda DeCherrie, Jennifer Hayashi, Bruce Leff, Theresa Soriano

Fig. 4.2 (continued)

juggling multiple other health care provider roles. Medicare now covers the cost of point-of-care INR monitors for home use, but patient safety requires a consistent, reliable method of ensuring that the data are communicated to the clinician who is managing the warfarin dosage and monitoring. The current evidence base for point-of-care INR monitoring supports weekly monitoring for patients who are clinically

Review of Systems
- ☐ Unable to obtain due to _____ ☐ All others negative except as noted

GEN   ☐Weight loss ☐Appetite change ☐Temp intolerance ☐Fatigue ☐Pain

EYES   ☐Vision change ☐Eye pain ☐Eye discharge

ENT   ☐Dysphagia ☐Hearing change

CV   ☐Chest pain ☐Palpitations ☐Edema ☐Orthopnea

RESP   ☐Cough ☐SOB ☐DOE

GI   ☐Abdominal pain ☐Constipation ☐Diarrhea ☐BRBPR

GU   ☐Dysuria ☐Frequency ☐Odor/color change

MSK   ☐Joint pain ☐Back pain

DERM   ☐Rash ☐Wound (Type: ☐Pressure ☐Venous stasis ☐Arterial ☐Other)

NEURO   ☐New memory problem ☐New movement problem

PSYCH   ☐Change in mood ☐Anxiety ☐Hallucinations

HEME   ☐Bruising ☐Bleeding

OTHER

Health maintenance   Date
Pneumonia vaccine
    PPSV23
    PCV13
Flu vaccine
Tdap vaccine
Colo / sig / guaiacs
Mammo/prostate
DEXA
Advance directives
  Living will   Y   N
  Health care agent (proxy or POA)   Y   N
    Name:_____
    Relationship:_____
    Phone:_____
    Document verified   Y   N
  Medical Orders for Life-Sustaining Treatment (MOLST)   Y   N
  ☐DNR   ☐DNI   ☐DNH

© Linda DeCherrie, Jennifer Hayashi, Bruce Leff, Theresa Soriano

Fig. 4.2 (continued)

stable and cognitively intact or have a reliable caregiver and meet criteria for consistent adherence [2, 3]. This standard increases the usual monthly amount of information and communication with the patient that must be managed by the clinician and so potentially increases the risk of medical error, especially outside of the framework of a dedicated anticoagulation practitioner. Similarly, patients and

Physical exam
VS: Ht_____ Wt_____ T_____ P_____ R_____ BP_____ SpO2_____

General: □NAD □Alert □Oriented x 3 □Malnourished

Skin: □Rash □Wounds □Xerosis

Eyes: □Lids/conjunctivae/sclera normal

ENT: □Temporal wasting □No oral lesions □Poor dentition □Dentures □Cerumen impaction

Neck: □Supple □Adenopathy □Thyromegaly □Carotid bruit □JVD

Back: □Deformity □CVAT □Point tenderness

Resp: □CTAB □Wheeze □Rhonchi □Crackles (location: _____)

Cardiac: □Regular rhythm □Normal S1S2 □Murmur □Gallop □Rub □Displaced PMI

Breasts: □Mass □Dimpling □Nipple discharge □Nipple inversion

Abdomen: □Soft □Nontender □Nondistended □NABS □Organomegaly □Mass

Vascular: □Femoral bruit □Abdominal bruit □Pedal pulses 2+/symmetric □Diminished pulses

Extremities: □LE edema □Clubbing/cyanosis □Cool □Feet ulcers

Adenopathy: □Inguinal □Axillary □Epitrochlear

GU (M): □Normal □Penile lesions □Discharge □Inguinal hernia

GU (F): □Normal □Atrophic □Mass □Discharge

Rectal: □Normal tone □Hemorrhoids □Enlarged prostate □Heme (+) stool

MSK: □Joint effusions □Limited ROM

Psych: □Normal judgment/insight □Normal mood/affect □Agitation □Psychosis

Neuro: □CN II-XII intact □Strength grossly normal/symmetric □Sensation grossly normal
□Tremor □Normal DTRs

MMSE score____/_____

Mini-Cog ___/3 item recall
        CDT normal / abnormal

PHQ-2 score ___/2

© Linda DeCherrie, Jennifer Hayashi, Bruce Leff, Theresa Soriano

Fig. 4.2 (continued)

caregivers must be readily available to receive and confirm instructions about dosing changes and dates of rechecks. Commercial systems exist to facilitate the multiple steps involved but availability and logistics vary with geographic location and clinical practice structure.

Assessment/plan:

Referrals (*diagnosis/need*)
       □ Skilled home care
            Nursing _____
            PT _____
            OT _____
            SLPT _____
            MSW _____
     □ Hospice _____
     □ Community resources_____

Follow-up:

© Linda DeCherrie, Jennifer Hayashi, Bruce Leff, Theresa Soriano

Fig. 4.2 (continued)

4.4 Telephone Management

Although the primary focus of this chapter is the in-person visit, much of home-based medical care occurs over the telephone with a patient or caregiver. For clinicians who care for patients in inpatient settings or in an ambulatory practice, the ability to quickly examine a patient for a concern requires little more than walking down the hall of the hospital or "squeezing in" a patient on the clinic schedule. In practical terms, immediate examination is not feasible for many home-based medical providers. Telephone medicine is a specialized assessment skill that can bridge the gap between a patient's real or perceived needs and the home-based medical practice's capabilities to provide urgent visits. Without it, patients may suffer inconvenience, financial burden, or medical harm from avoidable emergency department visits and hospitalizations. The clinician can gather relevant history over the phone and make a decision about the urgency of the concern. Sometimes the safest course of action will be to ask the caregiver to call 911, but often the question can be safely addressed with a visit within a few days or with observation and follow-up phone calls. Medications can be prescribed if the potential benefit outweighs the potential risk for harm; a common example is the use of antibiotics for uncomplicated urinary tract infection.

In summary, home-based medical care affords unique opportunities for the clinician to understand aspects of the patient's life that may not be apparent in the office visit. In addition, for older adults who cannot routinely leave their homes for office visits, home visits can be a crucial link to medical primary care.

4.5 Screening and Preventive Care

Screening and preventive care are essential components of primary care. There are important factors to consider when making screening recommendations to homebound older adult patients, including prognosis of the patient, time to benefit from the screening test, and logistical considerations for tests that can only be obtained in a hospital setting.

In fact, the concept of preventive care for this population should focus on maintaining health as much as possible while preparing for functional decline and death. It is not uncommon for home-based medical practices to experience a 20 % mortality per year; traditional screening and disease management guidelines become less relevant in such a population.

Clinicians who have been trained to use standard guidelines for the general adult population may have difficulty reconciling the discrepancies between evidence-based recommendations and the real-life circumstances of frail homebound patients. Internal medicine residents beginning a longitudinal home-based primary care experience often return from their first home-based medical visits with a comprehensive list of screening tests prompted by the algorithm built into the electronic medical record. As they learn about prognosis, functional capabilities, and patient goals, their concerns for obtaining colonoscopies, mammograms, and Pap smears are appropriately replaced with discussions about preference for hospitalization and escalation of care, advance directives, and preferred place of death.

Although many screening tests are recommended for adults within a certain age range (e.g., colorectal or breast cancer screening), it is appropriate to recommend against screening for some patients, in particular for patients with limited life expectancy. Recommended ages at which to stop screening often depend on the specific test and guideline; in some circumstances, screening should be avoided as it may lead to more harm than good. The decision to recommend screening is made by the provider, but must consider the preferences of the patient, and, in many instances, the caregiver. Conversations about stopping screening can be challenging, and it may be useful to frame it in terms of the patient's preferences and the risks and benefits of a given test balanced against a patient's other medical problems.

In homebound patients, decisions regarding screening must also incorporate unique considerations of the burden of testing. The burden of screening may not only be related to completing the test but also to following up with diagnostic testing or treatments related to a positive finding. For example, performing a screening colonoscopy on a homebound patient might require ambulance transport to an endoscopy suite or hospitalization, which may not meet acute care criteria for medical necessity. False-positive results may occur with any preventive screening test and may lead to anxiety [4], as well as to recommendation for further testing, thus multiplying the burden to functionally impaired patients.

The US Preventive Services Task Force (USPSTF) is a commonly cited resource for preventive screening guidelines. An example of these recommendations for colorectal cancer screening is as follows: "The USPSTF recommends screening for colorectal cancer…beginning at age 50 years and continuing until age 75 years… The USPSTF recommends against routine screening for colorectal cancer in adults 76–85 years of age… For adults (between 76–85) who have not previously been screened, decisions about first-time screening in this age group should be made in the context of the individual's health status…" [5].

Though these guidelines highlight the need to individualize screening decisions in older adults, they do not provide guidance for the provider regarding how to assess individual health status. Ultimately, clinicians must consider a complex set of related factors when helping a patient make such decisions:

- Life expectancy
- Time needed to benefit from screening
- Burden of screening
- Burden of follow-up testing
- Burden of treatment if screening identifies the disease in question
- Patient preferences regarding potential treatments for the disease in question
- Potential benefit of treatment if undertaken
- Patient preferences regarding screening in general

If the patient's estimated life expectancy is shorter than the typical duration in which an asymptomatic patient develops the disease of interest and succumbs to it, then screening for that disease is likely not indicated. Knowing how to address the question of whether a patient will live long enough to develop and die from a screen-detectable disease requires an understanding of prognostication as well as disease and screening-test characteristics.

There are a number of factors to consider when estimating an individual patient's life expectancy, such as age, sex, comorbidities, and cognitive and functional status. The National Vital Statistics System [6] regularly maintains and updates this data, which is openly accessible.

While age is a strong determinant of life expectancy, it is necessary to recognize the distinction between age and life expectancy. Because there is often a wide range of life expectancy at any given age, this distinction is especially important for providers when considering who to stop screening for various diseases. For example, approximately 25 % of 75-year-old women will live at least 17 years, 50 % will live at least 11.9 years, and 25 % will live less than 6.8 years [7]. Though most guidelines still focus on a particular age at which to stop screening, as geriatric providers, it is more important to ask, "How healthy is *this* older adult sitting in front of me?" An 85-year-old woman might have a longer life expectancy than a 70-year-old man; however, guidelines might recommend screening the 70-year-old and to stop screening the 85-year-old. An approach that focuses on life expectancy is more appropriate. For this reason, it is important to factor in other variables that affect life expectancy [8].

Not surprisingly, comorbidities have an impact on life expectancy. The more comorbidities patients have, the lower their life expectancy [9]. Cognitive status is a strong predictor of life expectancy, and patients with more advanced stages of dementia have a clear decline in life expectancy [10]. Likewise, functional status has an impact on life expectancy, particularly in those who meet criteria for frailty. This is an important consideration when estimating life expectancy prior to screening [11].

Keeping track of all these variables to render a prognosis is quite complicated and may not be feasible within the confines of a patient encounter. For this reason, it may be best to utilize "calculators" that can assist in generating an estimated mortality or life expectancy. Many such calculators exist which vary in complexity and incorporated variables [12]. One commonly used website, http://eprognosis.ucsf. edu, allows users to identify appropriate prognosis calculators based on patient location (clinic, nursing home, or hospital), comorbidities, functional status, and time frame for which prognosis is being considered (1–10 years).

In addition to estimating life expectancy, it is also important to consider certain characteristics of the screening test. Perhaps most important in the case of elderly and infirm patients is the "lag time" to benefit. This is the expected time that it takes for a patient to benefit from screening or, alternatively, the time it takes from initial screening to benefit observed in study findings [13]. This information is not always easy to find and may not be included in the summary statement of screening guidelines. It may even require looking to the survival analyses in the studies that support and form the basis for evidence-based guidelines. In the case of most cancers that are screened (e.g., breast and colon), the lag time is generally considered to be on the order of 10 years [13].

Finally, it is also important to recognize that disease risk itself can change with age. This, in part, may be due to varying disease presentation (e.g., more indolent forms of breast cancer may be more common in older women) [14] but more likely is related to "competing risks." Older patients are more likely to die from causes other than the disease being screened. This concept is perhaps best exemplified by examining the number needed to screen to prevent one cancer death. These numbers go up dramatically as patients age, suggesting that it becomes increasingly more challenging to prevent death from screen-detectable disease in the geriatric population [7].

Given the burden of screening on the geriatric homebound, it is important to consider what can be tested in the home. Though screening tests that are hospital based (e.g., colonoscopy for colorectal cancer, CT scanning for lung cancer) are largely infeasible in homebound patients, there are some tests that can rather easily be performed in the home. The widespread availability of home-based phlebotomy allows for hyperlipidemia screening, for example. Fecal occult blood testing can easily be done at home for colorectal carcinoma screening, and the increased availability of home-based radiologic and ultrasonographic testing allows for some testing, such as abdominal aortic aneurysm screening. In addition, common vaccinations such as influenza and pneumococcal vaccines can be easily administered to most homebound patients, provided that the vaccine can remain stable for short periods without refrigeration.

Though screening patients who are seen at home is often more challenging and at times less indicated than in the general geriatric population, it is important to take an individualized approach in the home-based medical encounter. Screening decisions must be made in light of patient prognosis and likelihood of receiving benefit from testing and must take into account patient preferences and goals. Increased access to home-based screening tests and refined instruments for prognostication will continue to make screening and prevention an important part of home-based geriatric care.

References

1. Unwin BK, Jerant AF. The home visit. Am Fam Physician. 1999;60:1481–8.
2. Garcia-Alamino JM, Ward AM, Alonso-Coello P, et al. Self-monitoring and self-management of oral anticoagulation. Cochrane Database Syst Rev. 2010; 4: Art. No.: CD003839.
3. Matchar DB, Love SR, Jacobson AK, et al. The impact of frequency of patient self-testing of prothrombin time on time in target range within VA Cooperative Study #481: The Home INR Study (THINRS), a randomized, controlled trial. J Thromb Thrombolysis. 2015;40(1):17–25.
4. Tosteson AN et al. Consequences of false-positive screening mammograms. JAMA Intern Med. 2014;174(6):954–61.
5. United States Preventive Services Task Force. [Internet] Available from: http://www.uspreventiveservicestaskforce.org/
6. National Vital Statistics Reports. [Internet] Available from: http://www.cdc.gov/nchs/products/nvsr.htm
7. Walter LC, Covinsky KE. Cancer screening in elderly patients: a framework for individualized decision making. JAMA. 2001;285(21):2750–6.
8. Yourman LC et al. Prognostic indices for older adults: a systematic review. JAMA. 2012;307(2):182–92.
9. Fried LP et al. Risk factors for 5-year mortality in older adults: the cardiovascular health study. JAMA. 1998;279(8):585–92.

10. Larson EB et al. Survival after initial diagnosis of Alzheimer disease. Ann Intern Med. 2004;140(7):501–9.
11. Fried LP et al. Frailty in older adults: evidence for a phenotype. J Gerontol A Biol Sci Med Sci. 2001;56(3):M146–56.
12. ePrognosis. [Internet] Feb 2015. Available from: http://eprognosis.ucsf.edu/default.php
13. Lee SJ et al. Time lag to benefit after screening for breast and colorectal cancer: meta-analysis of survival data from the United States, Sweden, United Kingdom, and Denmark. BMJ. 2013;346, e8441.
14. Tew WP et al. Breast and ovarian cancer in the older woman. J Clin Oncol. 2014;32(24):2553–61.

Common Cognitive Issues in Home-Based Medical Care

5

M. Victoria M. Kopke, Cameron R. Hernandez, and Silvia Chavez

Abstract

Dementia is commonly seen in the elderly population, as it affects up to 40 % of people over 85 years old. The progressive decline in cognitive and physical abilities, often accompanied by behavioral changes, can be devastating. Delirium is a condition affecting cognitive function also encountered with greater frequency among the elderly, but is usually reversible with proper treatment. This chapter aims to assist medical professionals working in the home-based setting in diagnosing both conditions and treating them with both pharmacologic and nonpharmacologic means, while remembering that it is not only the patient but also the caregivers and family who require attention and interventions.

Keywords
Alzheimer's • Cognition • Confusion • Delirium • Dementia • Vascular

5.1 Dementia

Dementia is an acquired progressive deterioration in global cognitive abilities that impairs the successful performance of activities of daily living (ADL) due to an organic disease. In addition to loss of memory, other cognitive functions that may be impaired include communication, visuospatial recognition, executive function, and emotional regulation.

The disease can be devastating not only for the patient, but also for the family. Caring for loved ones with dementia is a significant cause of caregiver burden and

M.V.M. Kopke, M.D. (✉) • C.R. Hernandez, M.D. • S. Chavez, A.N.P.
The Mount Sinai Health System, One Gustave Levy Place, 1216, New York, NY 10029, USA
e-mail: victoria.kopke@mountsinai.org; cameron.hernandez@mountsinai.org; silvia.chavez@mountsinai.org

© Springer International Publishing Switzerland 2016
J.L. Hayashi, B. Leff (eds.), *Geriatric Home-Based Medical Care*,
DOI 10.1007/978-3-319-23365-9_5

burnout. Though curative treatments do not exist, the early recognition of dementia can help a patient and his or her family prepare for what is to come and make plans, such as getting finances in order, sorting out insurance issues and discussing health care wishes including goals of care and choosing a health care proxy while the patient is still able to participate meaningfully in the decision-making process.

5.1.1 Epidemiology and Risk Factors

Approximately 10 % of people over 70 years old have significant memory loss. The frequency of Alzheimer's Dementia (AD) increases with each decade of adult life, reaching 20–40 % of the population over 85 [1]. It is thought that by the year 2040, over 81 million people worldwide will suffer from dementia [2]. Dementia is the leading diagnosis associated with being homebound, with studies of homebound elderly populations showing the prevalence of dementia ranging from 29 to 52 % [3, 4].

The most common cause of dementia is Alzheimer's disease, representing approximately 60 % of patients with dementia. AD is the slow progression of dementia over time resulting in the loss of memory, thinking and language skills, and eventually behavioral changes. AD is the cause of more than half of all cases of dementia seen in Western countries [1]. The second most common cause of dementia is vascular dementia, usually the result of uncontrolled hypertension and cardiovascular disease. Vascular dementia usually affects reasoning, planning, judgment, memory, and other thought processes caused by impaired blood flow to the brain. Recurrent strokes may give the characteristic stepwise decrease in brain function associated with vascular dementia.

Together, AD, vascular dementia, and the combination of AD plus vascular dementia account for over 80 % of dementia cases. Approximately 4 % of dementia cases are due to Parkinson's Disease (PD) [5] and the rest are made up of the following, less common, forms of dementia: frontotemporal dementia (FTD), progressive supranuclear palsy (PSP), and dementia with Lewy bodies (DLB). FTD is caused by the progressive degeneration of the temporal and frontal lobes of the brain resulting in significant changes in decision making, behavioral control, emotion, and language [6]. PSP can result in a dementia that causes gait and balance problems, as well as visual disturbances [7, 8]. DLB is a progressive dementia that affects thinking, reasoning, and independent function and is characterized by visual hallucinations and occasionally, muscle rigidity [9].

Risk factors for dementia include increasing age, family history of AD, vascular disease, alcoholism, PD, diabetes, and vitamin deficiencies [1].

5.1.2 Differential Diagnosis/Etiology

An important reason to evaluate cognitive impairment thought to be caused by dementia is to exclude modifiable or treatable causes. Medications and their side effects are frequently culprits and should be reviewed and considered first. Table 5.1 lists medication classes known to affect cognition. The other common modifiable

Table 5.1 Medication classes affecting cognition

Anticholinergics
Antihistamines, including H2 blockers
Overactive bladder treatments
Antispasmodics
Anti-Parkinsonian agents
Antidepressants
Antipsychotics
Benzodiazapines
Nonsteroidal anti-inflammatory drugs (NSAIDs)
Opioids
Sedatives
Steroids

Table 5.2 Causes of non-AD-related cognitive impairment

Type of non-AD-related cognitive impairment	Related symptoms
Normal pressure hydrocephalus	Wide-based gait, urinary incontinence. Change in gait occurs well in advance of cognitive changes
Parkinson's disease	Resting tremor, stooped posture, masked facies
Dementia with Lewy bodies	Parkinsonian features with visual hallucinations, psychiatric features
Frontotemporal dementia	Changes in decision making, increased disinhibition, poor control of emotions, problems with language
Progressive supranuclear palsy	Gait and balance problems, as well as visual disturbances
Brain neoplasms	Seizures Focal findings on neurological exam
B12 deficiency	Ataxia, fatigue and easy bruising

causes of cognitive impairment are depression, hydrocephalus, alcohol dependence, and thyroid disease [1]. Brain neoplasm is a rare presentation of dementia. Certain symptoms accompanying memory loss may serve as clues for possible etiologies. Table 5.2 shows a list of symptoms frequently seen with non-AD-related cognitive impairment.

5.1.3 Diagnostic Approach in the Home

Evaluating a patient in the home environment presents a unique opportunity for the clinician to gather information not usually apparent during an office visit.

When evaluating a patient in the home for cognitive decline, the assessment will entail similar evaluation tools as in an office-based setting: a thorough medical history including reviewing all medications, a physical exam, and a formal cognitive assessment. Unique to home-based care, the effects of a person's cognitive dysfunction can be better assessed by observing how the patient functions in their own environment, the condition of the patient's home environment and being able to spend time speaking with their family caregivers. In the office setting, patients are often able to present their "best side," coming in well groomed and nicely dressed. Stepping into someone's home, you immediately begin to gather information about your patient before even laying eyes on them—clutter, dirty sheets on the bed, papers strewn about, an empty fridge, bare walls - all provide insight into how someone is functioning on a day-to-day basis.

5.2   History

When interviewing the patient, always consider that he or she may not be an adequate informant, and in a nonoffending manner, include family members and caregivers within and outside of the interview to obtain further history. With the patient's or proxy's consent, additional relevant history can be obtained from friends, home care workers, housekeepers, neighbors, home care nurses, previous medical providers, doormen, pharmacists, Meals on Wheels representatives, and home/community social workers.

In addition to the usual thorough review, some specific historical elements are particularly important in the evaluation of a patient with dementia:

– Cognitive history (worsening short-term memory, word-finding difficulty, behavior changes/emotional lability, difficulty with problem-solving, and complex tasks such as keeping track of appointments, driving or bill paying)
– Fall history (any previous history of gait disturbance)
– Head trauma (loss of consciousness)
– Stroke history (ischemic heart disease, hemiparesis, arrhythmias, hypertension)
– Seizure history
– Movement disorders history (tremor, parkinsonism)
– Work history (toxin exposure)
– Recreational habits (alcohol, smoking, drugs)
– Eating habits (eating food from garbage)
– Sexual history (HIV, hepatitis, syphilis)
– Psychosocial history (onset of behavior changes, visual changes, hallucination, depression, paranoia)
– Genitourinary history (any new urine/bowel incontinence)

5.3   Medication Review

Being in a patient's home affords you the opportunity to perform a thorough and accurate medication reconciliation. Seeing how your patients keep and manage their medications provides substantial information about their ability to manage their medical conditions. Ask permission to look in the patient's medicine cabinets, on the kitchen counter, dining room table, bedroom tables and drawers, etc. Call the patient's pharmacy to confirm questionable medications. Check dispense dates on prescription bottles, which will provide information regarding adherence to medications. Performing a "pill count"—emptying a bottle's contents and counting the number of pills inside, looking at the fill date on the bottle, and then calculating the number of pills that should be left - can lead to valuable information regarding your patient's ability to manage their medications. It is not uncommon to find several types of pills in one bottle, or several unused bottles of the same medication, as the pharmacy may report to you that they dispense the medication every month, not knowing that it is not being taken by the patient. Conduct a thorough review of all prescribed and over-the-counter medications, paying particular attention to medications that can alter cognition. See Table 5.1 for a comprehensive list of medication classes that may affect cognition.

5.4   Physical Exam

When conducting a thorough head-to-toe physical examination, be sure to gather the following information, which may also help determine if there is a modifiable cause for the memory loss:

- Vital signs: orthostatic blood pressures (especially if patient has a history of syncope/dizziness)
- Skin: assess for infected decubitus/abscess, shunts
- Eyes: cataracts, poor vision, double vision
- Ears: cerumen impaction, hearing loss
- Cardiac: murmurs, irregular rhythm, pacemaker/automated implantable cardioverter defibrillator (AICD)
- Neuro: cranial nerves, deep tendon reflexes, tremor, rigidity, bradykinesia, myoclonic twitching, agnosia, apraxia, aphasia, gait

5.5   Cognitive and Functional Assessment Tools

You should conduct cognitive and functional assessment tests without family or caregivers present, to avoid distractions or potential patient embarrassment. It is important to put the patient at ease and emphasize that there are no repercussions or consequences for wrong answers. Explain the findings and recommendations to the patient. Obtain consent to share findings with family members/caregivers. Choose the appropriate cognitive assessment tool based on your clinical findings and the amount of time you have available. Table 5.3 lists the most commonly used cognitive assessment tools available [10] and the amount of time they take to administer. These cognitive tools may be influenced by patient's age, educational level, language, attention, visuospatial ability, and reduced attention. Referral for neuropsychological

Table 5.3 Cognitive status assessment tools [10]

Test	Description	Scoring	Limitations	Time to administer
Clock drawing	Patient asked to draw a clock face with all the numbers and place a number and place hands at a stated time	12 must appear on top (3 points) 12 numbers must be present (1 point) Two distinguishable hands (1 point) Time must be correctly identified for full credit Score of <4/6 implies impairment	Quick screening test, not diagnostic	3 min
Mini-Cog	Consists of recall of three unrelated words and clock drawing test	If no words recalled, diagnosis is dementia If one or two out of three words recalled, look at the clock draw test. If abnormal, diagnosis is dementia If all numbers on the clock are presented in the correct sequence and the hands display the correct time, no dementia	Quick screening test, not diagnostic	5 min
Mini-mental state examination (MMSE)	Tests a broad range of cognitive functions including orientation, recall, attention, calculation, language manipulation, and constructional praxis	Maximum score is 30, score must be adjusted based on education, language, and age; <24 implies dementia	Limited by education level, literacy, and language. The patient should have at least an eighth-grade education and be fluent in English Test is copyrighted	10 min
Montreal cognitive assessment (MoCA)	Tests a broad range of cognitive functions including orientation, memory recall, visuospatial relations, sustained attention, verbal fluency and executive function	Maximum score is 30; <26 implies mild cognitive impairment or dementia (dementia diagnosis dependent on presence of associated functional impairment)		10 min

(continued)

Table 5.3 (continued)

Test	Description	Scoring	Limitations	Time to administer
Verbal fluency test	The test consists of giving the person 60 s to list out loud as many words as possible from a category, such as animals, vegetables or fruits; or words beginning with a certain letter	Fewer than 12 correct words in a minute is considered abnormal	Not diagnostic Schizophrenics do poorly at this test	2 min
Geriatric depression screening—15	It is a series of 15 yes/no questions	0–4 considered normal 5–8 indicates mild depression 9–11 indicates moderate depression 12–15 indicates severe depression	Successful in differentiating depressed from nondepressed	10 min
Bristol activities of daily living scale (BADLS)	This scale is a 20-item questionnaire designed to measure the ability of someone with dementia to carry out daily activities			5 min

testing, an extensive evaluation of multiple cognitive domains done over several hours by a licensed clinical psychologist, is not essential but may prove helpful in making the diagnosis in certain difficult cases, such as in the very early stages of the disease, when the patient or caregiver senses something is wrong but the usual cognitive assessment tools do not pick up any abnormalities.

5.5.1   Tests

The home-based medical provider should obtain appropriate lab work to diagnose modifiable causes of cognitive changes. Table 5.4 lists the labs to consider ordering and what each test evaluates.

Obtain consent to obtain medical records for any previous CT/MRI/angiograms/ EKG/EEG and lab results for comparison. Neuroimaging can be helpful in the exclusion of secondary causes of dementia, such as masses or normal pressure

Table 5.4 Laboratory tests for evaluating modifiable causes of cognitive changes

Laboratory test	Evaluating for
Complete blood count (CBC)	Possible infection, immune disorders, anemia, blood disorder
Comprehensive blood chemistry	Metabolic, kidney, liver disorders
Calcium level	Parathyroid problem
TSH level	Thyroid, endocrine disorders
Vitamin B12, folate, iron level	Nutritional, vitamin deficiency
Erythrocyte sedimentation level	Signs of inflammation
Syphilis	Brain infection
HIV, Hepatitis	Viral infections
Lyme	Affecting central nervous system
Urine analysis and urine toxin screening	Infection, drugs that can be affecting cognition
Drug levels: dilantin (phenytoin), digoxin	Drug toxicity affecting cognition

hydrocephalus [10], and a finding of medial temporal lobe atrophy on MRI supports a clinical diagnosis of AD [11] but a normal head CT or MRI does not rule out dementia. In cases where you cannot obtain past records or the patient has not had any past imaging, it is important to use your clinical judgment as to whether you think it is of value to obtain a head CT. In a patient with a history of high blood pressure and strokes, with a step-wise decline in cognition, imaging is highly unlikely to reveal anything other than vascular changes. NPH will present with clinical exam findings; you do not need a head CT to rule it out. Did you find a focal deficit on the neurologic exam? Is there something about the patient's presentation or history that points you away from thinking their cognitive changes are due to AD or vascular dementia? Are getting them out of the home to obtain imaging and keeping them calm or still enough for a study insurmountable challenges? Will the results change your management based on the goals of care? These are all issues you need to consider before deciding to recommend imaging. In patients with a history consistent with AD and nonfocal neurological examination, our practice is to forego head imaging if it would be difficult to obtain.

5.5.2 Pharmacologic Treatment

5.5.2.1 Alzheimer's Disease

Medications indicated for Alzheimer's dementia have been shown to have a minimal effect on slowing the progression of disease, so the mainstay of treatment is not pharmacological. Medications should be used cautiously under close monitoring [12]. The mantra "start low, go slow" should be considered when it comes to dosing of these medications. Medications for Alzheimer's dementia have shown to minimally improve scores on cognitive function tests but still have not shown improvement in the ability of patients to perform activities of daily living (ADL) or instrumental activities of daily living (IADL), which would be more likely to translate into improvement in the quality of life of these patients. Cholinesterase inhibitors (AChEI) and noncompetitive N-methyl-D-aspartate (NMDA) receptor antagonist are currently the medications approved for Alzheimer's dementia. There is no difference in the efficacies of the three cholinesterase inhibitors [13].

Medications approved for the treatment of dementia are described in Table 5.5 [14]. Often patients' family members will ask to start their loved one on one of the medications they have seen advertised to help people with dementia. We take this as an opportunity to educate them on the limited efficacy of these medications seen in our practice, not to "burst anyone's bubble" but to set realistic expectations. If it is the family's wish to try one of the medications, we review the potential major side effects of the medications (data in Table 5.5) and offer a 2-month trial, making it clear that they can stop the medication at any time if they are concerned about side effects. After 2 months, we review together whether any beneficial changes have been observed, and if not, we do not write a new prescription. The pharmacologic treatment of vascular dementia focuses on management of risk factors for hypertension and hyperlipidemia to avoid further deterioration of the vascular system in the brain.

5.5.2.2 Behavioral and Psychotic Symptoms of Dementia (BPSD)

Table 5.6 shows medications used for agitation in delirium and dementia. These medications are approved for use in delirium but are also used by many clinicians to manage the behavioral and psychotic symptoms in dementia. All use of these medications to treat behavioral disturbance associated with dementia is off-label.

As discussed below, the nonpharmacologic approach is the mainstay in symptom control in dementia, but providers do turn to antipsychotics when they are having great difficulty managing patients' behavioral problems nonpharmacologically or when they feel the patient or caregiver is unsafe due to the patient's behavioral issues. While some of these medications can be, at least initially, very sedating (which may offer caregivers some respite from an extremely agitated patient) they have not been shown to have great efficacy in ameliorating the behavioral disturbances they are used to treat [15, 16] and they each carry a black-box warning stating that elderly patients with dementia-related psychosis treated with conventional or atypical antipsychotic drugs are at an increased risk of death compared to placebo [17]. Prescribing an antipsychotic to treat psychosis, aggression or agitation in someone with AD must be done with caution and the understanding that overall, the adverse effects have been found to outweigh any benefits.

5.5.3 Nonpharmacologic Management

The current lack of effective treatment or cure for dementia is frustrating for patients, caregivers, and medical professionals. Caring for someone afflicted with dementia involves a multipronged approach to help improve the quality of life of the patient and caregivers, manage active symptoms, and plan for the future.

Table 5.5 Pharmacological treatment for dementia [14]

Medications	Dosing	Major side effects
Cholinesterase inhibitors		
Donepezil (Aricept)	Mild to moderate dementia	Neuro: seizures, syncope, altered sleep with vivid dreams
	5 mg PO QHS for 4–6 weeks, then increased to target dose of 10 mg PO QHS	Cardiac: bradycardia
		MSK: muscle cramps
	Moderate to severe dementia	GI: nausea, diarrhea, cramping
	5 mg PO QHS for 4–6 weeks, increased to 10 mg PO QHS for 3 months, and then increased to target dose of 23 mg PO QHS	GU: urinary frequency, urinary obstruction
Rivastigmine (Exelon, Exelon patch)	Mild to moderate AD	Neuro: seizures, syncope, depression, hallucinations
	1.5 mg PO BID, increased by 1.5 mg PO BID Q2 weeks as tolerated to target dose of 6 mg PO BID	Cardiac: bradycardia, hypotension
		GI: vomiting, diarrhea, peptic ulcer, GI bleeding
	Transdermal Patch:	
	4.6 mg patch daily for 4 weeks, increased to 9.5 mg patch daily for 4 weeks, and then increased to target dose of 13.3 mg patch daily	
	Mild to moderate PDD	
	1.5 mg PO BID, increased by 1.5 mg PO BID Q4 weeks as tolerated to target dose of 6 mg PO BID	
	Transdermal Patch:	
	4.6 mg patch daily for 4 weeks, increased to 9.5 mg patch daily for 4 weeks, and then increased to target dose of 13.3 mg patch daily	
Galantamine (Razadyne and Razadyne ER)	Mild to moderate AD	Neuro: syncope, dizziness
	Regular:	Cardiac: bradycardia
	Start 4 mg PO BID, increased to 4 mg PO BID Q4 weeks as tolerated to maximum of 12 mg PO BID	GI: vomiting, nausea, anorexia
		Renal: renal impairment or failure
		Liver: hepatotoxicity
	ER:	
	Start 8 mg PO QAM, increased by 8 mg PO QAM Q4 weeks to maximum of 24 mg PO QAM	
	If either form is stopped for more than 3 days, medication must be restarted at 8 mg and retitrated up	
	Medication needs to be renally dosed, not advised for patients with liver problems	

(continued)

Table 5.5 (continued)

Medications	Dosing	Major side effects
Noncompetititve *N*-methyl-D-aspartate (NMDA) receptor antagonist		
Memantine (Namenda)	Moderate to severe AD	Neuro: dizziness, headache, somnolence, anxiety
	Start 5 mg PO daily, increased to 5 mg PO BID at 1 week as tolerated, and then increased by 5 mg weekly to a maximum of 10 mg PO BID	Pulm: dyspnea
		GI: vomiting, constipation
		GU: urinary incontinence
		MSK: back pain

AD Alzheimer's dementia, *BID* twice a day, *ER* extended release, *GI* gastrointestinal, *GU* genitourinary, *MSK* musculoskeletal, *PO* by mouth, *PDD* Parkinson's Disease with Dementia, *QAM* every morning, *QHS* at bedtime

Table 5.6 Pharmacologic treatment for agitation associated with delirium and dementia [36]

Medications	Dosing	Major side effects
Typical antipsychotic		
Haloperidol (Haldol)	Start 0.5 mg PO BID, titrate to lowest effective dose first by increasing frequency to max of q4h, then increasing dose with a maximum of 10 mg PO q4h	Neuro: TD, dystonia, EPS, NMS, seizures
		Cardiac: hypotension, hypertension, QT prolongation, torsades de pointes, arrythmias, sudden death
		Pulmonary: Pneumonia
		Heme: agranulocytosis, neutropenia, leukopenia
Atypical antipsychotics		
Olanzapine (Zyprexa, Zyprexa Zydis)	Start at 2.5 mg daily, increase to BID as needed, titrating up to a maximum of 5 mg BID	Neuro: NMS, TD, EPS, stroke syncope, seizures
		Endocrine: severe hyperglycemia
		Cardiac: hypotension, hyperlipidemia
		GI: hepatotoxicity, pancreatitis
		Pulmonary: dysphagia, aspiration
		Heme: anemia, thrombocytopenia, agranulocytosis, neutropenia, leukopenia
		Renal: rhabdomyolysis
		Heme: agranulocytosis, neutropenia, leukopenia
Risperidone (Risperdal)	Start at 0.25 mg PO daily, titrate to lowest effective dose first by increasing frequency to BID, then by increasing dose by 0.25 mg per week, with a maximum of 4 mg total daily	Neuro: EPS, TD, NMS, seizure, syncope
		Cardiac: TIA, stroke, hypotension, QT prolongation
		Endocrine: severe hyperglycemia
		Psych: suicidality
Quetiapine (Seroquel, Seroquel XR)	Start at 25 mg PO BID, titrate to lowest effective dose, to a maximum of 100 mg BID	Neuro: EPS, TD, NMS, dystonia, seizures, syncope
		Endocrine: hyperglycemia
		Cardiac: TIA, stroke, hypotension
		Psych: suicidality, depression
		Heme: agranulocytosis, neutropenia, leukopenia

BID twice daily, *EPS* extrapyramidal symptoms, *NMS* neuroleptic malignant syndrome, *PO* by mouth, *TIA* transient ischemic attack, *TD* tardive dyskinesia

5.5.3.1 Managing the Behavioral and Psychotic Symptoms of Dementia (BPSD)

Though medications cannot be relied upon to help reduce or eliminate unwanted physical or verbal behaviors associated with dementia, there are at-home nonpharmacological interventions to recommend to benefit the caregiver/family by alleviating the unwanted behaviors.

Careful clinical observations often reveal environment-related causes of problem behaviors. Some of the prevalent behavioral and psychological symptoms among community-dwelling residents with dementia are repetitions, apathy, depression, agitation, aggression, delusions, anxiety, hallucinations, and wandering [18].

It is important to assess the patient's, their family's, and caregivers' knowledge about the cognitive disease. Ask the patient, family, and caregivers to explain in their own words what their understanding of the cognitive disorder is and how it is affecting them. Educating caregivers, family, friends, and homecare workers about the disease process will assist in improving communication for timely interventions to reduce or eliminate disruptive behaviors. Placing an early referral to any of the following resources can give needed support to families caring for loved ones with dementia: social workers within your own practice, in a Medicare-certified home health agency, or in the community; the Alzheimer's Association, or the Department of Aging. These resources help reinforce your teaching in the home and may offer support groups as well.

Effective communication with the patient is a mainstay in managing disruptive behaviors due to cognitive impairment, especially in the early stages of the disease process. Be sure to allow adequate time for the patient to communicate his or her thoughts. Communication can be facilitated through visual cues, by remaining at the patient's eye level and speaking softly and slowly in a quiet place. If the patient uses glasses or hearing aids, be sure to make them available [19].

Agitation, aggression, confusion, irritability, delusions, and hallucinations are common and persistent unwanted behavioral problems that may have multiple etiologies. The most frequent cause of the behavioral change may be related to acute delirium, discussed later in this chapter or to modifiable environmental factors.

Finding the trigger is essential in reducing or eliminating the unwanted behaviors. A three-step ABC approach may be used to identify the behavior disturbance.

1. What are the triggering events, "antecedents," to minimize or eliminate?
2. Describe the "behavior" in detail. How often does it occur, how and where it is most likely to happen, and how long does it last?
3. What are the "consequences" of the behavior? How does the caregiver, family member or home care worker react to reinforce or deter the activity, and what happens when the activity ceases?

Identifying trigger events can help prevent them, or intervene to reduce or eliminate the unwanted behaviors.

Table 5.7 Unwanted behaviors seen in dementia, possible environmental triggers, and suggested interventions [19]

Unwanted behavior	Trigger	Therapeutic intervention
Sleep deprivation	Bright light during nighttime	Make living area bright, preferably with natural light, during the daytime
		Turn off TVs and radios at night
		Lower shades/curtains at night
		Use night lights
Pacing	Dark room/poor lighting	Add upward-facing light fixtures
	Sensation of confinement	Place pictures over doorways to prevent wandering
	Shadows can trigger visual hallucination	Place stop signs as visual cues
		Paint the walls with neutral colors
Refusing to shower	Fear of falling	Place a colorful bathmat in tub so the patient can see there is a bottom to the tub
Overstimulation	Elevated noise level	Reduce noise level
Restlessness	Room temperature too cold or too hot	Monitor and adjust room temperature to comfort level

Conduct a home environment assessment, as unwanted behaviors can be brought on by triggers from the home environment. Table 5.7 shows interventions to improve unwanted behaviors that are responses to the home environment.

Structured activities can also decrease unwanted behaviors. Write out a prescription with one personal care goal for the patient who refuses to bathe or accept personal care. Provide visual or sensory cues, such as colorful calendar, to indicate events, bathing, toileting, meals, exercise, or bedtime.

Sensory stimuli intervention, such as doll therapy, music, and reminiscing therapy can be done in the home by caregivers to help to reduce or eliminate unwanted behaviors.

– Doll therapy enhances participation in activities of daily living and personal care. Dolls have been found to be useful in reducing anxiety, withdrawal behaviors, depression, and mild agitation [20]. The Alzheimer's Association has an online Alzheimer's store where therapeutic products such as dolls can be purchased. Family members, caregivers, nurses, and home care workers can use the therapeutic object during unwanted behaviors and to engage participation.
– Music therapy has demonstrated decreases in overall agitation during personal care. Ask family members to choose the music and to monitor the patient's reactions to the music being played. Classical, nature, and instrumental music may be soothing during meals, sleep, or when agitated [21].
– Reminiscing therapy is used to decrease unwanted behaviors such as agitation, anxiety, or confusion. Patients become engaged as open-ended questions about their life are asked. Using open-ended questions allows the patient to tell their

story. If available, have them look at a picture album and describe the events in the pictures. An enjoyable event in their past is not confusing to them and they often become engaged.

Supportive care for family and caregivers is invaluable [12]. Spending time in your patients' homes lets you see the depth and breadth of supportive care provided to your patients by those around them, and at the same time gives you a fuller sense of which caregivers may need more support than others. Acknowledge all the work they do in the home and ask how they find time for themselves, what they do to relax and whom they turn to for support. Most caregivers have unmet needs for resource referrals and caregiver education. Encourage caregivers to educate themselves about the disease by providing resources and problem-solving skills. The number one resource is the Alzheimer's Association. Home medical providers should refer appropriate patients to home nursing agencies for home safety evaluations and caregiver education. A referral to social work can be used to educate caregivers about community resources such as day or night programs, as well as potential options for respite care arrangements. See Further Reading at the end of the chapter for additional information.

5.5.4 Prognosis

Discussing prognosis with patients and their families is important to accomplish. While the decline of a patient with dementia tends to follow a known course, the timeline is often difficult to predict. Dementia is a terminal illness. The prognosis for AD is typically 7–10 years after diagnosis but can range from 1 to 25 years [1], However, once a patient has advanced dementia and is bedbound, relying on others for all their care, the 6-month mortality rate is 25 %, with a median survival of 1.3 years [22]. The cause of death for either usually stems from difficulty in moving, eating, and swallowing—pressure ulcers, aspirations, and pneumonia. Over 50 % of patients with advanced dementia who have an episode of pneumonia will die in the next 6 months [22].

At one time it was thought that inserting feeding tubes in patients with dementia who can no longer feed themselves would prevent aspirations, however, it has been shown that not only do feeding tubes not prevent aspirations, but also they provide no mortality benefit and may cause undue pain. Talking with families about these findings helps them understand why we do not recommend artificial nutrition for patients with dementia [23]. Patients with vascular dementia tend to die from stroke, heart disease, or infection. Patients suffering from FTD and PSP have a shorter life expectancy given earlier age of onset and worse prognosis [24]

Regular discussions with caregivers concerning likely future events in the course of dementia should be undertaken. At each visit thereafter, it is helpful to end by giving them a brief summary of where you see the patient at this point of time and what interventions may help them remain comfortable at home. End-of-life issues, including palliative care and hospice referral, are discussed in Chap. 12.

5.6   Delirium

Delirium is a clinical syndrome characterized by an acute and fluctuating change in cognition and attention. Delirium, both in its hyperactive and hypoactive forms, is distressing for family and patients and associated with increased caregiver burden [25]. Hyperactive delirium is the more recognizable form of delirium, noted for mood lability, hallucinations, delusions, and agitation. Hypoactive delirium is more frequently missed or misdiagnosed, as it usually presents as lethargy; family and medical professionals often mistake it for depression or fatigue. Both forms of delirium are associated with increased morbidity and mortality. Treatment is focused on treating the underlying condition causing the delirium.

While the literature mainly focuses on delirium in the hospital setting, it is a common occurrence among homebound patients in the form of "sundowning"—patients whose behavior acutely and dramatically changes in the late afternoon or evening, becoming more confused, anxious, and agitated. This phenomenon is not well understood but is highly prevalent among people with dementia [26] and both challenging and distressing for their caregivers.

5.6.1   Risk Factors

Risk factors for delirium include dementia, advanced age (over 65), illness, and polypharmacy. It is estimated that 30–40 % of cases of delirium are preventable [27]. Up to two-thirds of elderly patients with delirium have underlying dementia [28].

5.6.2   Etiologies

The etiologies of delirium are diverse and multifactorial, often reflecting the consequences of an acute medical illness or effects of a drug [28]. Common underlying causes of delirium include the following:

- Medication side effects (See Table 5.1)
- Infection
- Volume depletion/dehydration
- Pain
- Constipation
- Sleep deprivation
- Metabolic imbalances—such as calcium, sodium, or glucose
- Hypoxia
- Ischemia
- Sensory deprivation—e.g., are they missing their glasses or hearing aids?
- Environmental changes—e.g., a recent move, a hospitalization, change in caregiver
- Drug withdrawal—from the above medications or alcohol, illicit drugs [25, 28–30]

5.6.3   Investigations at Home

Delirium is a clinical diagnosis; there is no lab test or imaging study that provides greater accuracy in the diagnosis of delirium than the confusion assessment method (CAM) algorithm. The diagnosis of delirium can be made quickly at a patient's bedside without any lab tests or studies. The CAM algorithm is a quick, validated screening tool, with a sensitivity of 94 % and specificity of 89 % [31].

The confusion assessment method algorithm assesses the patient for the following conditions: acute onset of confusion with a fluctuating course, inattention, disorganized thinking, and altered level of consciousness [32].

See Table 5.8: Confusion assessment method algorithm [32–34].

5.6.3.1   History

If the cause of the delirium is due to a general medical condition, a good history, thorough physical examination, and basic laboratory testing can often make the diagnosis.

The history should focus on the reversible risk factors listed above, including a thorough review of prescribed and over-the-counter medications in the home, looking for high-risk medications as listed above.

5.6.3.2   Physical Exam

Examination of the patient should focus on the potential causes, including looking for signs of infection, pain, shortness of breath, constipation, and urinary retention.

5.6.3.3   Tests

Labs should be ordered, guided by physical exam findings as warranted. Consider ordering a complete blood count (CBC), basic metabolic panel (BMP) including calcium, urinalysis, and/or chest X-Ray (CXR). Base your labwork choices on specific symptoms; for example, treatment of asymptomatic bacteriuria in delirious patients is not recommended unless a urinary catheter is present [35] and a head CT is not warranted in the absence of focal findings.

5.6.4   Nonpharmacologic Management

Successful treatment of delirium requires correction of all remediable factors. Given the multifactorial nature of delirium, especially in the elderly, it may not be possible to identify a single cause. Most often, nondrug therapy is a key to treatment and should be the initial course of action [36].

One of the most important nonpharmacologic treatments is frequent reorientation and socialization for patients with delirium or who are at risk for delirium. Take advantage of the home setting by having caregivers present patients with familiar photos and objects found in the home. Instruct the caregiver to ask the patient to

Table 5.8 Confusion assessment method algorithm [32]

Criteria	Assessment method
1. Acute onset and fluctuating course	Caregivers and family members are often the best sources for this information. Did the confusion present over hours to days? Do the symptoms fluctuate during the course of a day?
2. Inattention	Observe the patient—are they easily distracted, or over-absorbed in a task, such as picking at the bed sheet? [33]
	Two ways to test attention are as follows:
	Asking the patient to recite the months of the year backwards (abnormal if unable to do so correctly)
	Digit Span Test: Having the patient repeat a series of random numbers presented at a rate of 1 per second. First give a 2-number sequence and if the patient repeats the sequence correctly, then give a 3-number sequence. Continue adding one digit to each subsequent sequence. A digit span of less than 5 is considered to be abnormal [34]
3a. Disorganized thinking	Ask patient an open-ended question, such as "Describe your medical condition"
	Listen for rambling, incoherent speech, or tangential thought process [33]
3b. Altered level of consciousness	Do they respond to their name?
	Overall, would you rate this patient's level of consciousness as alert (normal), vigilant (hyperalert), lethargic (drowsy, easily aroused), stupor (difficult to arouse) or coma (unarousable)? Any answer other than "alert" counts

If patients have either 1 or 2 AND 3a or 3b, it is considered a positive screen for delirium, warranting further work-up and intervention

name the people in pictures, and if they cannot remember, to tell them who is in the pictures and ask about the person or event documented. If family members and friends live near, let them know how important it is to remain a presence in their loved one's life, visiting with consistency when possible.

Sensory deprivation can lead to delirium and is easily remedied by providing adequate sensory input. Make sure patients are wearing their eyeglasses and hearing aids, as appropriate. Encourage caregivers to sit with the patient at various times during the day, such as at meals and when watching television, and engage them in conversation.

Medication management may be as easy as removal of the offending agent and the observation of the patient. Nonpharmacologic treatment of severe pain includes massage or pressure point therapy. Hypoxia can be rectified by giving supplemental oxygen. Remind caregivers to pay careful attention to nutrition and hydration status, as older patients do not feel the same sense of thirst and/or may have difficulty accessing food and drink. Assistance with meals, including possible hand feeding and offering drinks, may be necessary to reverse hunger or volume depletion. Facilitate the adoption of healthy sleep–wake cycles in patients at risk for delirium, encourage night sleeping by reducing environmental stimuli within the home, including turning off televisions and radios at night and opening window blinds and increasing home light sources during the day.

Educate the patient's family and caregivers that recovery from delirium can be a long process even after the underlying cause is addressed and reversed. Patients may remain delirious for weeks to months despite resolution of the cause.

5.6.5 Pharmacologic Treatment

5.6.5.1 Treating the Underlying Cause of Delirium

As discussed above, delirium can be triggered by an infection or metabolic disturbance. Should the history, physical exam and tests point to an infectious or metabolic etiology, treat according to the underlying cause.

5.6.5.2 Treatment of Agitation in Delirium

If the patient is a threat to herself or others, it may be necessary to treat for delirium. Nonpharmacologic methods are the first line of management and are discussed above [37].

Typical and atypical antipsychotics are used to improve delirium and can be used in the home with proper supervision. In some small studies, low-dose haloperidol, risperidone, and olanzapine were shown to be equally effective in treating delirium. Higher dose of haloperidol resulted in an increase in Parkinsonian adverse effects [38].

Initiate drug therapy cautiously to manage agitation in delirium and do not hesitate to change medications if the patient's agitation does not respond. These medications are meant for short-term use; once the patient's agitation is well controlled and the underlying cause for the delirium addressed, begin to taper these medications down slowly until off.

Avoid the use of opioids, benzodiazepines, and cholinesterase inhibitors if possible in patients with delirium [34]. Sedating agents are thought to worsen or prolong delirium. Cholinesterase inhibitors have not been shown to be effective in improving delirium [39]. See Table 5.6 (Pharmacologic Treatment for Agitation Associated with Delirium [36]).

Given that approximately half of all homebound adults may have dementia, home-based primary-care providers are at the forefront of caring for this growing population. Both dementia and delirium are cognitive conditions that can be diagnosed and managed well in the home-based medical setting, especially given the primary role of nonpharmacologic management in these conditions. Recognizing, managing, and treating delirium in the home-based setting is a challenge and close work with patients' caregivers and family members is essential to keep these patients safe in their homes. Caregiver support and education goes a long way in giving families the tools they need to care for their loved one without sacrificing their own quality of life.

5.7   Further Reading

Alzheimer's Association: www.alz.org
Alzheimer's Association store: www.alzstore.com
American Delirium Society: www.americandeliriumsociety.org
Hospital Elder Life Program (HELP) for Prevention of Delirium: www.hospital-elderlifeprogram.org
National Association of Home Care: www.nahc.org
National Academy of Elder Law Attorneys: www.naela.org

References

1. Seeley WW, Miller BL. Harrison's principles of internal medicine [Internet]. 18th ed. New York: McGraw-Hill; 2012. Chapter 371, Dementia. Available from http://accessmedicine.mhmedical.com/book.aspx?bookId=331.
2. Ferri CP, et al. Global prevalence of dementia: a Delphi consensus study. Lancet. 2005; 366(9503):2112–7.
3. Qiu WQ, Dean M, Liu T, George L, Gann M, Cohen J, Bruce ML. Physical and mental health of the homebound elderly: an overlooked population. J Am Geriatr Soc. 2010;58(12):2423–8.
4. Kronish IM, Federman AD, Morrison RS, Boal J. Medication utilization in an urban homebound population. J Gerontol A Biol Sci Med Sci. 2006;61(4):411–5.
5. Aarsland D, Zaccai J, Brayne C. A systematic review of prevalence studies of dementia in Parkinson's disease. Mov Disord. 2005;20(10):1255–63.
6. Rosso SM, et al. Frontotemporal dementia in The Netherlands: patient characteristics and prevalence estimates from a population-based study. Brain. 2003;126:2016–22.
7. Bower JH, Maraganore DM, McDonnell SK, Rocca WA. Incidence of progressive supranuclear palsy and multiple system atrophy in Olmsted County, Minnesota, 1976 to 1990. Neurology. 1997;49(5):1284–8.
8. Schrag A, Ben-Shlomo Y, Quinn NP. Prevalence of progressive supranuclear palsy and multiple system atrophy: a cross-sectional study. Lancet. 1999;354(9192):1771–5.
9. Savica R, Grossardt BR, Bower JH, Boeve BF, Ahlskog J, Rocca WA. Incidence of dementia with Lewy bodies and Parkinson disease dementia. JAMA Neurol. 2013;70(11):1396–402.
10. Chai E, Meier D, Morris J, Goldhirsch S. Geriatric palliative care: a practical guide for clinicians. New York: Oxford University Press; 2014. p. 345–51. Chapter 67, Dementia.
11. Larner AJ. What's new in dementia? Clin Med. 2010;10(4):391–4.
12. Lyketsos CG, Colenda CC, Beck C, Blank K, Doraiswamy MP, Kalunian DA, Yaffe K, Task Force of American Association for Geriatric Psychiatry. Position statement of the American Association for Geriatric Psychiatry regarding principles of care for patients with dementia resulting from Alzheimer disease. Am J Geriatr Psychiatry. 2006;14(7):561–72.
13. Birks J. Cholinesterase inhibitors for Alzheimer's disease. Cochrane Database Syst Rev. 2006;1, CD005593.
14. Blass DM, Rabins PV, McCormick E, Ripp J. Dementia. In: Chick D, Korenstein D, Lazoff M, Lynn R, editors. ACP smart medicine. [Internet]. Philadelphia: American College of Physicians; 2014. Available from: http://smartmedicine.acponline.org/content.aspx?gbosId=164. Updated 2014 June 27.
15. Paleacu D, Barak Y, Mirecky I, Mazeh D. Quetiapine treatment for behavioural and psychological symptoms of dementia in Alzheimer's disease patients: a 6-week, double-blind, placebo-controlled study. Int J Geriatr Psychiatry. 2008;23(4):393–400.

16. Schneider LS, Tariot PN, Dagerman KS, Davis SM, Hsiao JK, Ismail MS, Lebowitz BD, Lyketsos CG, Ryan JM, Stroup TS, Sultzer DL, Weintraub D, Lieberman JA, CATIE-AD Study Group. Effectiveness of atypical antipsychotic drugs in patients with Alzheimer's disease. N Engl J Med. 2006;355(15):1525–38.

17. US Food and Drug Administration Information for Healthcare Professionals: Conventional Antipsychotics. http://www.fda.gov/Drugs/DrugSafety/PostmarketDrugSafetyInformationfor PatientsandProviders/ucm124830.htm

18. Lyketsos CG, Steinberg M, Tschanz JT, et al. Mental and behavioral disturbances in dementia: finding for the cache county study on memory in aging. Am J Psychiatry. 2000;157(5): 708–14.

19. Teri L, Rabins P, Whitehouse P, et al. Management of behavior disturbance in Alzheimer disease: current knowledge and future directions. Alzheimer Dis Assoc Disord. 1992;6(2): 77–88.

20. Fitzsimmons S, Barba B, Stump M. Sensory and nurturing nonpharmacological interventions for behavioral and psychological symptoms of dementia. J Gerontol Nurs. 2014;40(11):9–15.

21. Cohen-Mansfield J. Nonpharmacologic interventions for inappropriate behaviors in dementia. Am J Geriatr Psychiatry. 2001;9:361–81.

22. Mitchell SL, Teno J, Kiely DK, Shaffer ML, Jones RN, Prigerson HG, Volicer L, Givens JL, Hamel MB. The clinical course of advanced dementia. N Engl J Med. 2009;361(16): 1529–38.

23. Gillick M. Rethinking the role of tube feeding in patients with advanced dementia. N Engl J Med. 2000;342:206–10.

24. Kertesz A. Frontotemporal dementia/Pick's disease. Arch Neurol. 2004;61(6):969–71.

25. Chai E, Meier D, Morris J, Goldhirsch S. Geriatric palliative care: a practical guide for clinicians. New York: Oxford University Press; 2014. p. 190–5. Chapter 34, Delirium.

26. Khachiyants N, Trinkle D, Son SJ, Kim KY. Sundown syndrome in persons with dementia: an update. Psychiatry Investig. 2011;8(4):275–87.

27. Gonzalez M, de Pablo J, Fuente E, et al. Instrument for detection of delirium in general hospitals: adaptation of the confusion assessment method. Psychosomatics. 2004;45:426–31.

28. Fong T, Tulebaev SR, Inouye S. Delirium in elderly adults: diagnosis, prevention and treatment. Nat Rev Neurol. 2009;5(4):210–20.

29. Clegg A, Young JB. Which medications to avoid in people at risk of delirium: a systematic review. Age Ageing. 2011;40(1):23–9.

30. Young J, Murthy L, Westby M, Akunne A, O'Mahony R, Guideline Development Group. Diagnosis, prevention, and management of delirium: summary of NICE guidance. BMJ. 2010;28:341.

31. Wei LA, Fearing MA, Sternberg EJ, Inouye SK. The confusion assessment method: a systematic review of current usage. J Am Geriatr Soc. 2008;56:823–30.

32. Inouye SK, van Dyck CH, Alessi CA, Balkin S, Siegal AP, Horwitz RI. Clarifying confusion: the confusion assessment method. A new method for detection of delirium. Ann Intern Med. 1990;113(12):941–8.

33. Breitbart W, Alici Y. Agitation and delirium at the end of life "We couldn't manage him". JAMA. 2008;300(24):2898–910.

34. Strub RL, Black FW. The mental state evaluation in neurology. 4th ed. Philadelphia, PA: FA Davis Company; 2000.

35. McKenzie R, Stewart MT, Bellantoni MF, Finucane TE. Bacteriuria in individuals who become delirious. Am J Med. 2014;127(4):255–7.

36. Marcantonio A, Hernandez CR, Kopke MVM. Delirium. In: Chick D, Korenstein D, Lazoff M, Lynn R, editors. ACP smart medicine. [Internet]. Philadelphia: American College of Physicians; 2014. Available from: http://smartmedicine.acponline.org/content.aspx?gbosId=120. Updated 15 Mar 2014.

37. Roden M, Simmons BB. Delirium superimposed on dementia and mild cognitive impairment. Postgrad Med. 2014;126(6):129–37.

38. Lonergan E, Britton AM, Luxenberg J. Antipsychotics for delirium. Cochrane Database Syst Rev [Internet]. 2007 [cited 2015 Jan 17]. Available from: http://onlinelibrary.wiley.com/enhanced/doi/10.1002/14651858.CD005594
39. Overshott R, Karim S, Burns A. Cholinesterase inhibitors for delirium. Cochrane Database Syst Rev [Internet]. 2008 [cited 2015 Jan 17]. Available from: http://onlinelibrary.wiley.com/enhanced/doi/10.1002/14651858.CD005317.pub2

Common Neurologic Issues

6

Ritesh A. Ramdhani, Theresa A. Soriano, and Linda DeCherrie

Abstract

Neurological diseases are prevalent in homebound older adults and directly impact the quality of life. This chapter reviews some of the common neurologic issues that a home-based medical practitioner may encounter and provides a comprehensive diagnostic and treatment approach to managing such conditions in the home.

Keywords

Home-based primary care • Home-based palliative care • Home-based medical care • Home visit • Parkinsonism • Stroke • Multiple sclerosis • Amyotrophic lateral sclerosis • Spinal cord injury

R.A. Ramdhani, M.D. (✉)
Movement Disorders Division, Department of Neurology and Neurosurgery, Icahn School of Medicine at Mount Sinai, 5 East 98th St., First Floor, New York, NY 10029, USA
e-mail: ritesh.ramdhani@mssm.edu

T.A. Soriano, M.D., M.P.H.
Department of Medicine, Geriatrics, and Palliative Medicine, Icahn School of Medicine at Mount Sinai, One Gustave Levy Place, 1216, New York, NY 10029, USA
e-mail: Theresa.soriano@mountsinai.org

L. DeCherrie, M.D.
Department Geriatrics and Palliative Medicine, Icahn School of Medicine at Mount Sinai, One Gustave Levy Place, 1216, New York, NY 10029, USA
e-mail: linda.decherrie@mountsinai.org

© Springer International Publishing Switzerland 2016
J.L. Hayashi, B. Leff (eds.), *Geriatric Home-Based Medical Care*,
DOI 10.1007/978-3-319-23365-9_6

6.1   Key Points

1. Parkinsonism management should focus on the myriad of nonmotor features that can reduce a patient's quality of life, in addition to the motor complications.
2. Diagnosing an acute stroke in the home setting relies on understanding basic localization principles and conducting an efficient and effective neurological evaluation.
3. Understanding and distinguishing a multiple sclerosis attack from an exacerbation has both diagnostic and therapeutic implications.
4. Caring for a patient with amyotrophic lateral sclerosis (ALS) requires a multidisciplinary care team consisting of palliative medicine, a neurologist, a pulmonologist, physical and occupational therapists, social workers, and nurses.

6.2   Introduction

As the homebound geriatric population grows, the home-based medical practitioner will encounter patients with neurological diseases and conditions that are often superimposed on chronic medical conditions. An understanding of common neurological conditions both at an anatomical and functional level and the impact of medical conditions on the symptomatology will empower a home-based practitioner with the tools to provide optimal neurologic care to this population.

6.3   Stroke

Eighty-five percent of all strokes are ischemic in etiology—embolic, atherothrombotic, or a lacunar syndrome, while intracerebral hemorrhage and subarachnoid hemorrhage are responsible for the remaining 15 % [1]. In the home-based medical care setting, it is important to determine whether a patient has suffered an acute stroke and to implement secondary prevention measures for recurrent stroke, as such recurrences constitute close to 30 % of all preventable strokes; the average annual recurrent stroke risk of 4 % [2].

6.3.1   Diagnosing an Acute Stroke in the Home Setting

Assessment of a patient with stroke symptoms begins at the bedside with an evaluation of the patient's mental status.

6.3.1.1   Mental Status
A patient's level of consciousness is usually well-preserved during an ischemic stroke, while the presence of increased lethargy, stupor, or coma suggests diffuse cerebral hemispheric dysfunction stemming from increasing cerebral edema or a large expansive hemorrhage causing herniation, hydrocephalus, and/or seizure activity.

For those patients with intact consciousness, a home-based medical practitioner should begin a neurological assessment by obtaining a concise and pertinent history from the patient, family members, and/or caregivers:

When was the patient last seen in his/her usual state of health?

This question helps to determine approximate time of symptom onset. A patient whose symptoms started within the past 3 h may be a candidate for thrombolytic therapy to be administered in an acute tertiary care center.

Criteria for Intravenous Tissue Plasminogen Activator
- Onset of symptoms <3 h
- Contraindications: Systolic blood pressure >185 or diastolic >110, the presence of a hemorrhage on a head CT scan, blood dyscrasia (e.g., platelets <100,000/mm^3, INR >1.7), previous intracranial hemorrhage, history of an AVM, aneurysm or neoplasm, advanced heart failure, internal bleeding, myocardial infarction, or major surgery within the last 14 days.

Expanded TPA "Window" (4.5 h) Criteria
- Patient is <80 years
- Does not have diabetes mellitus *and* a history of a prior stroke

What are the symptoms? (Refer to Table 6.1)

Warning signs of stroke include sudden numbness or weakness on one side of the body or a limb, speech changes (i.e., dysarthria), language deficits (i.e., aphasia), sudden visual problems (i.e., diplopia, unilateral vision loss, or visual field defects), and sudden incoordination and gait difficulty.

Various brain regions are implicated based on the types of symptoms present. A change in the level of alertness accompanied by headache, nausea, or vomiting is highly suggestive of an intracerebral hemorrhage that can occur in the cortical regions, subcortical structures, such as the basal ganglia and thalamus, brainstem or cerebellum. Tables 6.1 and 6.2 contain detailed descriptions of specific localizing symptoms and stroke syndromes.

What medications is the patient taking?

Important medications to query about include use of anticoagulants, antiplatelet agents, antihypertensives, opioids, antihyperglycemic drugs, and anticonvulsants.

6.3.1.2 Conducting a Home-Based Stroke Assessment [3, 4]

1. Obtain vital signs (e.g., blood pressure, heart rate, temperature) and a bedside fingerstick glucose
2. Perform a basic neurological exam

Table 6.1 Localization of stroke symptoms

Brain region	Hemisphere	Functional region	Stroke symptom
Cortex	Left	Language	Speech fluency or language (Aphasia)
		Vision	Visual field defects
		Sensorimotor	Right-sided sensory impairment and/or hemiparesis or hemiplegia
		Cognition	Inability to read and/or write
	Right	Sensorimotor	Right-sided sensory impairment and/or hemiparesis or hemiplegia
		Vision	Visual field defects
		Higher sensory processing	Neglect of left side of body Inability to recognize body parts and depth perceptual problems
	Structures	**Stroke symptoms**	
Subcortex	Internal capsule	Lacunar syndrome (Table 6.2)	
	Basal ganglia/thalamus	Lacunar syndrome (Table 6.2)	
	Brainstem	Cranial neuropathies and unilateral or bilateral weakness (e.g. locked-in syndrome)	
		Lacunar syndrome (Table 6.2)	
Cerebellum		Headache	
		Vertigo	
		Nystagmus	
		Truncal or appendicular ataxia	

Table 6.2 Types of lacunar stroke syndromes

Lacunar syndrome	Clinical manifestations
Pure motor hemiparesis	Unilateral motor weakness of the face, arm, and leg
Pure hemisensory deficit	Unilateral numbness or paresthesia of face, arm and leg
Mixed sensorimotor	Unilateral weakness and numbness in face, arm, and leg
Dysarthria—clumsy hand	Unilateral lower facial weakness with slurred speech and impaired coordination with ipsilateral hand
Ataxia—hemiparesis	Mild unilateral weakness in leg greater than arm with ipsilateral cerebellar signs that are out of proportion to the weakness

(a) Evaluate patient's orientation
(b) Have patient repeat a sentence: "Today is a sunny day."
(c) Have patient follow three simple commands: Raise your right arm, stick out your tongue, show me two fingers with your left hand.

These tasks will enable the examiner to identify an aphasia or dysarthria. Common aphasias include the following:

Broca's aphasia—speech is nonfluent with impaired repetition and preserved command-following.

Wernicke's aphasia—speech is fluent, nonsensical with impaired repetition and command-following.

Conduction aphasia—speech is fluent with preserved command-following, but impaired repetition.

(d) Have patient follow your finger with their eyes in all cardinal directions.
A gaze preference to one side, while at rest, suggests the presence of a visual field defect that is consistent with a hemispheric stroke. Patient's eyes tend to look toward the side of the brain affected by the stroke. A centered gaze at rest with impaired eye movement(s) indicates a brainstem lesion.

(e) Have patient close their eyes tightly and smile
Check for eye closure weakness by gently pulling up on their upper eye lids against resistance. Carefully observe their lower face for an uneven smile. A stroke affecting the motor system produces lower facial asymmetry and the presence of both eye closure and lower face weakness with the absence of limb weakness is likely a Bell's palsy.

(f) Have patient raise both arms in front of them and count to 10. Have them do the same for each leg separately. Drifting downward or difficulty elevating the limb confirms weakness.

(g) Test tactile sensation by using a cotton swab or pinprick on both sides of the face, arms, and legs with patient's eyes closed.
Afterward, simultaneously test sensation on both arms and legs to determine whether patient is demonstrating extinction to one side. Neglect or inattention of the left hemibody is a higher sensory modality related to right cerebral cortex impairment.

(h) Conduct finger–nose–finger and heel–shin tests on both sides to determine the presence of limb ataxia. Overshooting or past-pointing and clumsiness during these tests suggest cerebellar involvement. It should be noted that marked weakness or confusion may limit the findings on this test.

6.3.1.3   What Is a Transient Ischemic Attack?

A transient ischemic attack (TIA) is a reversible focal neurological deficits occurring in any cerebral vascular territory that last less than 1 h and completely resolve in 24 h with no objective neurological findings.

6.3.2   Advanced Directives and Stroke Management

Based on a patient's care preferences and or advance directives, expedited transfer to an acute care center would be warranted in those eligible for TPA or in a stupor or coma. Studies have shown that stroke patients who receive TPA have a greater chance of returning home as opposed to requiring high-level nursing home care.

If a patient's preferences discourage hospitalization, a palliative and home stroke care support approach should be instituted based on the wishes of the patient and family members.

6.3.2.1 Strategies for Home-Based Management of Acute Stroke

1. Elevated blood pressure (BP) in the setting of a stroke is a compensatory mechanism to maintain cerebral perfusion. Rapid reduction can worsen the patient's symptoms. Systolic BP >185 and <220 is usually permissible for the first 48 h of a stroke, before it can slowly be reduced. Hypotension is unusual during an acute stroke and other etiologies for patient's symptoms should be explored. SBP should be maintained closer to 140–160 if an ICH has occurred or there is suspicion for it.
2. Check fingerstick glucose as hypoglycemia or hyperglycemia are stroke mimics and are reversible following rapid glucose correction.
3. Obtain electrolytes, a complete blood count, and PT/PTT to evaluate renal and liver function, coagulopathies, and blood dyscracias.
4. Obtain ECG if atrial fibrillation or other arrhythmias are suspected. Anticoagulation therapy is recommended in cases where cardiac arrhythmia is found (e.g., persistent or paroxysmal atrial fibrillation). Start an antiplatelet agent on the first day, if the stroke is deemed to be ischemic.

Initial Therapy Alternatives
- Aspirin (81–325 mg) daily
- Aspirin 25 mg/extended release dipyridamole 200 mg daily
- Clopidogrel 75 mg (preferable for patients with an aspirin allergy) daily

5. Check swallowing function by having patient drink 3–5 ml of water. The presence of coughing or a "wet" voice may warrant placing patient on an NPO status to reduce their aspiration risk until a formal home-based swallow evaluation is done by speech therapy, depending on the patient's goals of care and the extent of the stroke. Some patients with dysphagic stroke can recover swallowing function over several weeks, so may benefit from hospitalization for temporary placement of a percutaneous feeding tube. Hydration support will be important in these cases as well until nutrition status is established. If home-based clinicians lack staffing and equipment for home IV fluids, urgent transfer to a higher level of care should be considered. Patients who are obtunded or in a stupor may require a nasogastric tube to be placed for nutrition and medications unless otherwise stipulated by advanced directives or their health care proxy.
6. Comfort measures should be enacted immediately if a patient shows signs of cerebral herniation (e.g., irregular breathing, decerebrate or decorticate posturing, downward gaze deviation).

6.3.2.2 Home-Based Management of TIA [5]

If a patient's neurological deficit is not resolving within 1 h or has not completely resolved over 24 h, it is recommended to send the patient to the emergency department for evaluation or manage his/her condition as an acute stroke in the home setting.

Complete resolution of the neurologic deficit necessitates determining patient's stroke risk factors. The ABCD2 score [6], which takes into account age, blood pressure, and clinical symptoms, can be used to risk stratify TIA patients for the likelihood of having a stroke.

Risk Stratify Based on ABCD2 Score
- Age ≥60 (1) point
- BP >140/90 (1) point
- Clinical symptoms with focal weakness (2) points
- Speech impairment w/o weakness (1) point
- Duration ≥ 60 min (2) points or 10–59 min (1) point

Scores greater than 6 suggest a greater than 10 % stroke risk within 1 week and closer to 20 % chance in 90 days. Therefore, patients suspected of having a TIA should be screened for obesity, hypertension, diabetes, hyperlipidemia and managed aggressively. Based on a patient's goals of care and projected life expectancy, a pragmatic approach to managing the following risk factors should be employed to sustain an optimal quality of life:

1. Begin treatment with an antiplatelet agent, either aspirin (81–325 mg), aspirin 25 mg/extended release dipyridamole 200 mg, or clopidogrel (75 mg)
2. Aim for BP <140/90, which can be lowered with antihypertensive agents within 24 h.
3. Aim for glycemic control—AIC <7.0
4. Aim for total cholesterol <200, LDL <100,
5. Aim for BMI <25; obese patients should also be considered for evaluation of the presence of sleep apnea as it can increase the risk of cardiovascular disease and stroke.

Though no one risk factor(s) is greater than another, ensuring that hypertension and glycemic control are achieved can minimize complications from an acute stroke while directly reducing risk of an intracerebral hemorrhage and hyperglycemic/hypoglycemic induced stroke-like symptoms.

6.3.2.3 Management of Homebound Chronic Stroke Patients

Determine patient's level of disability and tailor therapy based on residual symptoms. Physical, occupational, and speech therapists are often required for management and retraining of limb movements, gait, cognitive, and speech/language deficits. Such therapy in an enriched interactive environment reduces overall disability and provides opportunity for stroke patients to regain a level of independence. Worsening of chronic stroke symptoms should prompt an evaluation for infectious, metabolic, or epileptic causes by the home-based provider.

Management of Spasticity: (*See Spasticity section in Spinal Cord Injury*)

6.4   Movement Disorders

6.4.1   Parkinsonism

The cardinal symptoms of Parkinsonism are a constellation of bradykinesia along with muscle rigidity, tremor, and postural instability.

Bradykinesia is most important for the diagnosis and is characterized as a decrease of rapid sequential movement on examination with lack of spontaneous, automatic movements. Its clinical manifestations include small handwriting that tends to trail off (micrographia), reduced facial expression (masked facies), and/or reduction in vocal intonation (hypophonia).

Rigidity, or muscle stiffness, is related to increased muscle resistance during passive limb movement that produces a ratcheting feeling similar to a "cogwheel." Very mild rigidity usually requires coactivation maneuvers of the contralateral limb in order to elicit it.

Parkinsonian tremor is primarily present at rest involving the fingers, usually the thumb and index, to produce the characteristic pill-rolling tremor. Tremor abates during action and tends to re-emerge after a brief delay.

Postural and gait changes in parkinsonism are characterized by a stooped posture, reduced stride length producing a shuffling appearance to the gait, and multi-pivot turning. In addition, impairment or loss of postural reflexes places many of these patients at risk of falling. A pull test, in which the examiner stands behind the patient and pulls them backwards while monitoring the number of steps they need to recover without assistance is often utilized. Greater than 2 steps to recover or the need of the examiner to prevent them from falling is abnormal.

Furthermore, these patients can develop gait freezing, whereby they stutter step in place or one or both feet suddenly seemed pasted to the floor when walking normally or through small spaces such as doorways, turning, and/or upon initiating walking. Failure to compensate by holding on to someone or an assistive device increases the risk of falling. This can be seen late in the disease course for Parkinson's disease (PD), but rather early on among the atypical parkinsonism syndromes.

6.4.1.1   Classification and Treatment of Parkinsonism

Parkinson's Disease

Parkinsonism results from either a degenerative disease or an acquired etiology (e.g., medications, toxins, infections, vascular). Among the degenerative causes, Parkinson's disease is the most common and an accurate diagnosis is predicated upon a clinical assessment, which clinic-pathological studies [7] have shown to have a greater than 90 % accuracy. This is based on the presence of an asymmetric bradykinesia with at least 1 concomitant symptom: muscle rigidity, tremor, and/or postural and gait instability. Further supportive features include a slow progression with sustained, robust levodopa response.

Distinguishing PD from atypical parkinsonism has both treatment and prognostic implications, as the latter conditions do not respond well to levodopa, and have a more rapid and deleterious clinical course. The atypical parkinsonism syndromes include progressive supranuclear palsy (PSP), corticobasal degeneration (CBD), multisystem atrophy (MSA), and dementia with Lewy Body (DLB) [8].

6.4.1.2   Treatment of Parkinson's Disease

The treatments for PD are symptomatic with levodopa being the gold standard. It is reasonable to start symptomatic treatment in the early stages of the disease when the level of severity is starting to adversely impact quality of life and daily activities. See Table 6.3.

Motor Symptom Management

- Levodopa is considered the first line therapy in patients older than 70 years. Providers should initiate levodopa in immediate-release formulations with a titration to at least three times per day. Nausea related to levodopa can be treated with extra carbidopa or domperidone taken with each dose of levodopa. Should patients develop levodopa-induced hallucinations or psychosis, incorporating quetiapine or clozapine into the regimen is often efficacious.

Table 6.3 Pharmacological treatment for Parkinson's disease

Medication class	Formulations	Initial doses	Clinical considerations
Levodopa	Carbidopa/levodopa, Carbidopa/levodopa ODT	Start 25/100 mg three times per day	Nausea
			Lightheadedness
			Hallucinations
Dopamine agonists	Pramipexole	Start 0.25 mg three times daily, max 4.5 mg daily	Impulse control disorders
			Hypersomnolence
			Cognitive deficits
	Pramipexole extended release	Start 0.375 daily, max 4.5 mg daily	Hallucinations
	Ropinerole	Start 0.25 mg three times daily, max 24 mg daily	
	Ropinerole extended release	Start 2 mg daily, max 12 mg twice daily	
	Rotigotine TD	Start 2 mg daily, max 16 mg/24 h	
MAO-B inhibitors	Selegiline	5 mg twice daily	Dizziness, headache, dyspepsia
	Rasagaline	1 mg daily	

- The dopamine agonist class or monamine oxidase (MAOB) inhibitors can be utilized early on in patients less than 70 years who are cognitively intact. Short-acting dopamine agonists are administered three times per day. Long-acting formulations exist for both pramipexole and ropinerole and can be used once a day, but oftentimes are dosed two to three times daily The rotigotine patch is utilized daily and should be changed and applied on different body regions (e.g., upper limbs, torso, back) at the same time each day to ensure continuous benefit. There are no clinical data demonstrating superiority of one agonist over another. Dopamine agonists can cause excessive sedation, sleep attacks, hallucinations, and impulse control disorders (e.g., gambling, hypersexuality, shopping). It is important to screen patients for these potential side effects, as reduction in dose or discontinuation the medication is ameliorative.

Patients on longstanding levodopa therapy can develop "wearing-off" episodes also known as motor fluctuations. As the disease progresses, the hours of good motor response ("on" time) per dosing interval decrease, while precipitous "off" periods increase. This along with the emergence of dyskinesia, involuntary muscle movement flowing from one region of the body to another, reduces a patient's quality of life.

Dystonia is involuntary contraction of muscle groups that cause abnormal twisting or repetitive movements or postures. Common focal dystonias that can develop in PD include the following.

- Cervical dystonia
- Blepharospasm (involuntary eyelid closure or spasms) or eyelid opening apraxia
- Hand dystonia
- Lower limb dystonia (e.g., toe curling or foot dystonia)
- Camptocormia (abnormal anteroflexion of the trunk)
- Pisa syndrome (lateral flexion of the trunk)

In order to manage motor fluctuations, dyskinesia, and other involuntary movements such as dystonia, it is important to initiate discussions with a neurologist who is willing to offer management guidance, even if the patient is unable to come in to a neurology office visit. The pharmacological strategies that are oftentimes considered are listed in Table 6.4.

There is little to no superiority data for the different classes of antidystonic agents. Uses of these therapies are based on the patient's tolerance and the existence of other underlying medical comorbidities. Botulinum toxin injections have emerged as the first line treatment choice for many of the focal dystonias, due to its targeted clinical efficacy and minimal risk of constitutional and cognitive adverse effects.

Surgical Strategies
As the disease progresses, pharmacological permutations not only become more complex, but the propensity for side effects increases.

Table 6.4 Management approaches for motor complications and dystonia in Parkinson's disease

Motor fluctuations/ wearing "Off"	Increase levodopa dose and/or dosing frequency
	Add COMT-I
	Add MAOBI
	Switch levodopa formulation to carbidopa levodopa extended release capsules (Rytary)
	Add a dopamine agonist
	Utilize apomorphine SC injections
Dyskinesia	Reduce dose or frequency of levodopa
	Discontinue COMTI
	Discontinue MAOBI
	Add amantadine 100 mg three to four times daily
Focal dystonia	
Cervical	Baclofen (Start 5 mg three times daily, max 80 mg daily divided)
Blepharospasm/eye-lid opening apraxia	Low dose benzodiazepines (clonazepam, diazepam, lorazepam) dosed two to three times daily
Hand dystonia Camptocormia Lower limb	Trihexyphenidyl (2 mg twice to thrice times daily, max 12–15 mg daily divided)
Pisa syndrome	Botulinum toxin injections

Deep Brain Stimulation
- Deep brain stimulation (DBS) is an effective treatment for the management of the cardinal Parkinson's motor symptoms, including refractory tremor. It should be considered in patients who have idiopathic PD and not atypical variants, demonstrate robust levodopa response, lack dementia or signs of atypical parkinsonism, and have motor complications (e.g., motor fluctuations, dyskinesia) requiring higher dopaminergic dosages.

Compared to best medical therapy, DBS produces longer "on" time for patients with dramatic reductions in wearing offs, dyskinesia, and medication burden. It can also benefit focal dystonia that emerge as a consequence of disease progression or levodopa complication.

Carbidopa/Levodopa Intestinal Gel
- This specially formulated enteral gel is particularly useful for a patient with advanced PD with motor complications, who also has cognitive dysfunction and/ or dysphagia that affects oral intake. It significantly increases "on" time while reducing dyskinesia by continuously infusing carbidopa/levodopa through a gastrostomy–jejunostomy tube (PEG-J) 16 h per day.

6.4.1.3 Nonmotor Symptom Management (Refer to Table 6.5)
Autonomic Dysfunction
- Constipation should be managed with stool softeners and increased daily water and fiber intact. Enemas, suppositories, and/or lubriprostone may be utilized in severe cases.

Table 6.5 Nonmotor symptom management in Parkinsons' disease

	Symptom	Treatment	Adverse effects
Autonomic	Constipation	Refer to Table 6.10.	
	Orthostatic hypotension	Midodrine 2.5 mg three times daily, can titrate to 10 mg three times daily	Hypertension, nausea, headache
		Fludrocortisone 0.1 mg daily, max 0.3 mg daily	Hypertension, electrolyte abnormalities
		Droxidopa 100 mg three times daily, titrate to max 600 mg three times daily	Hypertension, headache
	Urinary incontinence	Refer to Sphincter Dysfunction in Spinal Cord Injury	
Sleep disorders	REM behavioral disorder	Clonazepam 0.25 mg at bedtime, titrate to max 1 mg at bedtime	Sedation and confusion
	Fragmented sleep	Improve sleep hygiene	
		Melatonin 6–15 mg at bedtime	Somnolence
		Mirtazapine 7.5 mg–15 mg at bedtime	Same as melatonin
		Trazodone 25–50 mg at bedtime	Somnolence, headache, dizziness
Sialorrhea		Botulinum toxin injections to salivary glands	Dysphagia, pain at injection site
		Glycopyrrolate 1–2 mg two to three time daily, max is 8 mg daily	Anticholinergic effects
Neurobehavioral	Depression	SSRI	Gastrointestinal symptoms sexual dysfunction
		Venlafaxine 37.5 mg daily and can titrate to 225 mg daily	Same as SSRI
		Nortriptyline 25 mg daily, can titrate to 150 mg daily	Anticholinergic effects, heart block, gastrointestinal symptoms
	Anxiety	Benzodiazepines	Daytime sleepiness, confusion
		Change dosing of levodopa if symptom correlated with timing of medication	

(continued)

Table 6.5 (continued)

Symptom	Treatment	Adverse effects
Hallucinations/agitation	Quetiapine 12.5 mg at bedtime, can titrate to max 400 mg daily or divided	Sedation, extrapyramidal symptoms
	Clozapine 6.25 mg at bedtime, can titrate to 100 mg	Agranulocytosis, seizure, sedation, cardiomyopathy
	Donepezil 5 mg daily, max 10 mg daily	Gastrointestinal symptoms, heart block, bradycardia
	Rivastigmine: Oral 1.5 mg twice daily, can titrate to 6 mg twice daily	Same as Donepezil
	Rivastigmine: Transdermal 4.5 mg daily, can titrate to 9.8 mg daily	
Cognitive impairment or dementia (PDD)	Donepezil 5 mg daily, max 10 mg daily	Gastrointestinal symptoms, heart block, bradycardia
	Galantamine 4 mg daily, can titrate to 12 mg daily	Same as Donepezil
	Memantine 5 mg daily, can titrate to 20 mg daily or divided	Dizziness, headache, confusion
	Rivastigmine: oral 1.5 mg twice daily, can titrate to 6 mg twice daily	Same as Donepezil
	Rivastigmine: Transdermal 4.5 mg daily, can titrate to 9.8 mg daily	

- Orthostatic hypotension and urinary incontinence can emerge in advanced stages of Parkinson's disease. Refer to Treatment of Multiple System Atrophy (MSA) for further review.
- Sialorrhea—Refer to Botulinum Toxin Treatment for Parkinsonism.
- Urinary incontinence from detrusor hyperreflexia is prevalent in the PD population and must be distinguished from benign prostatic hyperplasia, which is also common in men above 65 years. Detrusor hyperactivity can be treated with medications such as oxybutynin or tolterodine (refer to "Sphincter Dysfunction in Spinal Cord Injury"). Dysphagia—Presence or history of dysphagia should prompt the home based clinician to recommend that patients wait to be in the medicated "on" phase before eating, change their food consistency to soft or puree, take small portions, and do a chin tuck with gentle cough after swallowing.

If these strategies are unsuccessful, an evaluation by speech-language therapy to investigate extent of swallowing difficulty and risk for aspiration will be important to obtain. Severe cases necessitate artificial nutrition if such measures are in keeping with the patient's overall condition and goals of care.

Sleep Disorders
- REM behavioral disorder (RBD) is a sleep disorder where by a patient acts out his/her dreams during REM sleep. Vocalizations or flailing arm and/or leg movements are common symptoms of RBD. Treatment with low dose clonazepam at bedtime is efficacious.
- Fragmented sleep or incomplete nonrestful sleep is common among PD patients. Conservative therapies such as relaxation methods, reduction in daily caffeine intact, avoiding watching television, or using a computer at night are recommended. Pharmacological agents to consider include melatonin, mirtazapine, or trazodone.

Neurobehavioral
- Serotonin reuptake inhibitors (SSRI), tricyclic, or serotonin norepinephrine reuptake inhibitors (SNRI) antidepressants may be used for treatment of depression, anxiety, and/or apathy.
- Quetiapine or clozapine are atypical neuroleptics for managing hallucinations or emotionally dysregulated behaviors (e.g., paranoid delusions) that can emerge late in the disease course.

Botulinum Toxin Injections for Parkinsonism
Botulinum toxin injections are very effective in treating a wide spectrum of symptoms in Parkinsonism, such as dystonia, sialorrhea, and bladder dysfunction. These injections should be done by a trained physician. They are covered by most commercial insurances, Medicare, and Medicaid. Its effects are realized over 7–10 days after the injection(s) and benefit can last up to 12–16 weeks. In order to minimize the development of antibodies to the toxin, low doses are used initially, treatment intervals are 3 months, and booster injections are avoided.

Dystonia
Botulinum toxin (BoNT) injections are the first line treatment for cervical dystonia, blepharospasm, eyelid opening apraxia, and focal hand dystonia and a treatment of choice for lower limb dystonia. Cranial and cervical injections can be conducted in the patient's home environment. Limb injections may require use of electromyography (EMG), ultrasound, or electric stimulation guidance to identify the muscles to be injected and therefore, should be done in a hospital or clinic setting.

Sialorrhea

BoNT injection to the parotids/submandibular glands is considered the treatment of choice for sialorrhea, especially when oral anticholinergic (e.g., glycopyrrolate) medications have limited benefit and/or not well tolerated. It can be done in the patient's home.

Neurogenic Bladder

BoNT injection to the bladder's detrusor muscle has been shown to be effective in reducing detrusor overactivity and improving incontinence and bladder capacity in medication refractory neurogenic bladder. The injections oftentimes require anesthesia, but the benefits can last up to 9 months before a repeat treatment is needed.

6.4.2 Multiple Sclerosis

Multiple sclerosis (MS) is a chronic, progressive, neurologic disease that, in its primary form, causes patients great morbidity and functional compromise. Characterized by attacks of neuronal inflammation, demyelination, and degeneration at different times and in differing locations of the central nervous system (CNS), MS affects over 2.5 million people worldwide, and about 350,000 in the United States [9]. While the patient's diagnosis of MS will likely be known and a primary reason for referral for home-based medical services, understanding the clinical type, baseline symptoms and general prognosis/course is important for a provider to best provide anticipatory guidance and recognize symptoms that may signify acute exacerbation and/or progression of disease.

Because the lesions of MS can affect any part of the CNS, the clinical symptoms vary widely in type and severity, including both motor and autonomic systems (see Table 6.6). The most common clinical type of MS, relapsing/remitting MS (RRMS) affects 85 % of patients and is usually characterized by recovery after an attack. However, a subset of those with RRMS may develop secondary progressive MS (SPMS) in which there is progressive deterioration in function with every attack. Together with primary progressive MS (PPMS), characterized by later age at onset and lack of discrete attacks, and progressive/relapsing MS (PRMS), which overlaps with PPMS and SPMS, these types collectively make up 15 % of all diagnoses and are those most likely to experience significant disability and benefit most from medical and personal care services in the home.

While prognosis varies by clinical type, in general, patients with clinical diagnoses of MS experience progressive neurological and functional disability and about 80 % of patients have some functional limitations 15 years after onset. In some studies, 80 % of patients required assistance with ambulation by 25 years after onset. Death from MS rarely occurs from the diagnosis itself but rather due to complications of the resulting debility (e.g., aspiration pneumonia or infection). Management of patients with MS as they age, whether in a traditional or home-based setting, can also be challenging as their functional disability may be compounded by other chronic conditions associated with overlapping symptoms, such

Table 6.6 Common symptoms of multiple sclerosis

Weakness of limbs
Spasticity
Optic neuritis
Visual blurring
Diplopia
Sensory symptoms (e.g., paresthesia, hyperesthesia)
Pain
Ataxia
Bladder dysfunction
Constipation
Cognitive dysfunction
Depression
Fatigue
Sexual dysfunction
Facial weakness
Vertigo
Heat sensitivity
Lhermitte's symptom
Paroxysmal motor and/or sensory symptoms
Cranial neuropathies V, VII, IX neuralgias and/or spasms
Facial spasms or contracture

as cerebrovascular disease or diabetes mellitus. Exacerbations of these chronic conditions may also cause worsening of their MS symptoms [9].

6.4.2.1 Disease-Specific Management of MS

Several agents have been shown to reduce rates of attacks, severity of disease, and new or total number of lesions on MRI (Table 6.7). Little is known, however, about long-term efficacy of these treatments. In general, patients with MS who are receiving home-based medical care and have been in the care of a neurologist are either already taking a disease-modifying agent or have stopped because of lack of response or inability to tolerate appropriate options.

The timing, selection, titration, and response monitoring of specific agents should always be made in consultation with a neurologist, as certain medications are more effective with specific clinical types of MS and many have contraindications or adverse effects that may worsen other chronic conditions. Some medications such as the INF-b treatments require monitoring of liver function tests and white blood cell count, so coordination of home-based labs and communication of results with the neurologist is ideal to reduce burden on the patient.

Table 6.7 Therapies for multiple sclerosis

Agent	Clinical considerations
Interferon-b	Subcutaneous injection
	Injection site reactions
	May cause flulike symptoms
	Monitor LFTs, CBC for hepatotoxicity, lymphopenia
Glatiramer acetate	Subcutaneous injection
	Injection site reactions
	Systemic reactions after injections (15 %)
	Lipoatrophy
Mitoxantrone	IV infusion
	Cumulative dose limitation due to cardiotoxicity
	Amenorrhea
	Risk of acute leukemias
Natalizumab	Monthly IV infusion
	Risk of PML with long-term treatment
	Hypersensitivity reactions
Fingolimod	Oral dosing
	Monitor LFTs, CBC for hepatotoxicity, lymphopenia
	First degree heart block or bradycardia

The home-based medical provider should advise the patient regarding feasibility of treatment administration, as traveling for monthly infusions (if home-based infusion services are unavailable) may not be possible for a sufficiently debilitated patient, who will need specialized travel arrangements or alternate therapies. Additionally, a caregiver, rather than the patient, may need to be trained to administer subcutaneous injections such as INF-b or glatiramer. As with all patients taking any immunosuppressant therapy, patients and their caregivers should be aware of their higher risk for infection, and providers vigilant for indicative signs and symptoms.

For patients who have progressive neurologic deterioration with the absence of relapses, experience unwanted side effects, or determine that the burden of a treatment is outweighing its benefits due to the severe stage of MS or another condition, and/or changes in prognosis or goals of care, it is reasonable to discuss discontinuation of disease-modifying therapies.

6.4.2.2 Management of MS Exacerbations

When an acute deterioration in function occurs, the first consideration is to ascertain whether the acute clinical worsening is due to an MS "attack" or "flare" signifying new disease activity (i.e., a new neurologic lesion), or attributed to an

MS exacerbation from a metabolic, infectious or environmental process (e.g., temperature change).

MS exacerbation typically manifest as worsening of underlying residual deficits or reemergence of past symptoms related to a known demyelinating lesion. Resolution of the medical trigger oftentimes improves the symptoms without need for glucocorticoids.

Therefore, a patient or caregiver who report an acute change in baseline function a thorough history, physical and appropriate labwork and/or imaging should be performed looking for a non-MS etiology such as an infection, new or changed medications, a pressure ulcer or other evidence of traumatic injury, evidence of organ dysfunction, new urinary retention, fecal impaction, exacerbation of a concomitant chronic condition, or even change in recent activity or location.

If there is no other identifiable cause of the acute decline and symptoms are new and/or severe enough to cause dysfunction, then glucocorticoid treatment is the standard management, though there is little evidence of long-term benefit. If home-based intravenous (IV) services are available, methylprednisolone 500–1000 mg/day via IV for 3–5 days, possibly followed by a 2-week taper of oral prednisone (starting at 60–80 mg/day) is preferred. Equivalent doses of oral dexamethasone or methylprednisolone can be substituted for the IV portion of therapy, but are associated with increased risk of GI complications such as gastritis or ulcers. Especially if patients have other chronic conditions, it is important to anticipate and manage common side effects of even short-term glucocorticoid therapy such as hyperglycemia, fluid retention, GI complications as already described, electrolyte disturbances (e.g. hypokalemia), and emotional lability. Acute symptoms of MS that are refractory to glucocorticoid therapy may require hospital admission for plasma exchange therapy.

6.4.2.3 Management of MS Symptoms

Whether or not patients with MS are receiving disease-modifying therapy, aggressively managing symptoms related to the motor, sensory, and functional effects of MS is important to maintain function, improve quality of life, and prevent complications. Management in the home setting is ideal as therapies can be delivered by multiple disciplines, tailored to be most appropriate to the patients' home setting and reinforced by training caregivers if capable. The management rationale for each symptom are general and do not modify this incurable disease; certain symptoms are also more responsive to treatment than others. Therefore, constant symptom assessment, titration of dosing or intensity of symptom management, and patient education is important and necessary in managing expectations [10]. The type of symptom and optimal management are summarized in Table 6.8.

6.4.2.4 Palliative Care and Hospice

In addition to assessing and managing symptoms in a patient whose MS has progressed, the home-based medical provider should effectively communicate the current status and possible course of the disease to the patient and caregivers [11, 12]. Furthermore, excluding other diagnoses, discussing treatment options, and providing resources for emotional and spiritual support are also important.

Table 6.8 Management of multiple sclerosis symptoms

Symptom	Management
Sensory	
Pain:	
• Neuropathic	Gabapentin (1200–3600 mg/day, divided doses)
	Pregabalin (300–600 mg two times/day)
	Duloxetine (60–120 mg daily)
	Venlafaxine extended release (150–225 mg daily)
	Tricyclic Antidepressants (25–150 mg one to times/day)
	Acetaminophen; NSAIDs; opiates
Nystagmus	Gabapentin (300–600 mg four times/day); memantine (5–10 mg four times/day)
Temperature Intolerance	Environmental modification; adequate room ventilation
Motor	
Cerebellar ataxia/tremor	Clonazepam (0.5–2 mg/day, divided doses); mysoline (25–150 mg/day); propranolol (60–320 mg/day, divided doses if not extended release); trihexyphenidyl (2–15 mg/day, divided doses); occupational therapy; deep brain stimulation
Dysphagia/dysarthria	Speech/language therapy; nutritional aids; artificial nutrition/hydration
Spasticity (See "Spasticity" in "Spinal Cord Injury" section of this chapter)	Physical therapy; botulinum toxin A injections; systemic oral drugs (e.g. tizanidine (2 mg two to three times/day, max. 36 mg/day), baclofen (5–10 mg three times/day, max 80 mg/day), gabapentin (100–300 mg three times/day, max. 3600 mg daily), diazepam (2–5 mg one to two times/day, max. 60 mg/day); intrathecal baclofen pump
Functional	
Fatigue/weakness	Workup for associated conditions; physical therapy; dalfampridine (10 mg two times/day); amantadine (100 mg two or three times/day); methylphenidate (5–10 mg two times/day)
Bladder dysfunction (See "Sphincter Dysfunction" in "Spinal Cord Injury" section of this chapter • Detrusor hyperreflexia • Detrusor dyssynergia/atony	Behavioral techniques; oxybutynin (2.5–5 mg, two or three times/day); tolterodine (2 mg two times/day); intravesicular botulinum toxin Terazosin (1–20 mg daily); bethanechol 10–50 mg three or four times/d, max. 150–200 mg daily); intermittent urinary catheterization
Constipation	Stepwise bowel regimen
Depression	Antidepressants; talk or behavioral therapy
Cognitive dysfunction	Management of associated conditions; donepezil (5–10 mg daily)

As symptoms become severe, difficult to treat, and/or a patient's overall clinical status is declining, it is appropriate to review a patient's prognosis, their goals of care and discuss referral to hospice, and even an inpatient hospice admission to control certain symptoms more aggressively.

6.5 Spinal Cord Injury/Traumatic Brain Injury

6.5.1 Management of Spasticity

Spasticity is a velocity dependent increase in muscle tone resulting from an upper motor neuron (UMN) lesion due to spinal cord and/or traumatic brain injury (SCI/TBI), stroke, multiple sclerosis, and other chronic neurological conditions causing motor dysfunction. The clinical manifestations can range from a subtle increase in resting tone on examination, to hyperexcitability of antigravity muscles causing impaired dexterity and restricted joint mobility.

Clinically, the pattern of increased muscle tone of spasticity presents in the upper extremity with excessive flexion of fingers and adduction of thumb, resulting in a "thumb in palm" clenched fist deformity, often with flexion and pronation of the larger muscles of the arm. In the lower extremity, adduction of the hips, knee and plantar flexion, inversion of ankles, and hyperextension of the big toe are the most common findings. Clonus, exaggerated tendon reflexes, muscle weakness, and spasms as a result of spastic co-contraction (inappropriate activation of antagonistic muscles during voluntary activity) are also seen. Sudden worsening of a known diagnosis of spasticity can be due to many factors including noxious somatic or visceral stimuli (see Table 6.9), primary disease progression, or a new neurological process. Therefore, the home-based medical provider should do a thorough evaluation to treat and/or refer for further diagnostic workup.

Chronic spasticity can lead to contractures, which tend to restrict movement of joint, ultimately fixing it in a deformed painful position. Timely diagnosis and management of spasticity are important to prevent such complications and optimize function. Furthermore, complications result from both unaddressed spasticity, as well as from associated debility such as falls, pain, pressure ulcers, infections, and contractures. There is little robust evidence to base clinical guidelines for spasticity management; current recommendations are based on expert recommendations for a multidisciplinary approach that combines both pharmacologic and non-pharmacologic agents.

6.5.1.1 Nonpharmacologic Management of Spasticity

While evidence is lacking to support passive manual stretching as management of spasticity, it is often recommended as part of a home management regimen to maintain flexibility and prevent permanent contractures. Furthermore, passive stretching 2–3 times per day serves to limit the amount of antispasmodic agents utilized in the management of the spasticity. Education of both patient and caregivers by physical and occupational therapists can occur in the home. There is weak evidence to support the use of rigid or Lycra-based splints to simulate a prolonged stretch to spastic limbs; however, some criticize that splinting holds the joint in only one position and does not provide the dynamic movement as with manual stretching.

Table 6.9 Potential triggers
of worsening spasticity

Visceral: constipation/impaction, UTI, dysmenorrhea, renal colic, urinary retention
Drugs: abrupt discontinuation of antispasmodic drugs, malfunction of intrathecal pump
Skin: pressure ulcers, ingrown toenails, rash, cellulitis
Environmental: improper seating, poorly fit orthotics, extremes of temperature
Others: physical or emotional trauma/stress; DVT, infections

Regardless, splinting can reduce skin breakdown and infection, especially in patients with spasticity in their wrist and finger, ankle and toe flexors.

Postural management involves devices or maneuvers to ensure proper alignment when sitting, standing, or laying in a bed. Standing frames may be customized to allow people to stand for prolonged periods of time by providing support for the affected limbs. Collaboration with physical or occupational therapists is necessary, as well as with involved caregivers. Small trials of postural management in patients with SCI and MS showed reduced spasticity in lower extremities.

Exercises to strengthen core muscle groups like the pelvic, trunk and shoulder girdle, or treadmill training have been shown in small studies to improve strength and stability and control over affected distal muscle groups. Physical therapy should be consulted and a patient should be evaluated for general ability to exercise, with caution in patients with severe osteoporosis, severe limitation in passive range of motion, or those who are in the immediate postoperative period.

6.5.1.2 Pharmacologic Treatments of Spasticity

Oral antispasmodic agents, with baclofen as first line and tizanidine and dantrolene as second line, have been used for several decades and are a mainstay in management, despite lack of robust trials to provide evidence for these agents' effectiveness. Benzodiazepines, such as clonazepam (0.25–1 mg at bedtime) can also be used, but the dose may be limited due to drowsiness. Timing of dosing should be tailored to a patient's lifestyle and function; for example, patients who are somewhat ambulatory should take lower doses during the daytime to allow spasticity and to provide stability. Bedtime dosing and immediately after awakening may be helpful as spasticity often increases with position change and reduced spasticity may facilitate personal care, respectively. Doses of these medications should be started at the lowest dose, especially in those who are still walking, as risk for falls can increase if spasticity unmasks underlying muscle weakness. For some, muscle spasticity provides some postural stability and reduction of spasticity may result in increased weakness or falls right after starting treatment. There is no evidence for combination therapy with oral antispasmodics and should only be reserved for patients who can only tolerate small doses of one drug and with little improvement in symptoms with one drug.

Cannabinoids, the pharmacologically active compound in marijuana, are available as oromucosal sprays in some countries and have been shown in multiple trials to result in subjective improvement in spasticity in up to 30–40 % of patients (without objective improvement in spasticity measures). There is a long side effect profile, and long-term effects on cognition, mental health, and behavior are unknown.

Botulinum toxin A injections into selected skeletal muscles result in focal reduction in spasticity without systemic side effects of weakness or sedation, though usually no improvement in function. Its use is recommended for patients with focal spasticity that has not responded to nonpharmacologic interventions and should be performed only by trained physicians. Therapeutic effect is seen within 1 week of administration, with peak effect in 4–6 weeks, and duration of effect about 12 weeks. If effective, planned injections every 12 weeks are appropriate.

If a patient with severe spasticity does not respond to adequate doses of oral antispasmodic drugs, they should be referred and evaluated for an intrathecal baclofen pump. When administered intrathecally, a small dose of baclofen can result in effective muscle relaxation without the systemic side effects.

6.5.1.3 Management of Sphincter Dysfunction

Bowel dysfunction: After a traumatic brain injury or spinal cord injury, constipation, impaction, and fecal incontinence due to overflow often occur. In addition, the decrease in mobility of the patient exacerbates this issue. It is important for the patient's quality of life that stool regularity is reestablished. Increased dietary fiber and fluid can help ambulatory patients, but for less ambulatory patients these interventions can exacerbate the problem. For those patients, medications are often necessary (see Table 6.10 [13]. Initial treatment is often with stool softeners and stimulant laxatives with the addition of a suppository, osmotic agents and enemas can be added. Determining the best regimen for each patient that is acceptable often takes a while to determine with trial of multiple agents till the preferred regimen is

Table 6.10 Pharmacological treatment for constipation for patients with spinal cord injury

Suppositories	Bisacodyl suppository 10 mg PR daily Glycerin suppository
Stool softeners	Docusate 100 mg orally twice a day, can increase to 500 mg per day
Stimulant laxatives	Sennosides 17.2 mg orally at night, max 34.4 mg twice daily Bisacodyl 5–10 mg orally daily
Osmotic	Polyethylene glycol 1 capful orally as needed Lactulose 15–30 ml orally daily, may increase to twice daily
Enemas	Saline enema Mineral oil enema

found. A visiting nurse with as needed medication orders can be especially helpful in this process. These nurses can see the patient frequently for a period of time to help determine the best medication and help teach how to administer a suppository or enema.

Urinary dysfunction: Most spinal cord or traumatic brain injury patients have urinary retention ("neurogenic bladder") which can lead to overflow incontinence. Urinary continence requires complex control of brain, brain stem, spinal cord, and peripheral nerves where any injury to the brain or spinal cord can cause dysfunction. The most important decision is the drainage mechanism. Clean intermittent catheterization every 4–6 h is recommended [14], but requires manual dexterity that, depending on the type of injury, some patients do not have. For these patients, chronic urethral or suprapubic catheterization may be necessary. Clean intermittent catheterization has the same rates of infection as sterile technique and thus is recommended [15]. However, indwelling catheters can lead to more urinary tract infections, especially in the home setting where it may be more difficult for the patient to follow evidence-based recommendations to minimize the risk of infection. Patients with bladder and sphincter spasms can benefit from any of the many anticholinergic medications that exist for urinary urgency, but need to be aware of the side effects such as dry eyes, dry mouth, confusion, falls, and constipation.

Crede's Method is the application of suprapubic pressure to cause bladder drainage. It also can be enhanced with valsalva at the same time. It can lead to high intravesicular pressures and reflux, so monitoring by the provider is needed if complications occur [14].

Overflow incontinence causes skin maceration and breakdown, and the distended bladder can stimulate autonomic dysreflexia [14] with hypertension, sweating, and flushing. The hypertension is severe and can lead to cardiac problems. In addition, long-term urinary retention leads to hydronephrosis, urine reflux, and urinary tract infections [14].

6.6   Amyotrophic Lateral Sclerosis

ALS is a progressive neurodegenerative disease that is seen by most home-based primary care providers at the later stages of the disease. Annually, 5000 people are diagnosed with ALS in the USA, with age of onset between 40 and 60 years [16]. Most patients die of ALS within 2–5 years [17] of the diagnosis and the home-based medical providers need to be able to manage symptoms and end-of-life care. Approximately, 10–20 % of patients survive more than 10 years [18]. Patients suffer from progressive weakness without sensory symptoms [16] with bulbar, upper motor neuron, and lower motor neuron signs and symptoms. Patients presenting with bulbar signs such as dysphagia, dysarthria, and sialorrhea often have a shorter life expectancy [16]. There is no cure for ALS; therefore, treatments are directed at improvement of quality of life (QOL).

Most home-based medical providers will not be diagnosing ALS, and thus the focus in this section will be evaluation and management of symptoms related to more advanced stages of ALS.

6.6.1 General Management

Specialized multidisciplinary clinics have improved outcomes, including increased survival and less hospitalizations [17] for the care of patients with ALS. However, as the disease progresses, it may become difficult or impossible to access these clinics. Home-based medical providers should have relationships with these clinics to identify recommendations that can be implemented without bringing the patient into the office.

Riluzole is the only medication that is FDA approved for ALS treatment [19]. It has been shown to increase tracheostomy-free survival, possibly by 2–3 months. It is expensive but generally well-tolerated and should be offered to all patients as an option to prolong survival [20].

Most deaths from ALS are the result of respiratory failure and noninvasive ventilation with BiPAP prolongs survival [20]. Close monitoring of respiratory function and symptoms is necessary. Forced vital capacity (FVC) declines at a consistent individual rate [16] and should, therefore, be assessed every 3 months. Once the FVC is less than 50 % predicted value, the patient should be considered for BiPAP or invasive ventilation [16]. When the BIPAP is ordered for the home, respiratory therapists can assess in the home for the right mask type and adjust the machine to the right settings with orders from the provider.

Most patients also develop dysphagia and dysarthria as weakness in muscles of the throat and mouth develop. They have an increased risk of aspiration and weight loss. Changes in a patient's speech may be the first sign of weakness [16] and should prompt a speech therapy consultation. Speech therapists can help work to improve speech and recommend assistive devices such as communication devices (alphabet boards, electronic communication devices). Gastrostomy tubes have been shown to prolong survival in ALS and should be considered in the context of the patient's overall condition and goals of care. The timing of the procedure can be challenging, as it can be difficult when the respiratory status is compromised [20]; it is therefore best to have the PEG placed before the patient's FVC is less than 50 % predicted value [16].

Mobility deteriorates as muscle weakness and spasticity in the limbs progress. Referrals to physical therapists and occupational therapists through a home care agency can be helpful. There are many assistive devices that can be of use to patients and the home-based medical provider is uniquely able to assess for the need. These include canes, ankle-foot orthoses, walkers, wheelchair, headrests, and eating utensils.

Caregiver support is an important aspect of the management of a patient with ALS especially when they are homebound. If possible, an interdisciplinary approach with social workers can help the caregiver identify and access support groups and other community resources.

One of the most important interventions for any provider who cares for patients with ALS is to address goals of care and other advanced directives. These issues need to be readdressed often, as choices may change and patients may not be able to fully address on the first conversation. Especially important are discussions regarding respiratory and nutritional choices.

6.6.2 Symptom Management in ALS

- Sialorrhea is a common embarrassing symptom. It is also associated with aspiration pneumonia. Home suction machines are helpful and are covered by most insurances at least partially. Aides, funded through Medicare (Home Health Aides) or state Medicaid programs usually cannot operate the machine, but private help or family can. First line treatments include anticholinergic medications (see Table 6.11). Injections of botulinum toxin or radiation to the parotid and submandibular glands are often helpful at reducing or eliminating the drooling in refractory cases [16]. These injections are usually done in the ALS multidisciplinary clinic or neurology office.
- Psuedobulbar effect is characterised as laughter or crying devoid of emotionality. It affects 20–50 % of patients with ALS. Antidepressants are often employed but fixed-dose combination of dextromethorphan/quinidine reduced symptoms but can cause side effects of dizziness, nausea, and somnolence [17] (See Table 6.11).
- Fatigue is very common in patients with ALS, and some of the medications including riluzole can contribute. Fatigue can also be a symptom of depression, immobility, or respiratory dysfunction [17].

Table 6.11 Symptomatic treatments in amyotrophic lateral sclerosis

Symptom	Treatment
Spasticity	Baclofen 5–10 mg orally two to three times daily, can titrate to 20 mg four times daily
	Tizanidine 2–4 mg three times daily, can titrate to 24 mg daily
Pseudobulbar affect	Dextromethorphan-quinidine (20 mg/10 mg) orally once daily, can increase to two times daily
	Sertraline 50–100 mg orally at bedtime
	Amitriptyline 10–75 mg orally at bedtime
Sialorrhea	Atropine eye drops 0.4 mg orally every 4–6 h
	Glycopyrrolate 1–2 mg orally four times daily
	Scopolamine 0.125 mg SC three times daily
Depression	Sertraline 50–100 mg orally at bedtime
	Paroxetine 10–40 mg orally daily

- Spasticity is a painful symptom and it impairs mobility. There are few studies of spasticity treatments in ALS, but it can be treated with benzodiazepines and baclofen [17] (See Table 6.11).
- Pain is usually related to spasticity or neuropathy, but patients may have contractures or arthritis as well. Position change, padding, stretching, and massage are all nonpharmacological treatments. Otherwise treatments should include NSAIDS, acetaminophen, and then escalation to opioids [21].
- Cognitive impairment and behavioral disorders are common in later stages of ALS, occurring in 10–75 % of patients [17]. Therefore, screening for cognitive issues through neurocognitive testing and caregiver interviews may be warranted based on the clinical circumstances.
- Depression is common in ALS patients and should be assessed by the home care provider. Many of the common screening tools can be used. Pharmacological treatment is mostly with selective serotonin reuptake inhibitors (See Table 6.11).

6.6.3 Referral to Hospice

- ALS patients are not routinely enough referred to hospice. Many who do not meet hospice criteria die within 6 months. The US-based ALS Peer Workgroup [22] has suggested specific criteria for referral of these patients to hospice (see Table 6.12).

Chronic neurological conditions can be debilitating for patients at a physical, cognitive, and psychiatric level. Understanding the manifestation of these conditions—their progression and the influence that other medical problems and medications can have on them—builds an integral foundation for a home-based medical practitioner to exact a treatment plan. The management of these conditions oftentimes requires a multidisciplinary team who can work in synergy to address the varied symptom spectrum of these conditions. The home-based medical practitioner's ability to conceptualize the neurologic sequelae of the conditions discussed in this chapter will enable them to orchestrate the necessary diagnostic and management plan efficiently and effectively, giving homebound patients and their caregivers the best achievable quality of life.

Table 6.12 Amyotrophic lateral sclerosis peer workgroup hospice referral triggers [21]

1. Forced vital capacity (FVC): 60 % predicted (or rapid decline in FVC (more than 20 %) over 2–3 months
2. Clinical signs or clinical symptoms of respiratory insufficiency
3. Respiratory weakness requiring noninvasive positive pressure ventilation
4. Nutritional decline requiring enteral feeding
5. Severe pain or psychosocial distress requiring intensive palliative care interventions (including opioid medication)
6. Rapidly progressive paralysis (over 2–3 months) in two body regions

References

1. Murray CJ, Lopez AD. Mortality by cause for eight regions of the world: global burden of disease study. Lancet. 1997;349(9061):1269–76.
2. Hardie K, Hankey GJ, Jamrozik K, Broadhurst RJ, Anderson C. Ten- year risk of first recurrent stroke and disability after first-ever stroke in the Perth Community Stroke Study. Stroke. 2004;35(3):731–5.
3. National Institute of Neurological Disorders and Stroke (NINDS). NIH stroke scale [Internet]. 2013. Available from: http://www.ninds.nih.gov/doctors/nih_stroke_scale.pdf
4. Brazis P, Masdeu JC, Biller J. Localization in clinical neurology. 6th ed. Philadelphia: Lippincott Williams & Wilkins; 2012.
5. Johnston SC, Nguyen-Huynh MN, Schwarz ME, Fuller K, Williams CE, Josephson SA, et al. National Stroke Association guidelines for the management of transient ischemic attacks. Ann Neurol. 2006;60(3):301–13.
6. Rothwell P, Giles M, Flossmann E, Lovelock C, Redgrave J, Warlow C, Mehta ZA. A simple tool to identify individuals at high early risk of stroke after a transient ischaemic attack: the ABCD score. Lancet. 2005;366(9479):29–36.
7. Hughes AJ, Daniel SE, Kilford L, Lees AJ. The accuracy of clinical diagnosis of idiopathic Parkinson's disease: a clinicopathological study. J Neurol Neurosurg Psychiatry. 1992;55(3):181–4.
8. Stamelou M, Bhatia KP. Atypical parkinsonism: diagnosis and treatment. Neurol Clin. 2015;33(1):39–56. doi:10.1016/j.ncl.2014.09.012.
9. Hauser Stephen L, Goodin Douglas S. Multiple sclerosis and other demyelinating disease. In: Harrison's principles of internal medicine. 18th ed. McGraw-Hill; New York. 2011 (Chapter 380).
10. Thompson AJ, Toosy AT, Ciccarelli O. Pharmacological management of symptoms in multiple sclerosis: current approaches and future directions. Lancet Neurol. 2010;9:1182–99.
11. Strupp J, Romotzky V, Paed D, Galushko M, Golla H, Voltz R. Palliative care for severely affected patients with multiple sclerosis: when and why? Results of a Delphi survey of health care professionals. J Palliat Med. 2014;17:1128–36.
12. Lorenzl S, Nubling G, Perrar KM, Voltz R. Palliative treatment of chronic neurologic disorders. In: Bernat JL, Beresford R, editors. Handbook of clinical neurology, vol. 118. 3rd ed. Amsterdam: Elsevier; 2013. Chapter 10.
13. Tramonte S, Brand MB, et al. The treatment of chronic constipation in adults. J Gen Intern Med. 1997;12:15–24.
14. Francis K. Physiology and management of bladder and bowel continence following spinal cord injury. Ostomy Wound Manage. 2007;53:18–27.
15. Shekelle PG, Morton SC, Clark KA, Pathak M, Vickrey BG. Systematic review of risk factors for urinary tract infection in adults with spinal cord dysfunction. J Spinal Cord Med. 1999;22:258–72.
16. Davis M, Lou J. Management of amyotrophic lateral sclerosis (ALS) by the family nurse practitioner: a timeline for anticipated referrals. J Am Acad Nurse Pract. 2011;23:464–72.
17. Miller RG, Jackson JC, et al. Practice parameter update: the care of the patient with amyotrophic lateral sclerosis: multidisciplinary care, symptom management, and cognitive/behavioral impairment (an evidence-based review). Neurology. 2009;73:1227–33.
18. Eisen A, Schulzer M, MacNeil M, et al. Duration of amyotrophic lateral sclerosis is age dependent. Muscle Nerve. 1993;16:27.
19. Bensimon G, Lacomblez L, Meininger V. A controlled trial of riluzole in amyotrophic lateral sclerosis. N Engl J Med. 1994;330:585–91.
20. Bedlack R. Amyotrophic lateral sclerosis: current practice and future treatments. Curr Opin Neurol. 2010;23:524–9.
21. Blackhall L. Amyotrophic lateral sclerosis and palliative care: where we are, and the road ahead. Muscle Nerve. 2012;45:311–8.
22. Mitsumoto H. Promoting excellence in end-of-life care in ALS. Amyotroph Lateral Scler. 2005;6:145–54.

Adult Psychiatric Care in the Home

7

Peter A. Boling, Lyons T. Hardy, and Ericka L. Crouse

Abstract

Nearly a third of patients seen by providers in home-based primary care are likely to have significant mental health problems, the most common of which is major depression. In general, these conditions are under-recognized and under-treated. Providers should screen for common mental health conditions, understand basics of diagnosis for key types of illnesses, and be familiar with the options for treatment, including community resources and medications. This chapter reviews practical approaches including assessment, diagnostic criteria, interplay of medical and psychiatric conditions, tables to guide medication selection, how to manage difficult situations, and patient and provider safety.

Keywords

Home health care • Mental health disorders • Psychopharmacology • Home-based primary care • Depression • Dementia • Community-based care

7.1 Introduction

The home-based medical practitioner and treatment team often encounter psychiatric issues in the home-based medical care setting. These include the common problems of anxiety, depression, and grief that are prevalent in longitudinal medical practices, plus the need to help manage what are called serious mental illnesses (SMI) such as schizophrenia, bipolar disorder, and major depressive disorder, often

P.A. Boling, M.D. (✉) • L.T. Hardy, N.P. • E.L. Crouse, Pharm.D.
Virginia Commonwealth University, 2116 West Laburnum Ave, Richmond, VA 23227, USA
e-mail: peter.boling@vcuhealth.org

© Springer International Publishing Switzerland 2016
J.L. Hayashi, B. Leff (eds.), *Geriatric Home-Based Medical Care*,
DOI 10.1007/978-3-319-23365-9_7

for individuals who lack access to regular health or psychiatric care and become increasingly homebound and isolated by virtue of their mental health problems. This chapter will take a practical approach to guiding practitioners in this work.

7.2   Patient Population, Screening, Assessment

Mental health disorders are common. Lifetime prevalence is approximately 4 % for bipolar disease, 0.5–1 % for schizophrenia, and 15 % for anxiety disorders. Most importantly, major depression occurs in 5–10 % of the population at some point. In those who are home limited, these conditions are more common. Depression is particularly important with 10–12 % of patients with chronic physical illness experiencing depression and prevalence of depression as high as 27 % in the home-limited population [1].

Difficulty navigating in society leads individuals with SMI diagnoses to become home limited at higher rates than those recorded for the general population, so home medical care providers are likely to have patient populations with prevalence of significant mental health problems at 25 % or higher.

Since many mental health problems are responsive to treatment, detection is important. The provider in the home is often best positioned to detect these problems. Standardized screening and diagnostic assessment are best practices. The PHQ-2 [2] and PHQ-9 tools are gradually taking precedence over older validated screening tools such as the Geriatric Depression Scale (GDS) which comes in 15-item short form and 30-item versions. There are also psychiatric subscores in the Medical Outcomes Study SF-36 (Short Form-36). PHQ-2 [2] and PHQ-9 [3] scores are validated tools, useful for efficient screening. PHQ-9 scores range 0–27; a cut point of 9 has a sensitivity of 95 % and specificity of 84 % for the existence of depression; scores above 15 identify moderate or severe depression. The authors write: "The PHQ-2 includes the first two items of the PHQ-9. The stem question is, "Over the last 2 weeks, how often have you been bothered by any of the following problems?" The two items are "little interest or pleasure in doing things" and "feeling down, depressed, or hopeless." For each item, the response options are "not at all," "several days," "more than half the days," and "nearly every day," scored as 0, 1, 2, and 3, respectively. Thus, the PHQ-2 score can range from 0 to 6." A cut point of 3 on the PHQ-2 is considered as a positive screen for depression that should be followed up with the PHQ-9. The PHQ-9 is shown below in Table 7.1.

An example of case finding using structured in-home screening assessment is the GRACE trial where nurse practitioners visited at-risk adults in their homes and found depression in about 10 % of cases; compared with usual office-based primary care, patients seen at home were at least twice as often charted as having depression, started on antidepressants and seen as outpatients for depression [4].

Comprehensive assessment of patients in home-based medical care should include inquiry about prior episodes of serious mental illnesses (SMI) such as

Table 7.1 Nine symptom checklist, PHQ-9

Over the *last 2 weeks*, how often have you been bothered by any of the following problems?	Not at all	Several days	More than half of the days	Nearly every day
1. Little interest or pleasure in doing things	0	1	2	3
2. Feeling down, depressed, or hopeless	0	1	2	3
3. Trouble falling or staying asleep, or sleeping too much	0	1	2	3
4. Feeling tired or having little energy	0	1	2	3
5. Poor appetite or overeating	0	1	2	3
6. Feeling bad about yourself—or that you are a failure or have let yourself or your family down	0	1	2	3
7. Trouble concentrating on things, such as reading the newspaper or watching television	0	1	2	3
8. Moving or speaking so slowly that other people could have noticed? Or the opposite—being so fidgety or restless that you have been moving around a lot more than usual	0	1	2	3
9. Thoughts that you would be better off dead or of hurting yourself in some way	0	1	2	3
(For coding: Total score ____ = ____ + ____ + ____)				

schizophrenia and bipolar disorder. Clues that might indicate the presence of one of these disorders include inpatient psychiatric care by history, history of suicidal ideation or suicide attempts, history of psychosis, multiple psychiatric medications, antipsychotic or anticonvulsant medications, or finding tardive dyskinesia on physical exam. More detailed questions should then be asked. Starting in the 1970s, many individuals with SMI whose conditions had stabilized were relocated from long-term psychiatric hospitals to community settings. Due to the lack of resources in the community, many of these people did not have adequate follow-up care. Due to the lifelong nature of most of these conditions, these individuals have ongoing needs for psychiatric care and medications.

Avoid the trap of taking for granted the labels that now appear in electronic health records. If the patient does not fit the typical picture for this sort of condition, check twice. An unfortunate consequence of electronic record use is that it can lead to the immortalization of inaccurate diagnostic labels inferred from medication records, second hand comments, or for other reasons. These may not be well-substantiated or they may be outdated. One clue may be the presence of multiple conflicting diagnoses of different serious mental illnesses. Call family members or other providers who have known the patient, search out appropriate records, and verify information related to SMI. Obtaining an accurate assessment of the patient right at the start of care can avert problems that may appear later. For example, quetiapine or haloperidol may have been added during an acute hospitalization to treat delirium or agitation but then are inaccurately labeled as being indicated for "schizophrenia."

Practically speaking, the examiner's skills are also important. Be observant for tears shed, withdrawn or flattened affect, bizarre or unusual behavior or comments, and inattention to self-care or hygiene. Start with open-ended approaches and allow time for patients to answer. Sometimes taking an indirect angle is helpful, asking about the family, the new caregiver, life in general, about things the patient would like to do, rather than asking specifically about depressed mood and using diagnostic terms that may connote "mental health" problems.

7.3   Family and Social History as Part of the Assessment

Family history is an important aspect of the evaluation for mental illness. Many mental illnesses are known to have a genetic component. Major depression and occasionally schizophrenia or bipolar disorder can present initially in middle or later life. These conditions are more common in people with a family history of psychiatric disorders. Obtaining a thorough family history helps with making an accurate diagnosis. Assessing family history of drug and alcohol use is also an important component.

Social history   is also important. In older age, as health declines and as death and losses of family members increase, situational grief, depression, and the sometimes serious problem of pathological grief all become more common. Moving from home, loss of a key caregiver (even if it is a paid worker), loss of a body part, or loss of function and independence can be major stressors. Be alert to depression as a diagnosis when patients' mental status or mood and affect change. Sometimes you will have to probe gently but persistently to learn what has happened to cause a depressive episode. Depression can be differentiated from a normal grief reaction by the severity of symptoms and the length of time they persist. In addition, assessing an individual's history of witnessing or experiencing traumatic events is crucial. Trauma reactions can be related to long-standing psychiatric symptoms including full-blown post-traumatic stress disorder as well as depression, anxiety, and other psychiatric symptoms. Trauma reactions are by no means limited to people who have served in the military. A simple question that can be used to assess trauma is "In your life, have you ever had any experience that was extremely frightening, horrible, or upsetting?" Current symptoms and functional problems related to past traumatic experiences should be assessed further in the event of a positive response.

Because psychiatric services and resources for home-limited patients are sometimes limited, the home care providers may find themselves working out probable psychiatric diagnoses on their own. Table 7.1 offers some general guidelines to help navigate this complex field.

7.4   Psychosis, Hallucinations, Delusions, and Paranoia

Hallucinations are common in severe mental illnesses, but they also accompany other conditions and are not necessarily diagnostic of a primary psychosis. Auditory hallucinations that are related to a primary psychiatric disorder are often experienced as voices talking or whispering. These may or may not be intelligible or recognizable to the individual. Often the content is very upsetting and disturbing. Auditory hallucinations such as hearing a song playing may be more likely to be related to neurological conditions. Some types of hallucinations are normative such as hearing the voice of a deceased relative after the person's death. Visual hallucinations can reflect drug side effects, Lewy body dementia, and delirium due to medical illness; some are unique and specific such as seeing cats in patients with late stage Parkinson's disease who take dopaminergic medication. Paranoia and delusions occur in primary psychotic disorders like schizophrenia but are also common in dementia and delirium. Major depressive disorder can be associated with psychosis. Rapid intervention is indicated in the case of psychotic depression. Do not forget to consider Charles Bonnet syndrome: visual hallucinations in patients with severe visual loss who otherwise lack psychiatric diagnoses; this is common in the elderly population.

7.5   Suicidality

Providers should be alert to the possibility of suicidal ideation in patients with psychiatric disorders. Older white males have a high rate of suicide. Depression, bipolar disorder, substance abuse disorders, and schizophrenia are all associated with higher rates of suicide. Do not be afraid to specifically assess suicidal thoughts. A good introductory question is "Do you ever feel like life is not worth living?" A positive response should elicit a more in depth assessment of the quality of the thoughts and whether the patient has had any specific thoughts or plans to harm him or herself. Patients will need further psychiatric evaluation and stabilization if they do have specific suicidal thoughts.

7.6   When Medical and Psychiatric Illness Symptom Overlap

Consider both physical health problems and mental health conditions in your differential diagnosis and assessment (see Table 7.2). Medical problems can simulate mental health disorders and vice versa; and in a given case, symptoms and signs that suggest medical illness and those that indicate psychiatric illness often intermingle. Delusions and hallucinations may be from medications, delirium, encephalopathy, or from dementias like Lewy body disease rather than primary thought disorders and psychoses. Weight loss, sleep cycle changes, and cognitive function changes

Table 7.2 Overlap between medical and psychiatric symptomatology

Medical causes of changed mood or cognition
Medication side effects (many)
Uncontrolled pain
Constipation
Infection (UTI, other)
Thyroid function abnormality (high or low)
Low or high serum sodium (>150, <130)
Impaired renal function (est. GFR <30 mL/min)
Poor liver function (asterixis, high ammonia, or INR)
Severe anemia (hemoglobin <8)
Sleep apnea and/or restless legs syndrome
Uncontrolled diabetes (blood sugars >400, <60)
Subclinical seizures
Brain lesion (tumor, stroke, subdural hematoma)
CNS infection such as neurosyphilis
Psychiatric causes of physical symptoms
Depression or other psychiatric disorder causing
Weight loss
Fatigue
Altered sleep–wake cycle
Anorexia
Pain, localized (e.g., abdomen) or diffuse
Conversion disorder
Munchausen syndrome

often indicate depression in older patients. Fatigue, lethargy, and anhedonia can be related to anemia, hypothyroidism, sleep apnea, or diabetes. Somatic complaints that seem "organic" such as abdominal pain or chest pain may resolve when patients are treated for depression. Chronic pain can also lead to psychiatric symptoms such as depression and anxiety. Persons with sleep complaints may be screened for sleep apnea or restless legs syndrome. Narcolepsy is rare but should be considered if there is excessive, overwhelming sleepiness during the day and may respond to psychostimulant medication. Neurosyphilis is rare in advanced old age but is a treatable cause of neuropsychiatric disease in middle-aged adults.

7.7 Recluses

This is a special category. There are individuals in every community who have gradually separated themselves from society and keep to themselves. Some have mental illness and many have unusual ways of dressing, grooming, and keeping house. Often they hoard things and are not careful about personal hygiene or dress. Many hermits are cognitively intact and have no defined mental health disorder.

Be careful to avoid labeling these unique individuals with dementia or mental illness until after you have thoroughly evaluated them. Some may have personality disorders as defined by the DSM-5 (Diagnosis and Statistical Manual, Edition 5). One of the more difficult dimensions in mental health is the category of personality disorders (10 of them in DSM-5) that share as common features. (1) Distorted thinking patterns; (2) problematic emotional responses; (3) over- or under-regulated impulse control; and (4) interpersonal difficulties. Among "cluster A" or the odd, eccentric clusters are: Paranoid Personality Disorder, Schizoid Personality Disorder, and Schizotypal Personality Disorders.

7.8 Concurrent Chemical Dependency and Mental Illness

Dependency on or heavy misuse of alcohol, cocaine, and other chemical substances make it difficult to diagnose and treat mental illness. Often the chemical dependency must be addressed before progress can be made with depression, anxiety, or other mental illness; this usually requires the help of people who are specialized in the care of addiction disorders and psychiatric care resources. If you are on your own, be careful to address the substance abuse problems first and foremost. You may get more information if you ask patients specifically about commonly used names for street drugs and various alcoholic beverages. Performing comprehensive urine drug screen testing may also be indicated. Patients may abuse prescription drugs that they obtain from others or from their own prescriptions.

7.9 Managing Controlled Medications in Home-Based Medical Care

In the setting of concurrent mental illness and chronic medical conditions, a frequent challenge is management of controlled medications. Because of diversion and accidental deaths, this is a national focus. Many patients at home suffer from chronic pain or anxiety, for which opiates and other controlled medications are needed and should be prescribed. Careful documentation about diagnosis, about numbers of pills that are prescribed, pill counts, patient contracts related to controlled substances and in some cases regular use of urinary drug screens are all important. Keep track of current local and national regulations and remain compliant. Be alert; in the home you may find that drugs needed by older patients with pain are diverted and sold to pay for needs of other household members, which is a form of abuse and a crime. Providers must take care to be thorough in determining the appropriateness of medication use. Signed paper prescriptions are needed for each new and refilled prescription for Schedule II medications. Since our patients are not mobile, this can present problems between visits. In our practice, we have found local pharmacies that will send a driver to our office to pick up prescriptions for patients. In selected circumstances, providers must ultimately refuse to continue prescribing controlled medicines. This may be difficult, particularly when there is a genuinely painful condition and concern about elder abuse and neglect, yet the older patient refuses to leave the situation for what we would consider to be a safer alternative. Lock boxes and other strategies may allow the prescriber to continue providing medications that are truly indicated for the patient. For additional guidance on managing controlled substances prescriptions in home-based palliative care, please see Chap. 12: "Palliative Care."

7.10   Managing Mental Health Problems Using Nonmedication Resources

Managing conditions without medications is always a good initial goal. In some conditions, such as depression, there is evidence that cognitive behavioral therapy (CBT) is equivalent to or better than antidepressant medication in some cases. Many older individuals respond well to CBT. One of the problems in home care is finding a mobile resource for this kind of treatment, but when resources exist providers should offer them. This does not require a psychiatrist or a psychologist, but may be provided by a licensed clinical social worker (LCSW), licensed professional counselor (LPC), or advanced practice psychiatric nurse. Some episodes of depression are situational and transient and should not result in medication management. Improved socialization may help, as may reassurance and effective management of concurrent symptoms like pain that can lead to depression [5]. Another important intervention that has good research support is the use of relaxation techniques such as deep breathing, progressive muscle relaxation, and guided imagery. These can be taught to patients in 10–15 min and can be very beneficial for managing pain, anxiety, and depression.

Patients with mental health disorders are better able to manage their symptoms when they are active and have something that brings meaning to their lives. This can be as simple as performing housework, spending time with family, and staying involved in a religious community. An important assessment question is "What do you spend your time doing?" Providers should be concerned when patients say they spend most of their time watching TV, sleeping, or sitting around. Physical activity and exercise are also important components of improving mental health. Even those who have mobility limitations can usually perform chair exercise or a stretching program. The importance of adequate sleep to mental and physical health cannot be overstated. Many patients who complain of difficulty sleeping will benefit from basic sleep hygiene interventions such as adhering to routine bedtime and wakeup times, increasing activity level during the day, removing TVs and electronics from the bedroom, avoiding any electronic devices for at least an hour before bedtime, and keeping the bedroom cool and dark.

7.11   Medications for Psychiatric Disorders

Assuming that nonmedication strategies have failed, use of medications for mental illness is a key skill in home-based medical care. A comprehensive discussion is impractical but general guidelines follow.

First, follow this time-honored axiom in geriatrics: "start low and go slow... but go." This means that caution should be taken with dosing but one should not under-treat. Some older patients do not improve until doses are raised to therapeutic ranges.

In depression, antidepressant medications are used as the first-line pharmacologic strategy. These include serotonin reuptake inhibitors (SRIs), serotonin norepinephrine reuptake inhibitors (SNRIs), and several atypical antidepressants such as bupropion and mirtazapine. Tricyclic antidepressants (TCAs) are still used in some cases; however, they have anticholinergic properties and should be used with caution in the elderly. Because of drug interactions and required diet restrictions, monoamine oxidase inhibitors (MAOIs) are used infrequently for treatment-resistant depression.

When selecting an antidepressant medication, be mindful of other symptoms that may benefit from that particular medication. For example, chronic neuropathic pain or migraine headaches may also respond to TCAs or SNRIs. Bupropion is also used for smoking cessation. Mirtazapine and TCAs may benefit those who have difficulty with insomnia. Mirtazapine may also increase appetite. Antidepressants that are commonly used in older patients include citalopram, mirtazapine, and sertraline. Side effect profiles and potential for drug interactions should be taken into consideration in medication selection. All antidepressants may increase the risk of falls, and elderly patients may be more susceptible to antidepressant-induced hyponatremia, particularly with serotonergic agents (SSRI, SNRI, other)—so check the sodium level routinely after starting these drugs.

Patients usually require at least a 4–6 week trial on a given antidepressant to determine benefit. Doses must be increased to a therapeutic range before concluding the drug is not effective. It is helpful to target and quantify the specific symptoms being treated and evaluate those systematically when deciding whether a medication is effective. While the patient's subjective experience is important, simply asking patients if they feel "better" may provide an inaccurate assessment. Additionally, with major depression, research clearly indicates that a treatment period of 6–12 months or longer is usually needed. Early withdrawal of medication is not advisable unless there are side effects.

In active bipolar disorder, patients usually have a psychiatric care provider involved. If the nonpsychiatric home-based medical care provider is the only provider involved, continuing maintenance medications is important to prevent manic and depressive episodes. Commonly used now are the anticonvulsants like valproic acid, carbamazepine, and lamotrigine. Lithium is another effective mood stabilizer but may be less often preferred due to the side effects and a narrow therapeutic window. Second generation antipsychotics (SGAs) are also effective as mood stabilizers for patients with bipolar disorder. Do not let these medications expire, and do not let patients with known mania talk you out of continuing their drugs. Often patients with significant bipolar disorder are taking multiple medications, and in these cases trained psychiatric providers are an important part of the treatment team.

In disorders like schizophrenia and schizoaffective disorder, there is a subpopulation of older individuals whose psychiatric disease has stabilized and who are now able to function with less intensive psychiatric interventions. There may be chronic fixed delusions or hallucinations that are not particularly disturbing to the patient, and these can be managed by acknowledging the existence of symptoms, tracking them, and maintaining the patient on some medications to limit exacerbations. Nonpharmacological techniques such as distraction can also be very helpful. These patients can remain stable in the community for years without many changes to their regimen. If the problems are less stable or more complex, psychiatrically trained providers should be involved. Regular review for the development of tardive dyskinesia should be performed for any patient on long-term antipsychotic medication therapy.

7.12   Psychiatric Medication Pharmacology and Prescribing

Table 7.3 provides information and guidelines regarding the more commonly used prescription medications [7, 8].

Among the first rules of prescribing for geriatric patients is to minimize anticholinergic burden, particularly in those with dementia. First generation TCAs such as amitriptyline should be avoided. TCAs may occasionally be used when SRI or SNRI medications have failed and the patient still has significant depressive symptoms. If a TCA is used, *N*-demethylated versions such as desipramine and nortriptyline are less anticholinergic and are preferred. Because TCAs overdose can be fatal, they should not be given to patients with active suicidal ideation. Among SRI drugs, paroxetine is relatively more anticholinergic.

Knowing whether drugs are cleared by liver or kidney and whether the patient has problems with clearance in either of these areas is important. Doses should be adjusted as appropriate.

For insomnia and anxiety, sedating agents such as benzodiazepines and nighttime sedative hypnotics sometimes are necessary but should be limited, and patients should be informed about risks. Falls and related injuries are common side effects. Research links long-term use of benzodiazepines and hypnotics to the development of dementia, and these drugs also seem to increase the risk of sudden death. Additionally, the combination of benzodiazepines and opiate pain medications can be deadly and should be avoided if possible. Benzodiazepines are also highly habit-forming and may actually increase anxiety when the effects wear off, leading to a cycle of requiring more and more medication to obtain the same effect. If benzodiazepines must be used, choose agents with a shorter half-life such as lorazepam (6–8 h) and limit the duration of use. Antidepressant medication is considered the first-line pharmacological treatment for anxiety disorders; however, it does take time to obtain a therapeutic benefit. At bedtime, trazodone has become a favorite of clinicians, though without much evidence. Sedation is a side effect of trazodone, and it is relatively safe to use for sleep. Chronic insomnia is not particularly responsive to medication and we are often treating the caregiver as much as the patient by helping the patient to sleep. Our general practice is to avoid sedatives for insomnia; use nonpharmacologic

Table 7.3 Commonly used psychiatric medications, dosing, adverse effects, clearance, and kinetics [6]

	Initial dose for elderly (per day)	Dose range in elderly	Timing	Half-life (hours)	Clearance/elimination	Adverse effects	Additional considerations
Antidepressants							
Citalopram	10 mg	10–20 mg	Daily	35 50 % higher in elderly	Primarily hepatic	Nausea, insomnia, sedation, sexual dysfunction, QTc prolongation, hyponatremia; occasionally tremors and some fall risk	Maximum dose in elderly 20 mg due to QTc prolongation; and in hepatic impairment or if combined with CYP2C19 inhibitors May be sedating due to histaminic activity
Escitalopram	5 mg	5–10 mg	Daily	27–32 50 % higher in elderly	Primarily hepatic	Nausea, insomnia, sedation, sexual dysfunction, hyponatremia, less QTc effect than citalopram	
Sertraline	25 mg	25–200 mg	Daily	26	Primarily hepatic	N/V, insomnia, sedation, sexual dysfunction, hyponatremia	Less drug interactions than other SSRIs

(continued)

Table 7.3 (continued)

	Initial dose for elderly (per day)	Dose range in elderly	Timing	Half-life (hours)	Clearance/ elimination	Adverse effects	Additional considerations
Fluoxetine	10 mg	10–40 mg	Daily	24–72 (acute use) 96–144 (chronic use)	Primarily hepatic	Activating SSRI, weight loss, nausea, insomnia, sexual dysfunction	Prolonged half-life in elderly Active metabolites' half-life is longer than parent drug CYP 2C19+2D6 inhibitor
Paroxetine	10 mg	10–40 mg	Daily	21	Primarily hepatic, metabolites cleared by kidney	Sedation, weight gain, more anticholinergic than other SSRIs	Levels can be elevated: (2×) if hepatic or (4×) if renal impairment CYP 2D6 inhibitor
Venlafaxine XR	37.5 mg daily	37.5–225 mg	Daily	3–7	Primarily hepatic, metabolites cleared by kidney	Dose-dependent hypertension, nausea, sexual dysfunction, insomnia	Withdrawal syndrome can occur when stopping med
Duloxetine	20–30 mg daily	30–120 mg	1–2×/day	12	Primarily hepatic, metabolites cleared by kidney	Nausea, insomnia, sexual dysfunction	Not recommended if Cr Cl<30 mL/ min Also FDA approved for pain syndromes
Mirtazapine	7.5–15 mg at bedtime	7.5–45 mg	Bed	20–40	Both hepatic and renal	Sedation and weight gain	45 mg should be dosed in the morning; reduce dose in renal impairment

Bupropion	100–150 mg	100–450 mg daily	IR: TID SR: BID XL: daily	12–30	Primarily hepatic, metabolites cleared by kidney	Insomnia, anxiety, tremor, weight-neutral	Do not use in bulimia, anorexia, seizure disorders Reduce dose in renal disease CYP 2B6 and D6 inhibitor
Trazodone	25–50 mg at bedtime	25–150 mg	Bed	7–10	Primarily hepatic	Sedation, orthostasis	Used primarily off-label to treat insomnia
Nortriptyline	10 mg	10–100 mg	Bed		Primarily hepatic, metabolites cleared by kidney	Sedation, weight gain, orthostasis	Drug levels, target 50–150 ng/mL
Second generation antipsychotics							
Risperidone	0.25–0.5 mg	0.5–2 mg	1–2×/day	3–20	Primarily hepatic, metabolites cleared by kidney	Metabolic, orthostasis, EPS, sedation, high prolactin level, dysphagia, osteoporosis, sedation	
Quetiapine	12.5 mg-25 mg	12.5–300 mg	1–3×/day	6	Primarily hepatic, metabolites cleared by kidney	Orthostasis, sedation, metabolic, QTc prolongation, less EPS, constipation	May be considered in persons with Parkinson's disease Lower doses more sedating—histaminic properties

(continued)

Table 7.3 (continued)

	Initial dose for elderly (per day)	Dose range in elderly	Timing	Half-life (hours)	Clearance/elimination	Adverse effects	Additional considerations
Olanzapine	2.5 mg	2.5–10 mg	Bed	21–54	Primarily hepatic, metabolites cleared by kidney	Metabolic (more than other agents in class), sedation, dysphagia, anticholinergic, constipation	Smoking can reduce olanzapine concentration
Aripiprazole	2 or 2.5 mg	Not clear Adults: 2–15 mg	Daily	75	Primarily hepatic, metabolites cleared by kidney	More activating, insomnia, akathisia	
Clozapine	12.5 mg	12.5–200 mg	Bed – BID	4–12	Primarily hepatic, metabolites cleared by kidney	Agranulocytosis, seizures, constipation, orthostasis, sedation, QTc prolongation, drooling, weight gain	Monitor ANC (absolute neutrophil count) weekly for 6 months; every 2 weeks next 6 months; and then monthly Seizure risk is dose-dependent If misses more than 48 h return to initial dose and retitrate. May be preferred in movement disorders

First-generation antipsychotics							
Haloperidol	0.5 mg	0.5–4 mg	1–3×/day	18	Primarily hepatic, metabolites cleared by kidney	EPS, sedation	Avoid in Parkinson's disease
Mood stabilizers							
Valproic acid/ divalproex (VPA)	250–375 mg	500–2000 mg	SR: BID ER: QD IR: TID	9–19	Primarily hepatic, metabolites cleared by kidney	Sedation, hyponatremia, falls, low platelet count, elevated ammonia, diarrhea, increased LFTs, pancreatitis, alopecia, edema, weight gain	Elderly patients using VPA for behavior may respond at low levels
Lithium	150–600 mg[a]	150–1200 mg Based on serum level	1–3×/day IR + ER forms avail	24 Extended in elderly	Renal	Weight gain, nausea, nocturia, psoriasis, hypothyroidism, hyperparathyroidism, nephrogenic diabetes insipidus	Hydration is important Narrow therapeutic range, blood levels must be monitored regularly Monitor renal function Target lower end of dose range in elderly Drug interactions (e.g., NSAIDs, ACE-I, thiazide diuretics)

(continued)

Table 7.3 (continued)

	Initial dose for elderly (per day)	Dose range in elderly	Timing	Half-life (hours)	Clearance/ elimination	Adverse effects	Additional considerations
Carbamazepine	100–200 mg	200–800 mg based on serum level	BID-TID	25–65 (initial use) 12–17 (chronic use)	Primarily hepatic, metabolites cleared by kidney	Hyponatremia, increased LFTs, agranulocytosis, aplastic anemia, rash	Potent inducer of CYP1A2, 2B6, 2C19, 2C8, 2C9, 3A4
Lamotrigine	25 mg[b]	25–400 mg	IR: BID XR: Daily	Depends on interacting medications	Hepatic and renal	Nausea, rash, edema, insomnia, sedation, dizziness	Risk of adverse effects increased with rapid titration and when taken concurrently with divalproex sodium. Follow strict slow titration schedule to minimize risk of rash

IR immediate release, *SR* sustained release, *XL* extended release, *OH* orthostatic hypotension, *EPS* extrapyramidal symptoms, *N/V* nausea and vomiting, *metabolic* weight gain, diabetes, increased cholesterol, *LFTs* liver function tests, *NSAID* nonsteroidal anti-inflammatory, *ACE-I* angiotensin converting enzyme inhibitors

[a]Lithium initial doses should be based on renal function and drug interactions; elderly patients require lower doses than healthy young adults

[b]Initial lamotrigine level depends on concurrent meds. As monotherapy 25 mg daily; with concurrent valproic acid 25 mg every other day; with concurrent carbamazepine, phenytoin, or phenobarbital 50 mg daily

measures first. As discussed previously, sleep hygiene interventions can be very effective and unfortunately are rarely discussed.

When prescribing psychiatric medications, attention is needed to emerging pharmacologic problems, including serotonin syndrome, neuroleptic malignant syndrome, hyponatremia, and QT prolongation on EKG. Serotonin syndrome is a serious but rare condition that involves a serotonergic crisis which may be related to a combination of several serotonergic agents. Presenting symptoms include mental status changes, nausea, vomiting, malaise, and autonomic instability. More advanced symptoms may include hyperreflexia, muscle rigidity, and myoclonus. Neuroleptic malignant syndrome is most commonly related to antipsychotic medications and may include mental status changes, autonomic instability (especially hyperthermia), and eventually muscular rigidity. Caution should be exercised when combining serotonergic antidepressants with linezolid. Hyponatremia is a side effect to antidepressant medications that occurs more commonly in the elderly. Monitor patients for mental status changes after starting an antidepressant, particularly if they take other agents that can put them at risk for hyponatremia (e.g., thiazide diuretics).

QT prolongation is an increasing focus, particularly with certain agents and combinations, such as antipsychotics (e.g., quetiapine, ziprasidone, haloperidol) and some antidepressants (e.g., citalopram). The Federal Drug Administration (FDA) suggests a maximum dose of citalopram 20 mg in patients 60 years and older. Yet, drugs that are very effective for patients get flagged as possible contributors to QTc prolongation. Guidelines suggest concern when QTc intervals exceed 460 ms. Serious, even fatal arrhythmias may be the first indication of this problem. Usually the dangerous arrhythmias occur in patients with underlying heart disease or with greater increases in QTc (500 ms or more). Best practice is to monitor the QTc by EKG after starting and periodically, ensure electrolytes (i.e., potassium and magnesium) are within normal limits, take appropriate precautions, and weigh burden and benefit. Important here is that these rhythm problems are known to occur but are relatively rare. Sometimes the stability of the psychiatric condition outweighs the unknown risk of a potential rhythm problem.

When newly prescribing medications or when nonspecific but potentially significant side effects like nausea, altered mentation, weakness, falls, or constipation are reported, check for relatively common problems like hyponatremia, caused by inappropriate secretion of antidiuretic hormone (SIADH) due to the medication. If present, confirm the diagnosis with a concurrent urine osmolality and serum osmolality—in SIADH the urine osmolality will be higher than serum. Be aware that use of diuretics invalidates this testing algorithm.

When tapering or switching medications, give consideration to potential for duplication of neurotransmitter effects (serotonin toxicity) or re-emergence of depression, and keep a careful watch during these transitions, checking on patients every few weeks.

In some cases of refractory psychosis or nonadherence, injectable depot medications are effective. These situations should involve a psychiatrically trained person, at least for periodic review. Injectable medications given without an incapacitated patient's permission should be established on the basis of well-documented authority (guardian, POA). Haloperidol, fluphenazine, risperidone, paliperidone, aripiprazole, and olanzapine are available in a long-acting formulation. Also, electroconvulsive therapy can be effective in severe cases where drugs are not adequate.

7.13 Home-Based Services Covered by Insurance (Medicare Part a Home Health Agency Psychiatric Care)

An underused resource in psychiatric home care is the home health agency. In part this is because many agencies have not developed the needed team which includes nurses with special qualifications in psychiatric care and licensed clinical social workers. When the teams exist, Medicare covers psychiatric diagnoses for skilled home healthcare episodes, and there is evidence of improved outcomes such as in patients with more severe forms of depression [7]. Inquire among local agencies to see if these resources exist. In addition, for patients who have had at least one psychiatric hospitalization in their lifetime, who have a serious mental illness, who have the potential to improve functioning, and who have Medicaid, mental health skill building is an available service. This benefit provides up to 12 h per week of in-home mental health support provided by trained personnel who are supervised by licensed mental health professionals.

7.14 Behavioral and Psychological Symptoms of Dementia (BPSD)

One of the most common problems for home-based medical care providers is managing troubling behaviors associated with dementia. BPSD are noted in 60 % or more of community-dwelling patients with dementia. Management can be organized in categories: assessment; caregiver education and support; respite and social support; medication management; and placement. A stepwise approach to this vexing issue is best and a nice summary article in 2015 is available [8].

In assessment, look first for the potential causes of behavior changes among medications, particularly new medications; any intercurrent illnesses, including the notorious urinary tract infection but not forgetting others such as constipation, sensory isolation, and undertreated pain; and changes in the home situation or related social stressors. Pay careful attention to recent changes in the home environment including review of individuals recently been directly involved in giving care. Often, understanding the causes of worsened behaviors averts use of nonspecific medications to treat the behaviors.

BPSD includes many phenomena including wandering, repetitive behaviors, calling out, day/night reversal, and rejection of care including medications, bathing and grooming. These are difficult for families, but they are often less responsive to medication. Symptoms that are more psychotic in nature, like paranoia, delusions, hallucinations, and aggression are better indications for medications.

Before you start treating, specifically characterize the behaviors and identify any patterns as to when they occur—are they at certain times of day, in response to certain stimuli, related to barriers that the patient may be trying to overcome (hunger, pain, need to use the bathroom) or conflicts with caregivers? What exactly are the key behaviors? Is the patient aggressive or emotional? Is the patient doing things that may hurt themselves or other people? Identify for treatment target behaviors the ones that are the most problematic and use those behaviors to evaluate the treatment plan.

Best practice in management is to first remove and reduce any contributing factors to BPSD, including educating caregivers about dementia and how to manage behaviors, redirection, use of adult day care for respite, daily activities to engage the person during the day and tire them out for night, and making the home safe to permit indoor wandering and harmless activities. The formal evidence from studies related to training of caregivers and improving social interactions is generally more impressive [9] than the evidence related to giving drugs [10]. For additional information on nonpharmacologic management of BPSD, please see Chap. 5: "Common Cognitive Issues in Home-Based Medical Care."

After nonmedication measures are tried, or when matters are urgently unstable, we may resort to medications. BPSD problems sometimes mirror psychotic disorders, so antipsychotic medications are tried. Controversy remains. There is evidence of efficacy in challenging cases—reduced intensity of symptoms—both with older first generation antipsychotics (FGA) such as haloperidol and with newer second generation antipsychotic (SGA) agents (e.g., risperidone, ziprasidone, quetiapine, olanzapine, aripiprazole) that cause fewer extrapyramidal side effects. Evidence of efficacy is mixed, and there is a concern about an increased risk of stroke, pneumonia, and death with all antipsychotics. Though the absolute risk of death is still small, retrospective data suggest an increase in relative death risk by about 1.7 that led to a 2005 "black box" warning on these agents which are not FDA-approved for treating BPSD. Because of the black box warning, providers should inform patients and families carefully about the choice to use these medications, and seek to use low doses if possible. When the safety issue first surfaced there was an initial focus on newer SGA medications where the FDA reported increased risk of deaths. At that time, a group led by Avorn then wrote a paper [11] suggesting that FGA medications like haloperidol were more likely to cause deaths than SGA medications. A group of national expert leaders in dementia research and neuropsychiatry that participated in the safety discussion addressed this complex subject in a review paper [12]. In brief, the evidence is inconclusive in several regards, and the challenges are real and difficult, so assess well, use nonmedication approaches first, if using medications for truly disruptive, agitated, or psychotic behaviors, pick target symptoms, inform patients and families about risk benefit, keep doses as low as possible, and periodically reassess.

Also tried when there is a strong affective component to the BPSD are drugs like valproic acid that is approved for bipolar disorder. Again, there is neither strong clinical trial evidence nor FDA approval when treating BPSD. Anecdotally, low dose valproic acid at 125–250 mg twice a day can help with BPSD when there are wide mood swings and a lot of emotion associated with behaviors. Be aware of sedation and of the occasional development of idiopathic edema.

Utilizing antidepressants to help with BPSD has become another treatment option. In a small study, citalopram reduced agitation and caregiver distress. Overall it was well tolerated, but citalopram was associated with more falls than placebo. Antidepressants may be a safer alternative to antipsychotics or valproic acid especially when targeting agitation associated with anxiety or depression [13].

There is some evidence that treatment with citalopram moderates the extent of BPSD in some cases and evidence of similar but modest beneficial effects from acetylcholinesterase inhibitors like donepezil, rivastigmine, and galantamine. Typically, this also becomes a trial-and-error exercise for individual patients. Benzodiazepines lack evidence of benefit and increase the risk of falls. Yet, individuals sometimes will respond to short term use of low dose medications such as lorazepam. As with all other medications that affect the central nervous system in this patient group, periodic attempts to reduce the medication burden are recommended.

Whatever you do, explain to patients and families that there is no one best answer, that there are burdens and benefits, and that it is best to try one thing at a time when managing behaviors with drugs, since there are so many different factors concurrently at play in these situations and because the medications themselves have side effects.

Use of the psychiatric inpatient unit to regulate BPSD is an option, but note that these hospital stays are short because of payment incentives, place patients in environments different from home, and often result in adding medications to the regimen that may or may not be the best long-term options.

7.15   Patient Selection for In-Home Psychiatric Care

If patients with psychiatric disorders are chronically home limited, or in some cases homeless, it is appropriate to see them in the community (at home) rather than in an office. Being home limited can result from either medical or mental health conditions. Like other diagnoses that lead to inability to visit the office, seeing psychiatrically incapacitated patients at home not only improves access but also gives more insight and sometimes increased effectiveness in treating. Examples of home-limiting psychiatric conditions are severe agoraphobia, severe depression, psychoses, and dementia. Conversely, when patients can leave home, they should. Home-based medical care providers should not foster dependency or reduce autonomy, and they should not see patients at home for convenience. In some cases, short-term in-home care for psychiatric conditions is all that the patients need, just as is the case for some medical home-based medical care conditions. When charting home visits for psychiatric conditions, you should write a few words about why the care is being rendered at home.

7.16 Useful Community Resources

One of the best solutions to alleviate impacts of psychiatric conditions including BPSD is adult day care. It helps to diminish caregiver's burden and makes for more sustained in-home caregiving. Finding the right day care is crucial. The other participants should be at a similar level of cognitive function, staff should be well trained, and activities should be suited to the patient's needs and preferences. Orienting the patient to the care setting and making sure they are comfortable is a key part of the initial process—think about the first day of school for children as an analogy. Unfortunately, the right resource may not exist and after some attempts adult day care may not work. Short-term respite care, in adult homes or in nursing homes, can also be important when caregivers need a break. This option also is prone to fail, sometimes dramatically so as patients can become agitated, dehydrated, or malnourished, and should be tested in advance of the actual departure of the primary caregiver.

The community mental health clinic or public health department in your community is an important resource, potentially offering a crisis intervention team who will provide in-home assessments and treatments either urgently or chronically depending on local funding. When placement into a facility appears necessary, either voluntary or involuntary, these mobile teams often play a central role. Engaging law enforcement may also be an unfortunate, but necessary intervention when community resources do not support the use of crisis intervention services in the home.

In many communities mobile psychological or psychiatric care practices are established. Experience suggests that these often focus on group care settings such as assisted living and nursing homes for reasons of efficiency, but sometimes these clinicians will visit private homes and apartments.

Personal care can help, funded by Medicaid, private pay, or long-term care insurance. This may give the primary caregiver some time to themselves or time to work and depending on the patient's economic status, can come to several hours per day. The key in these situations is to make sure that the paid caregiver is trained well in strategies to avoid conflict when caring for patients with dementia or serious mental illness. Once you have a strong aide, every effort should be made to keep them and this can be a role for a creative healthcare provider, as such situations are sometimes fluid and require work to maintain, for example, as aides change agencies and you may change agencies to keep the aide.

7.17 Patient Safety

The key issues here are abuse and neglect; risk of self-harm in patients with impaired cognition; and suicidal or homicidal concerns. Abuse and neglect are subjects for an entire book and are briefly addressed in Chap. 11: "Common Social and Ethical Issues in Home-Based Medical Care." The most important principle is to think of Adult (or Child) Protective Services as a helpful agency which can add resources and rather than a punitive entity. This is sometimes difficult particularly if the home care provider is the only healthcare professional involved, and the caregivers will know and may then resent who made the call. This could alienate the provider and leave a patient without an advocate. Patients often choose to remain in risky settings, and they may have or appear to have capacity for these decisions, making sticky situations even more difficult. Providers are mandated reporters and when in doubt, take the safest action for the patient and document your decisions well. Accidental self-harm is fractionally easier when it comes to removing dangerous objects including firearms, but never easy when it comes to impaired individuals being left along briefly because caregivers need to run errands. Risk of fire or sudden illness is always possible, and a burden-benefit calculation is needed when there are no easy alternatives and the patient's needs are best served at home.

Most critical is the need to recognize and react to a suicidal or homicidal patient. In general, calling 911 is the best course, unless there is another resource such as an emergency response behavioral health team. In our experience, suicide is rare in our chronically homebound patients that we see in home-based primary care. Patients who make brief references to suicidal ideation, without a plan or frequent perseveration are at lower risk than those who dwell on the subject, have severe depression, or are able to describe an intent and a plan. In any case, all firearms and other obvious weapons should be removed, and dangerous medicines should be secured.

In "gray zone" cases where the patient should leave home in most peoples' judgment, but refuses to leave and is not clearly incapacitated or judged incompetent, the role of the home care provider is to stand by, and be prepared for the day when everything suddenly falls apart, which it invariably will, keeping the patient as safe as possible in the meanwhile.

7.18 Provider Safety

Providing medical care in patients' homes is a fairly safe role, but there are tragic exceptions. Chemical dependency and severe mental illness in patients and family members raise the risk. Home-based medical care providers should remove themselves from situations that are volatile, particularly when drugs and alcohol are involved, and should arrange a chaperone or withdraw from a case if need be. The presence of weapons in the home likewise should be assessed. In tough neighborhoods, experienced clinicians go early in the day when violent criminals are often sleeping and generally should alert people in the home that they are coming.

7.19 When to Hospitalize

Other than suicidal or homicidal thinking, circumstances that require psychiatric hospital admission typically relate to depression, mania, or psychosis that are severe enough to prevent the patient from caring for themselves at their baseline level of functioning. Common indications are weight loss, behaviors that are unmanageable, and hallucinations or delusions that cannot be controlled with outpatient medication adjustment. When considering a psychiatric admission, make sure to first look for medical instability or factors. Laws regarding criteria and process for involuntary hospitalization vary by state. You should familiarize yourself with the regulations in your locality.

7.19.1 Capacity Determination and Competence

A common decision point in home-based medical care for patients with psychiatric problems is whether the patient has capacity to make decisions, which is something determined by experienced clinicians. Capacity comes into play when deciding about treatment, living situation, or use of resources. For a detailed discussion of capacity determination, please see Chap. 11, "Common Social and Ethical Issues in Home-Based Medical Care."

7.20 Acts: Intensive Team-Based Psychiatric Care at Home

In the 1980s and 1990s there were numerous studies, including many randomized trials of small, intensive community-focused teams, with the acronyms assertive community treatment (ACT), mental health intensive care management (MHICM), and program of assertive community treatment (PACT). This literature is summarized by Mueser [14]. Notably, caseloads in these intensive models were in the 10–30 patient range and enrolled subjects numbered fewer than 100, predominantly individuals with schizophrenia, bipolar disorder, and schizoaffective disorder. Teams functioned as a sort of "virtual hospital" with services as intensive as nurses administering medications in the home on a daily basis if needed. These models of home-based care are both effective and cost-effective and the studies are quite robust. However, this work requires funding and a team that includes staff with training to care for this very complex population. Typically, these teams include a psychiatrist or psychiatric advanced practice nurse, social workers, psychiatric nurses, and case managers. In many states, Medicaid does provide funding for PACT team services. Some PACT teams are provided by private agencies and some are provided by community mental health clinics. If psychiatric home care is a special interest, there is newer evidence that integrating mobile psychiatric home care with housing can be effective [6].

7.21 Med-Psych Comorbidity and Integrated Medical and Psychiatric Care Teams

Many homebound patients have both medical and psychiatric problems. In current parlance, the advanced medical-psychiatric medical home typically refers to a clinic, but there is every reason to establish the same sort of approach for patients who are not mobile. We are stronger together than we are apart. Look for opportunities to collaborate.

7.22   Workforce Issues

As health care evolves and home-centered care takes an ever larger role with stronger incentives, the relative lack of health professionals with psychiatric training available to see patients at home should improve. In the meantime, get to know those in your community who do this work, collaborate, and help one another. This is a precious resource that requires care and nurture.

References

1. Davitt JK, Gellis ZD. Integrating mental health parity for homebound older adults under the Medicare home health care benefit. J Gerontol Soc Work. 2011;54:309–24.
2. Kroenke K, Spitzer RL, Williams JB. The patient health questionnaire-2: validity of a two-item depression screener. Med Care. 2003;41(11):1284–92.
3. Kroenke K, Spitzer RL, Williams JB. The PHQ-9: validity of a brief depression severity measure. J Gen Intern Med. 2001;16(9):606–13.
4. Counsell SR, Callahan CM, Clark DO, et al. Geriatric care management for low-income seniors: a randomized controlled trial. JAMA. 2007;298:2623–33.
5. England MJ, Butler AS, Gonzalez ML. Psychosocial intervention for mental and substance use disorders: a framework for evidence-based standards. Institute of Medicine of the National Academies. Washington, DC: National Academies Press; 2015. Downloaded at http://books. nap.edu/openbook.php?record_id=19013&page=R1
6. Stergiopoulos V, Hwang SW, Gozdzik A, Nisenbaum R, Latimer E, Rabouin D, Adair CE, Bourque J, Connelly J, Frankish J, Katz LY, Mason K, Misir V, O'Brien K, Sareen J, Schütz CG, Singer A, Streiner DL, Vasiliadis HM, Goering PN, for the At Home/Chez Soi Investigators. Effect of scattered-site housing using rent supplements and intensive case management on housing stability among homeless adults with mental illness: a randomized trial. JAMA. 2015;313(9):905–15. doi:10.1001/jama.2015.1163.
7. Bruce ML, Raue PJ, Reilly CF, Greenberg RL, Meyers BS, Banerjee S, Pickett YR, Sheeran TF, Ghesquiere A, Zukowski DM, Rosas VH, McLaughlin J, Pledger L, Doyle J, Joachim P, Leon AC. Clinical effectiveness of integrating depression care management into Medicare home health: the depression CAREPATH randomized trial. JAMA Intern Med. 2015;175(1):55–64. doi:10.1001/jamainternmed.5835.
8. Kales HC, Gitlin LN, Lyketsos CG. Assessment and management of behavioral and psychological symptoms of dementia. BMJ. 2015;2015:350–69. doi:10.1136/bmj.h369.
9. England MJ, Butler AS, Gonzalez ML. Psychosocial intervention for mental and substance use disorders: a framework for evidence-based standards. Institute of Medicine of the National Academies. Washington, DC: National Academies Press; 2015. Downloaded at http://books. nap.edu/openbook.php?record_id=19013&page=R1 (Op Cit.).
10. Schneider LS, Tariot PN, Dagerman KS, Davis SM, Hsiao JK, Ismail MS, Lebowitz BD, Lyketsos CG, Ryan JM, Stroup TS, Sultzer DL, Weintraub D, Lieberman JA, CATIE-AD Study Group. Effectiveness of atypical antipsychotic drugs in patients with Alzheimer's disease. N Engl J Med. 2006;355(15):1525–38.
11. Wang PS, Schneeweiss S, Avorn J, Fischer MA, Mogun H, Solomon DH, Brookhart MA. Risk of death in elderly users of conventional vs. atypical antipsychotic medications. N Engl J Med. 2005;353:2335–41.
12. Jeste DV, Blazer D, Casey D, Meeks T, Salzman C, Schneider L, Tariot P, Yaffe K. ACNP white paper: update on use of antipsychotic drugs in elderly patients with dementia. Neuropsychopharmacology. 2008;33:957–70.

13. Porsteinsson AP, Drye LT, Pollock BG, Devanand DP, Frangakis C, Ismail Z, et al. Effect of citalopram on agitation in Alzheimer disease: the CitAD randomized clinical trial. JAMA. 2014;311(7):682–91.
14. Mueser KT, Bond GR, Drake RE, Resnick SG. Models of community care for severe mental illness: a review of research on case management. Schizophr Bull. 1998;24(1):37–74.

Common Functional Problems

8

Jonathan Ripp, Elizabeth Jones, and Meng Zhang

Abstract

In this chapter, we will discuss three common functional problems in the home-bound elderly: falls, incontinence, and unintentional weight loss. All three are associated with increased morbidity and mortality and decreased function and independence. The risk factors and etiologies for these problems are often more diverse and complex in the homebound elderly than in younger patients, with psychiatric and socioeconomic factors playing an important part.

Evaluation for these problems should focus on prevention and investigation of reversible causes. While some pharmacological treatment options exist, the optimal management of these problems requires a multidisciplinary approach and should always reflect the patient's preference and goals of care.

Keywords

Falls • Home-based medical care • Urinary incontinence • Unintentional weight loss

J. Ripp, M.D. • E. Jones, M.S.N., A.N.P.-B.C. • M. Zhang, M.D. (✉)
Mount Sinai Visiting Doctors Program, Mount Sinai Icahn School Medicine,
1 Gustave L. Levy Place, 1216, New York, NY 10029, USA
e-mail: jonathan.ripp@mountsinai.org; elizabeth.jones@mountsinai.org;
meng.zhang@mountsinai.org

© Springer International Publishing Switzerland 2016
J.L. Hayashi, B. Leff (eds.), *Geriatric Home-Based Medical Care*,
DOI 10.1007/978-3-319-23365-9_8

8.1   Falls

A fall is "…an event which results in a person coming to rest inadvertently on the ground or floor or other lower level" [1].

8.1.1   Prevalence

Falls in the elderly are common. Nearly one-third of all elderly adults will fall once or more on an annual basis [2]. In 2006, the Centers for Disease Control of the Behavioral Risk Factor Surveillance Survey, the largest continuous telephone-administered health survey in the world, found that nearly 6 million (over 15 %) of community-dwelling persons over the age of 65 had fallen in a 3-month period [3].

In 2013, falls were the most common cause of injury in elderly adults [4] and are the most common cause of accidental death in the home [5]; homebound elderly are at high risk. One study found that, of 228 homebound persons over the age of 60 who were evaluated by a nurse to identify individual- and environmental-level fall risk factors, nearly half (44 %) lived in a home that placed them at either moderate or high fall risk. The same study also identified individual-level factors that placed nearly a third (32 %) of the participants at a moderate or high fall risk [6].

8.1.2   Consequences

Falls exact a toll both in terms of morbidity and mortality, leading to decreased physical function, loss of independence, and subsequent institutionalization. In addition, falls result in death [6], fractures, and head injury (e.g., subdural hematoma). Up to 6 % of hospitalizations and 10 % of all emergency department visits from elderly patients are due to falls. Falls engender a vicious cycle; the majority of elderly patients, who have fallen or are at high risk for falls, experience a fear of falling which may lead to restricted activity, a further decline in independence, and possibly increased fall risk [7].

8.1.3   Risk Factors

There are multiple risk factors for falls. A history of previous falls places one at considerably higher risk for future falls. In one study of more than 300 community-dwelling elders over the age of 70 who were assessed in the home and followed for 36 weeks, one-third of all participants fell and nearly half of those who fell, fell more than once. Furthermore, having a history of two or more falls in the previous year conferred an increased risk of a future fall with an odds ratio of 3.1 (OR 3.1, 95 % Cl 1.5–6.7) [2].

While being homebound has not specifically been shown to be a risk factor for falls, it is possible to draw this inference from data on patients receiving skilled home

Common Risk Factors for Falls
- History of previous falls
- Medications [8]
  - Any combination of four or more medications [9]
  - Psychotropics (e.g., sedative-hypnotics, neuroleptics, antidepressants) [10]
  - Antihypertensives (e.g., diuretics) [11, 12]
- Urinary incontinence
- Vitamin D deficiency [13]
- Hyponatremia [14]
- Arthritis
- Cognitive impairment
- Low vision
- Needing home care within 1 month of hospital discharge [5]

health-care services after a hospital discharge, who have been found to experience increase fall risk [5]. In addition, homebound patients typically have numerous traditional fall risk factors and are likely, as a group, to have an increased risk of falls.

8.1.4 Screening and Prevention

The mainstay of fall prevention focuses on screening for risk and instituting a multi-faceted approach to fall prevention and reduction. Individual patient-level factors and environmental conditions are both important contributors to falls risk.

8.1.4.1 Individual Level

Given the importance of a fall history predicting future falls, it is recommended to simply ask patients annually if they have had a fall in the previous year [5]. Patients should also be screened for fear of falling, since the fear itself increases the risk for future falls [15]. The history should elucidate the circumstances of the fall and any contributing risk factors, such as new medications. Examination should focus on identifying physical risk factors, such as visual, cognitive, proprioceptive, and strength deficits. Orthostatic blood pressure should be measured. Laboratory tests should be limited to those that might uncover a suspected risk factor, such as serum vitamin B12 and D levels, to look for deficiencies that might predispose to balance or strength defects.

A host of bedside screening and assessment tools that can easily be performed in the home are available to assess for gait and balance abnormalities. Most of them have poor sensitivity and specificity. There is no one tool that is specifically recommended, although the "get-up-and-go" test is commonly used for its ease of administration. Participants are asked to stand unassisted from an armless chair, walk 10 ft, turn around, and return to their original position. The time in which the individual completes this task is used as a measure of fall risk. Greater than 12 s [16] is considered to place a patient at increased risk. Though easy to administer, its effectiveness at predicting falls in community-dwelling elderly patients has been called into question, so it is not recommended as an isolated instrument to assess fall risk in this population [17]. That being said, many providers gain great insight into their patient's fall risk by viewing their "Get-up-and-Go" test. Therapy can be tailored to the individual based on their performance and their specific areas of weakness (e.g., initiating gait, making turns, etc.)

Some fall assessment tools have specifically been studied in the homebound population and found to be effective in identifying homebound patients at risk for falling. In light of the variable efficacy of fall assessment tools, the US Preventive Services Task Force (USPSTF) indicates that "No single recommended tool or brief approach can reliably identify older adults at increased risk for falls" [18].

The approach to preventing falls on an individual level should be multifactorial. Any high-risk patient should be referred for physical therapy, as this intervention has been shown to be effective [5] with a USPSTF grade of "B" [18]. Simple exercise programs that can easily be taught and performed in the home have been shown to be effective in decreasing falls and fall-related injuries [19, 20].

In addition to a home exercise regimen, high-risk patients should be assessed for individual-level risk factor modification. Medication lists should be reviewed carefully. Medication that is not clearly needed should be eliminated. High-risk "culprit" medications, such as those that affect the central nervous system, should be discontinued unless absolutely necessary. Vitamin D or B12 deficiency should be treated [13, 18]. Orthostasis and hyponatremia should be corrected if possible. Pain should be adequately controlled. Implementing these changes can be challenging when concurrently trying to limit medication use; risks and benefits must be weighed on an individual basis.

8.1.4.2 Environmental Level

Assessing for environmental fall risks is as important as assessment of individual-level factors. The home assessment is a critical component of screening and strategies for fall reduction. Standardized home assessments of community-dwelling elders performed by physical or occupational therapists, which are then followed by recommended modifications, have been shown in randomized trials to reduce falls when compared with control groups that receive no such intervention. Though these standardized assessments are beyond the scope of most medical providers, common basic recommendations include optimizing lighting, the removal of loose mats and rugs, and the use of nonslip bath mats, shower chairs, grab bars, hand rails on both sides of a stairwell, and chairs with arms [21, 22]. The home-based medical clinician can play an instrumental role by conducting a visual inspection of the home focusing on these areas during an initial visit. The provider can also identify patient-level barriers to implementing recommendations, such as misconceptions about expense or emotional attachment to items that are household trip hazards, and try to negotiate compromises to reduce risk. Furthermore, it is important to follow up on whether suggested modifications are made, as many patients are reluctant to make changes in their home environment [23].

8.1.5 Summary and Recommendations

Falls are exceedingly common in homebound elderly population and are frequent causes of significant morbidity, mortality, and loss of functional independence. Homebound patients typically have multiple risk factors for falls, most notably a history of previous falls, polypharmacy, vitamin D deficiency, and abnormal gait, balance, or strength. Screening and prevention can be achieved in the home and should focus on both individual- and environmental-level risk factors identification and reduction. The most effective strategies to minimize falls include physical therapy, vitamin D supplementation, and home assessment followed by recommended modification. All of these measures are available to and can be implemented by the home-based medical provider.

8.1.6 Key Points

- Falls in the elderly are extremely common and homebound patients should be considered at high risk.
- Homebound patients are likely to have multiple risk factors for falls, including a history of previous falls, polypharmacy, vitamin D deficiency, and abnormal gait, balance, or strength.
- Home-based medical providers are uniquely able to screen their patients for both individual- and environmental- level fall risk factors.
- USPSTF guidelines recommend physical therapy and vitamin D supplementation to prevent falls in community-dwelling elderly who are at increased risk for falls.
- Physical therapy referral, vitamin D supplementation, and home modification are all interventions that can be implemented by home-based medical providers.

8.2 Further Readings

- Moyer, V.A., *Prevention of falls in community-dwelling older adults: U.S. Preventive Services Task Force recommendation statement.* Ann Intern Med, 2012. 157(3): p. 197–204.
- McCullagh, M.C., *Home modification.* Am J Nurs, 2006. 106(10): p. 54–63
- Tinetti, M.E., *Clinical practice. Preventing falls in elderly persons.* N Engl J Med, 2003. 348(1): p. 42–9.

8.3   Urinary Incontinence

Urinary incontinence (UI) is defined as the involuntary leakage of urine [24]. Older persons have the highest prevalence of UI of any age group [25], with about 75 % of older women experiencing some involuntary urine loss [26]. UI is among the top ten principal diagnoses among individuals receiving home health services [27]. Persons who are incontinent may experience anxiety, embarrassment [28], depression [29], and social isolation. Patients may not volunteer their symptoms due to embarrassment or the belief that UI is a normal part of aging [30]. UI increases caregiver stress due to the patient's wet clothing and bedding, urine odor, increased laundry needs, time and effort toileting the patient, and the cost of briefs and pads [31]. UI is associated with frailty [32], longer length of hospital stay [33], and an increased risk of death in community-dwelling adult [28]. UI also contributes to skin breakdown, including pressure ulcers and fungal infection.

8.3.1   Etiology/Differential Diagnosis

Many age-related changes in the physiology of the lower urinary tract can contribute to UI in older adults, but their presence does not always lead to UI [25]. These changes include detrusor overactivity with or without impaired contractility, decreased bladder sensation and bladder capacity, pelvic floor dysfunction, urogenital atrophy causing a decrease in normal flora and a subsequent colonization of urinary tract infection (UTI)-causing pathogens, decreased urethral closure pressure, and, in men, prostatic obstruction [24, 29]. Age-related changes in neurons that regulate bladder function may predispose the elderly to neurogenic bladder dysfunction even in the absence of neurologic conditions such as multiple sclerosis or spinal cord injury [28]. In addition, homebound adults who have functional and cognitive impairments are more susceptible to UI.

Types of UI are distinguished by their characteristic signs, symptoms, and underlying causes. In many patients, more than one mechanism exists. *Urge incontinence*, more common in older women, is characterized by a sudden urge to void which results in involuntary urine loss. Overactive bladder (OAB) is associated with urge incontinence in both men and women and is often associated with complaints of frequency and nocturia. *Stress incontinence*, more common in younger women, is characterized by an inability to hold urine during coughing or sneezing and is associated with impaired sphincter function and pelvic floor weakness. The most common type of UI in men is stress incontinence, most often following iatrogenic injury during surgery for benign prostatic hyperplasia (BPH) or prostate cancer [30, 34]. *Mixed incontinence* is a combination of both stress and urge incontinence and is the most predominant type of UI in older women [24, 26]. *Overflow incontinence* occurs when the bladder is overfull, yet normal bladder emptying does not happen, resulting in a periodic leakage of urine and a large post-void residual (PVR) volume of urine in the bladder [30]. Neurogenic bladder, caused by a lesion or disease of the central nervous system such as spinal cord injury, multiple sclerosis, stroke, or

Parkinson's disease, can lead to overflow incontinence [35, 36], as can BPH, the most common cause of overflow incontinence in men [30]. *Functional incontinence* is the result of physical, cognitive, or psychiatric disabilities and a common type of UI in homebound persons.

While the establishment of urine leakage is somewhat straightforward, medical providers should differentiate UI associated with underlying medical conditions, sometimes referred to as "transient" UI, from other types. "Transient" UI is present in up to one-third of community-dwelling older women [25], and conditions associated with it include UTI, fecal impaction, pelvic organ prolapse, medication side effects, atrophic vaginitis, hyperglycemia, volume overload, and excess fluid intake including caffeinated beverages, alcohol abuse, and delirium [24–26, 29]. In addition, functional or cognitive disability and fear of falling can also contribute to UI and should be addressed.

8.3.2 Investigations in the Home

8.3.2.1 History

All homebound adults should be screened for UI. Home-based medical care providers are ideally positioned to recognize UI that may not be evident in a primary care office visit by noting the smell of urine, disposable pads on furniture, or boxes of pads, diapers, or pull-ups in a corner. A patient may not volunteer symptoms of UI due to embarrassment or the belief that it is a normal part of aging, although a caregiver might provide this information. In one research study of UI, over one-quarter of potential research participants denied incontinence after being referred to the study by their home care nurses [27].

Review of systems should focus on acute versus chronic, timing, frequency, associated symptoms such as dysuria or coughing, and amount of leakage. Make note whether the patient is aware of the need to urinate and can verbalize this need to a caregiver. A voiding diary may help the patient or caregiver explain the circumstances and severity of UI episodes [24, 25]. Assess for a chronic cough as a contributor to stress UI. Keep in mind the transient causes of UI and contributing comorbidities when interviewing the patient and/or their caregivers. Evaluate all medications being taken for their impact on mental status, urinary retention, cough, polyuria, constipation, and other contributing factors to UI [25]. Ask about the impact of UI on quality of life and about goals of care. To further assess function, ask about history of falls, light-headedness or dizziness, and manual dexterity.

An assessment of the home environment can aid in the diagnosis and formulation of an effective treatment plan. Observe the patient in a "walk-through" of the steps in toileting, if feasible, including use of assistive devices and the need for assistance from a caregiver. Observe transfers, ambulation, and ability to manipulate clothing. Assess the accessibility of the toilet and any trip hazards present. Assess caregivers and their behaviors, including hours of availability, willingness and ability to help with toileting, and any physical and cognitive limitations. Note that other clinicians, notably physical therapists, occupational therapists, and visiting nurses, can contribute to a thorough assessment of both the home environment and a patient's functional capacity.

8.3.2.2 Physical Exam

A focused physical exam can reveal transient causes of UI and contributing comorbidities and may help to differentiate the type of UI [29]. Perform a visual exam of a female patient's genital area to assess for prolapse and evidence of atrophic vaginitis. Concurrently, assess the strength of pelvic floor muscles by observing the patient's attempt to contract them. Perform a digital rectal exam to assess fecal impaction or prostatic hypertrophy. Assess for contributors to nocturia such as lower extremity edema, obstructive sleep apnea, or congestive heart failure. Assess for orthostatic hypotension [24, 25, 37]. Test for stress incontinence by having the patient cough and note urine output into an incontinence pad. Assess the buttocks, genital areas, and the back to look for skin breakdown, pressure ulcers, and fungal infections as a result of sitting or lying in wet clothing or diapers. Assess psychological and cognitive status for alcohol abuse, dementia, or psychotic disorders and for delirium as either a cause or outcome of UI.

8.3.2.3 Labs and Tests

A variety of tests can be helpful for first-time evaluations of UI. Based on differential formulated through history and exam, labs such as urinalysis, urine culture and sensitivity to detect UTI or hematuria, and blood work to detect uncontrolled diabetes, hypercalcemia, renal impairment, B12 deficiency, or other comorbidities can assist with diagnosis.

Bladder post-void residual volume (PVR) measurement can diagnose urinary retention associated with the neurogenic bladder or the bladder outlet obstruction of BPH or prior prostate surgery. PVR can be measured in the home with a portable bladder scanner or by catheterization and should be measured in men especially [34]. A volume of less than 50 ml is considered normal; a volume greater than 100 ml may be cause for concern; and volumes between 50 and 100 ml may be acceptable for persons over 65 years of age, but not so for younger persons. However, current guidelines for treatment decisions based on PVR measurements have not been established [38]. Urodynamic testing, cystoscopy, diagnostic renal, and bladder ultrasound should not be used in the initial evaluation in an uncomplicated case [39] and are often not feasible for a homebound person. There is a lack of evidence that urodynamic testing of older women has a positive impact on diagnosis or treatment outcomes, and therefore some experts recommend against routine urodynamic testing of older women, especially those who are not surgical candidates [25, 26].

8.3.3 Treatment

Improvement in continence is possible for many patients, including those with cognitive and/or physical impairments and multiple comorbidities. Before embarking on a potentially time-consuming or expensive treatment plan, first consider if discontinuing or reducing an existing medication or changing the home environment for ease of navigation may help. Other treatment choices include behavioral therapy, medications, and invasive treatments including surgery. In many cases, behavioral and pharmacological therapies can be combined for optimal management. Consider the patient's comorbidities, functional and cognitive impairments, goals of care, polypharmacy, and susceptibility to adverse effects [24, 25].

While little is known about outcomes of surgical treatment of UI in frail elderly patients, perhaps reflecting a bias toward conservative therapy in patients with multiple impairments, age alone should not be a contraindication for surgical or invasive treatment [24, 30]. For women with stress UI who fail behavioral therapies such as pelvic floor muscle training as described below, one surgical option is a suburethral sling. However, homebound patients may have significant comorbidities or may be unwilling to undergo surgery. These women may benefit from a less invasive procedure done in an office or surgical setting in which bulking agents such as collagen are injected periurethrally, a method which has been found to improve incontinence in some elderly women with stress UI or mixed UI [40]. For some patients in whom improved continence is either unachievable or not priority in the goals of care, the best strategy may be management of incontinence to prevent skin breakdown, maintain quality of life, and relieve caregiver burden [24].

8.3.3.1   Nonpharmacologic Management

Behavioral treatments for UI include pelvic floor muscle training, urge and stress strategies, and bladder retraining. Behavioral strategies can reduce incontinence episodes in patients who are homebound with multiple comorbidities and significant functional impairment [27], in patients on diuretics, and in the elderly [41]. Studies show that behavioral strategies result in about a 75 % reduction in the frequency of incontinent episodes for both predominantly stress and urge UI [27, 41], although the interventions take significant time and attention that may not be practical for all patients. These conservative techniques should be tried for 8–12 weeks and then assessed for success [24]. Handouts that explain the behavioral technique may help the patient or caregiver with effective execution.

Pelvic floor muscle training (PFMT), or "Kegels," can reduce incontinence in cognitively intact homebound adults with stress, urge, or mixed UI, in men with postprostatectomy incontinence, although the benefit and duration may be modest [29], and in patients with OAB [39]. Data on the efficacy of PFMTs for frail elderly patients is lacking, although younger, cognitively intact patients who are homebound due to a physical or mental disability may benefit from this technique [24]. Patients can learn the technique by using portable biofeedback instruments which may enhance effectiveness [41], although the practicality of this in the home may be low. If biofeedback is not feasible, patients can practice to isolate the pelvic floor muscles aiming to stop urination midstream. Patients should do 10–15 muscle contractions three times a day. Once the technique is mastered, the patient can utilize the contractions to suppress both urge and stress incontinence, employing the technique as needed either at a strong urge to void or during a stress incontinence activity such as sneezing or coughing [27].

Bladder retraining is a method to consider for urge UI in non-frail adults [24] and for patients with OAB [39]. Advise patients to gradually increase the time between voids and to use pelvic floor muscle contractions to suppress the urge between voids [42]. This method is effective for cognitively and physically intact adults [43], both men and women [30], but may not be appropriate for cognitively impaired or frail homebound elders.

Prompted voiding, a potentially effective strategy for cognitively impaired patients, is a method in which the caregiver asks the patient if he or she is wet or dry every 2 h while awake. The caregiver praises the patient if he or she answers correctly. Then the caregiver asks the patient if he or she would like to use the toilet and encourages the patient to do so. If the patient does use the toilet correctly, the caregiver again praises the patient. For this strategy to be effective, a willing and able caregiver must be available for most of the waking hours. The time intervals can be adjusted to accommodate competing demands on caregivers or patients. In one study of cognitively impaired homebound older adults with an available caregiver, prompted voiding reduced the number of daytime incontinence episodes by about 25 % [31]. This method has been shown to be effective in both men and women [30].

Physical or occupational therapists can address functional incontinence and environmental barriers through gait and balance training and strength training. Therapists can assess the need for and order assistive devices, such as walkers, canes, Hoyer lifts, raised toilet seats, grab bars, and train patients and caregivers in their use. Other strategies that may improve continence in some situations include eliminating caffeine and alcohol and promoting smoking cessation to reduce chronic cough. For nocturia, strategies include limiting fluids in the evening, adjusting the timing of diuretics, and treating dependent lower extremity edema by elevating the legs for several hours before bedtime. Weight loss for obese persons may also be helpful [24, 31].

"Contained incontinence" through the use of pads, pull-ups, diapers, or catheters may be the most realistic option for some patients for whom other treatments are not effective or possible. Absorbent incontinence products are available specific to both male and female anatomy. Patient may be able to achieve the "social presentation of continence," and thus maintain quality of life and avoid complications such as skin breakdown and infection [27]. Information on prevention of skin breakdown can be found in the wound care section of this book.

Catheterization can relieve high bladder pressure, thus preventing renal damage, and maintain continence for patients with overflow incontinence from neurogenic bladder [35]. Catheterization can also manage functional obstruction from BPH if pharmacological treatments fail and the patient is not a good candidate for surgical therapy. Choice of catheter therapy depends on several factors, including individual preference and ability, prior surgical intervention, degree of obstruction, and patient gender. Intermittent catheterization, usually performed every 4 h, requires a willing and able patient or caregiver and may reduce the risk of UTI compared to an indwelling catheter [35]. An external or condom catheter is an option for men with many types of UI. Indwelling and suprapubic catheters may increase the risk of UTIs or bacterial colonization and need to be changed monthly by a clinician or trained family caregiver. A recent Cochrane review found no evidence to create guidelines for choosing among intermittent, external, indwelling, or suprapubic catheterization [35], so clinicians should base their decisions on urologist recommendations, patient preferences, and goals of care.

The most common treatment modalities for men with stress UI are surgical: the artificial urethral sphincter and the male sling [34], which may not be an option for those homebound men with multiple comorbidities who are not good surgical candidates.

8.3.3.2 Pharmacologic Management

The main pharmacological treatments for UI are anticholinergics and the beta-3 adrenoceptor agonist mirabegron, although these drugs are not indicated for all types of UI. A review by the Agency for Healthcare Research and Quality (AHRQ) found drugs are more effective than placebo in treating adult women, but that overall effectiveness is low. Complete continence was achieved less than 20 % of the time for all drugs reviewed, although reductions in frequency of UI episodes were often higher [27].

Patients with urge neurogenic bladder, urge UI, and/or OAB may find relief with anticholinergics that improve urine flow, lower bladder pressure, and prevent detrusor overactivity. Anticholinergics may also reduce urine leakage between intermittent catheterizations in patients with neurogenic bladder [44]. The AHRQ review found that the anticholinergics oxybutynin, solifenacin, tolterodine, darifenacin, fesoterodine, and trospium all resolved UI in a higher percentage of adult women treated compared to placebo [28]. A recent systematic review [45] found a small decrease of about half a leakage in a 24 h period in elderly patients taking anticholinergics for urge UI and found no positive effect of oxybutynin on urinary leakage in the frail elderly. When selecting an anticholinergic, an extended release preparation of oxybutynin or tolterodine may be preferred over an immediate release formula due to lower side effect profile, notably dry mouth. The newer generation anticholinergics, darifenacin, solifenacin, and trospium, are generally comparable in effectiveness to the older generation ones, while solifenacin may be better tolerated [30]. Providers should weigh the risk of anticholinergic side effects (notably dry mouth, risk for falls, confusion, orthostatic hypotension, constipation, and blurred vision) and heed recommendations for geriatric and renal dosing. Side effects may affect a third or more of elderly patients [45]. Anticholinergics should not be prescribed without a detailed discussion of risks and benefits for patients with urinary retention, narrow angle glaucoma, or impaired gastric emptying.

Mirabegron is a new medication that has a similar rate of effectiveness compared to anticholinergics at reducing incontinence episodes in person with urge UI and OAB, but with lower rates of dry mouth and constipation [34, 39]. There are no data on the use of mirabegron in the frail elderly or those with complex comorbidities and polypharmacy [39], so its use in the home-based medical care population may be limited. Any medication should be tried for 1–3 months to determine effectiveness.

For selected patients who experience neurogenic detrusor overactivity, especially those with multiple sclerosis or spinal cord injury, who fail anticholinergic or mirabegron therapies, benefit may be seen with botulinum toxin type A (Botox) injected either into the bladder wall or the external sphincter. A patient must be willing and able to leave home repeatedly for the procedure and for frequent PVR measurements and to perform self-catheterization if necessary. Therefore, botulinum toxin injections may not be an option for many homebound patients [34, 44].

Postmenopausal women with stress UI may benefit from low-dose vaginal estrogen. Another medication that has been tested for stress UI in this group is oral duloxetine, which is not better than placebo and carries a high risk of adverse effects [28].

8.3.4 Key Points

- UI is a common syndrome in homebound patients, and providers need to look for UI even in patients who deny complaints.
- Types of UI include urge UI which is often associated with OAB, stress UI, mixed UI, functional UI, transient UI, and overflow UI which is often associated with neurogenic bladder or outlet obstruction. Providers should try to determine type of UI through history, exam, and tests because the management varies by type.
- First-line treatment for many types of UI is nonpharmacological therapy, which includes PFMT, prompted voiding, catheters, physical or occupational therapy, or the contained continence of diapers and pads.
- Pharmacological treatments, which can be used in conjunction with nonpharmacological therapies, are the anticholinergic medications and the new beta-3 adrenoceptor, mirabegron. Use caution with these medications in the frail and elderly due to side effect profiles that include orthostatic hypotension and increased risk for falls.

8.4 Further Readings

- DuBeau CE. Beyond the bladder: management of urinary incontinence in older women. Clin Obstet Gynecol. 2007;50:720–734.
- DuBeau CE, Kuchel GA, Johnson T 2nd, Palmer MH, Wagg A. Incontinence in the frail elderly: Report from the 4th International Consultation on Incontinence. Neurol Urodyn. 2010;29:165–178.
- Bettez M, Tu LM, et al. 2012 Update: Guideline for Adult Urinary Incontinence Collaborative Consensus Document for the Canadian Urological Association. CAUJ. 2012;6(5):354–363.

8.5   Unintentional Weight Loss

Unintentional weight loss, or the involuntary decline in total body weight over time, is clinically defined as more than a 5 % reduction in body weight within 6–12 months [46]. It is common among elderly homebound patients and is associated with increased morbidity and mortality [47]. Studies have reported as many as 27 % of community-dwelling frail elderly people and 50–60 % of nursing home residents being affected [48], and the incidence in the elderly homebound population probably falls somewhere in between.

In the homebound population, unintentional weight loss may be associated with functional decline in the activities of daily living [49], increased risk of institutionalization [50], in-hospital morbidity [51], increased risk of hip fracture in women [52], decreased quality of life [53], and increased overall mortality [54]. At the extreme, cachexia (a complex metabolic syndrome associated with underlying illness and characterized by loss of muscle with or without loss of fat mass [55]) has been associated with increased infections, pressure ulcers, poor wound healing, and failure to respond to medical treatments [47]. While the etiologies of unintentional weight loss should be investigated and treated when appropriate, possible, and desired, it is also important to note that weight loss is an expected disease trajectory in dying patients with multiple morbidities.

8.5.1   Etiology

Substantial weight loss should never be attributed to the normal aging process [48]. However, several important age-associated physiologic changes do predispose the elderly person to weight loss, such as declining chemosensory function (smell and taste), reduced efficiency of chewing, slowed gastric emptying, and alterations to the neuroendocrine axis [56, 57]. These changes are associated with early satiety and a decline in both appetite and pleasure of eating. Involuntary weight loss may also be associated with the development of the frailty syndrome (defined as a clinical syndrome in which three or more of the following criteria were present: unintentional weight loss, self-reported exhaustion, weakness, slow walking speed, and low physical activity) [45].

While involuntary weight loss in younger adults often has a single medical cause, in older patients and especially the homebound elderly population, causes are more diverse and complex, with psychiatric and socioeconomic factors playing an important part. While the causes of unintentional weight loss in this population can be classified as organic (Table 8.1) [47, 58–61, 64, 65] and psychosocial, often a combination of factors coexist and all contribute to weight loss. A majority of homebound elderly patients have multiple chronic illnesses, take a variety of medications, have impaired cognition and mobility, and are socially isolated, all of which predispose them to weight loss.

Medication adverse effects are common but often overlooked causative factors for weight loss [62].

Table 8.1 Organic causes of unintentional weight loss in older adults [49, 58–63]

Malignancy (19–36 %)
Gastrointestinal: accounts for 50 %
Lung, lymphoma, prostate, ovarian, or bladder
Nonmalignant gastrointestinal disease (9–19 %)
Swallowing and motility disorders
Peptic ulcer disease
Malabsorption
Chronic diseases
Endocrine (4–11 %): hyperthyroidism, diabetes
Cardiopulmonary (9–10 %):
Cardiac cachexia from heart failure
Pulmonary cachexia from severe obstructive or restrictive lung disease
Alcohol-related disease (8 %)
Infectious disease (4–8 %): HIV, viral hepatitis, tuberculosis, chronic fungal, or bacterial infection
Neurologic (7 %): stroke, dementia, Parkinson's disease
Rheumatic disease (7 %)
Renal disease (4 %): cachexia in end stage of renal disease
Systemic inflammatory disorders (4 %)
Oral and dental problems
Poor dentition
Three fitting dentures
Xerostomia
Side effects of medication

Common medication side effects are [46]:

- Altered taste/smell: allopurinol, angiotensin-converting enzyme inhibitors, antibiotics, antihistamines, calcium channel blockers, levodopa, propranolol, selegiline, and spironolactone
- Anorexia: amantadine, antibiotics, anticonvulsants, antipsychotics, benzodiazepines, digoxin, levodopa, metformin, neuroleptics, opiates, selective serotonin reuptake inhibitors, and theophylline
- Dry mouth: anticholinergics, antihistamines, clonidine, and loop diuretics
- Dysphagia: bisphosphonates, doxycycline, gold, iron, nonsteroidal anti-inflammatory drugs, and potassium
- Nausea/vomiting: amantadine, antibiotics, bisphosphonates, digoxin, dopamine agonists, metformin, selective serotonin reuptake inhibitors, statins, and tricyclic antidepressants

Polypharmacy has been shown to interfere with taste and can cause anorexia [63]. Drugs such as sedatives and opiate analgesic may interfere with cognition and affect the patient's ability to eat. Many medications used in the elderly are also constipating which can lead to decreased appetite and early satiety. Any medication temporally related to the development of involuntary weight loss should be suspected. Published observational studies report that psychiatric problems, particularly dementia and depression, are the main cause of unexplained weight loss in 10–20 % of elderly patients. Depression can be the sole cause, or one of the many contributors, to weight loss. It is common in the elderly and often under diagnosed and under treated. Patients with cognitive impairments and dementia who are agitated or have a tendency to wonder can expend significant energy in pacing. Others may lose the skills to cook and feed oneself or simply forget that they have to eat. Unintentional weight loss has been reported in 30 % of community-dwelling elderly with mild to moderate Alzheimer disease [66]. Poverty and social isolation add further insult through the unavailability of nutritious and preferred foods, leading to inadequate food intake and malnutrition.

8.5.2 Evaluation

Unintentional weight loss is a nonspecific condition with multiple causes. While there are no published guidelines for its evaluation, there is consensus on how to proceed in the geriatric population. It is important to consider the context under which weight loss is occurring, as presence (or absence) of underlying disease states and associated syndromes will impact both the patient's clinical course and potential intervention. The extent of the workup should always be consistent with the goals of care of the patients.

8.5.2.1 History
The mainstay of evaluation for unintentional weight loss involves a detailed history, thorough clinical examination, and baseline laboratory investigations. It is important to first establish the extent of weight loss. While serial measurements of body weight offer the simplest screening tool, it may not always be possible, especially for frail patients who are no longer able to stand. If it is not possible to measure weight directly, a change in clothing size or corroboration of weight loss by a caregiver can be helpful. Questions about appetite may help elucidate whether the weight loss is caused by inadequate energy intake or has occurred despite an adequate intake. Several screening tools exist for identifying older adults at risk for poor nutrition.

Previous and current medical history can identify conditions that can lead to weight loss and drugs that may contribute via their side effects. Obtaining an accurate chief complaint is important, as it has been found to lead to etiology of weight loss in a considerable proportion of cases. A history that includes a review of systems may elicit additional symptoms (e.g., cough, nausea/vomiting, abdominal pain) that might direct further investigation. All elderly patients with weight loss should undergo screening for dementia and depression using standardized assessment tools [67]. A detailed social history can elicit information on alcohol intake and smoking and shed light on the patient's living situations. With whom does she live? Who buys and prepares the food? Is there any help from aides or family members? Home-based medical providers have a unique opportunity to obtain this information firsthand by speaking with the caregivers during home visits and doing "refrigerator biopsy" and direct surveillance of the home.

8.5.2.2   Physical Exam

In patients with unintentional weight loss, a full physical examination should aim to exclude major cardiovascular and respiratory illnesses, as well as abdominal masses, organomegaly, prostate enlargement, and breast masses that may indicate cancer. The physical examination can aid in evaluating concerns prompted by history findings. Evaluation of the oral cavity may indicate difficulty with chewing or swallowing. Baseline investigations should be guided by patients'/proxies' goals of care and findings from history and physical exam and aim to identify reversible and easily treated causes.

8.5.2.3   Diagnostic Testing

Recommended laboratory tests include complete blood count, basic metabolic panel, liver function tests, thyroid function tests, C-reactive protein levels, erythrocyte sedimentation rate, lactate dehydrogenase measurement, and urinalysis [48]. Chest radiography, fecal occult blood testing, and abdominal ultrasonography can also be considered in the home setting if history and exam suggest pulmonary or gastrointestinal involvement, respectively. In one prospective study of 101 patients with an average age of 64 years, the etiology of unintentional weight loss was established in 72 % patients with the basic evaluation described above [65]. Organic disease was identified in 57 patients, and 16 patients had a psychiatric diagnosis. More importantly, all of the 22 patients with malignant disease had abnormal results in the baseline assessment. Tests with the highest yield were C-reactive protein, hemoglobin, lactate dehydrogenase, and albumin measurements. None of the 25 patients with negative findings on baseline evaluation had a malignancy on additional workup, such as computed tomography, endoscopy, colonoscopy, magnetic resonance imaging, or radionuclide examinations.

Therefore, if baseline test results are normal, close observation for 3–6 months is justified [57, 67]. Continued watchful waiting is a reasonable strategy. Undirected pan-body scanning is not recommended. There are no clear guidelines for how to proceed in the assessment of a patient with weight loss and negative initial findings. The diagnostic yield of a thoracic/abdominal/pelvic CT examination to assess for occult or metastatic disease has not been determined. Incidental findings are common, the studies are costly, and they may be inappropriate or impossible to obtain in patients who are frail or who have multiple comorbidities. Clear and prompt communications with the patient and family regarding the initial evaluation are critical, and conversations regarding risks/burdens vs. benefits of further testing and goals of care should be ongoing.

8.5.3 Treatment

Management of unintentional weight loss in the elderly homebound requires a multidisciplinary approach to treat remediable causes. Physicians; dieticians; physical, occupational, and speech therapists; dentists; and social workers all have important roles to play. Management of chronic medical illness should always be optimized first. Depression should be aggressively treated.

8.5.3.1 Nonpharmacologic Management

Common strategies to address unintentional weight loss in older homebound adults are dietary changes, environmental modifications, nutritional supplements, and flavor enhancers [68]. Examples include:

- Minimize dietary restrictions and liberalize diet to enhance the palatability of the food.
- Optimize energy intake by maximizing intake with high-energy foods at the best meal of the day. Many elderly people consume most of their daily energy intake at breakfast [69, 70].
- Eat smaller meals more often, eat favorite foods and snacks, and provide finger foods for dementia patient.
- Avoid gas-producing foods to avoid early satiety.
- Optimize and vary dietary texture; enhancing chewing and palatability of foods may stimulate positive feedback to eat more and minimizes fatigue-associated chewing.
- Use flavor enhancers to counteract age-related increase in smell and taste thresholds.
- Ensure adequate oral health, as poor oral hygiene and dry mouth are risk factors for decreased oral intake through altered taste sensation and difficulty in chewing and swallowing.
- Take high-energy and nutritionally dense supplements or add fats or oils to usual foods.
- Take supplements between meals to minimize appetite suppressions and compensatory decreased intake of foods [71].
- For patients who live alone, eat in company may lead to enhanced enjoyment of meals and increased energy intake.
- Get assistance to help with grocery shopping, preparing food, and feeding for those with cognitive and physical impairment.
- Utilize community nutritional support services, such as Meal on Wheels programs.
- Home-based medical providers should reconcile medications regularly to reduce polypharmacy.

Physical therapy may help patients increase their amount of exercise, to thereby stimulate appetite and increase energy intake and muscle mass [72].

When weight loss becomes resistant to nutritional intervention at the end of life or when cachexia worsens as the underlying disease progresses, it is important to focus on the comfort measures that are consistent with the patient's goals of care. These measures can include careful hand feeding for pleasure eating while minimizing aspiration risk, treating pain and nausea aggressively, and proper oral care. Home hospice referral not only can provide the patients the necessary support but is also invaluable in educating and supporting the families and caregivers. Watching loved ones lose weight and stop eating is inevitably difficult for family members. If patients start having difficulty swallowing or no longer care to eat, feeding tubes are often considered as a way to prolong life. Since the benefit of feeding tube varies in different medical conditions and the discussion of artificial nutrition and hydration is complex and often emotionally charged, we will not discuss it in depth in this chapter. But the evidence shows that feeding tubes do not provide adequate nutrition, prolong life, prevent aspiration, or improve comfort in patients with advanced dementia [73, 74]. In these difficult situations, home-based medical providers can provide important guidance to allow patients and families to make decisions that reflect their preferences and goals.

8.5.3.2 Pharmacologic Management

Several medications to stimulate appetite are available, but limited evidence exists to support the use of any pharmacologic agent for the treatment of weight loss. The existing literature is mostly small, uncontrolled studies, and benefits are generally restricted to a small gain in weight without evidence of decreased morbidity and mortality or improved function and quality of life [75]. Most of these agents have significant side effects, particularly in frail elderly people, which limit their usefulness. Thus, home-based medical providers should weigh the risks and benefits carefully with the patient and family. It is our general practice not to use appetite stimulants.

Megestrol, a progestational agent, has been shown to improve appetite and increase weight gain in patients with cancer and AIDS cachexia. Its use in AIDS patients is also associated with higher mortality rates [63]. However, studies in older patients are limited, and there are insufficient data to define an optimal dose. Adverse effects of megestrol include gastrointestinal upset, insomnia, impotence, hypertension, thromboembolic events, and adrenal insufficiency.

Mirtazapine, a serotonin antagonist used to treat depression, is another possible treatment for unintentional weight loss in older patients because 12 % of patients who take this drug for depression report weight gain [76]. Although no literature exists to support its use for unintentional weight loss, mirtazapine may be a good choice for treatment of depression in older patients who also have unintentional weight loss. Because dizziness and orthostatic hypotension are possible adverse effects of mirtazapine, caution is warranted in patients at risk of falls [46]. Dronabinol has been shown to improve appetite in patients with AIDS [77], but is associated with significant adverse effects, particularly central nervous system toxicity (sedation, fatigue, hallucination).

8.5.4 Key Points

- Unintentional weight loss is common among elderly homebound patients and is associated with increased morbidity and mortality.
- While unintentional weight loss in younger adults often has a medical cause, in homebound elderly population, causes are more diverse and complex, with psychiatric and socioeconomic factors playing an important part.
- There are no published guidelines exist for the evaluation and management of unintentional weight loss. The extent of workup and treatment should target reversible causes and align with patient's goals of care. Watchful waiting after an initial targeted workup is a reasonable strategy.
- Management of unintentional weight loss in the elderly homebound requires a multidisciplinary and multi-faceted approach and should reflect patient's preference and goals of care. Appetite stimulants are not recommended.

8.6 Further Readings

- McMinn J, Steel C, Bowman A. Investigation and management of unintentional weight loss in older adults. *BMJ.* 2011; 342:d1732
- Gaddey H, Holder K. Unintentional weight loss in older adults. *Am Fam Physician.* 2014; 89(9): 718–722
- Lankisch PG, Gerzmann M, Gerzmann JF, et al. Unintentional weight loss: diagnosis and prognosis. *J Intern Med.* 2001;249(1):41–46.

References

1. World Health Organization. Falls fact sheet. Oct 2012 [cited 1 July 2015]. Available from: http://www.who.int/mediacentre/factsheets/fs344/en/
2. Stalenhoef PA, et al. A risk model for the prediction of recurrent falls in community-dwelling elderly: a prospective cohort study. J Clin Epidemiol. 2002;55(11):1088–94.
3. Stevens JA, Mack KA, Paulozzi LJ, Ballesteros MF. Self-reported falls and fall-related injuries among persons aged ≥65 years--United States, 2006. MMWR Morb Mortal Wkly Rep. 2006;57(9):225–9.
4. Centers for Disease Control, N.C.f.I.P.a.C. 7 July 2014 [cited 7 Jan 2015]. Available from: http://www.cdc.gov/injury/wisqars/
5. Stevens JA, et al. The costs of fatal and non-fatal falls among older adults. Inj Prev. 2006;12(5):290–5.
6. Tanner EK. Assessing home safety in homebound older adults. Geriatr Nurs. 2003;24(4):250–4. 256.
7. Salkeld G, et al. The cost effectiveness of a home hazard reduction program to reduce falls among older persons. Aust N Z J Public Health. 2000;24(3):265–71.
8. Field TS, et al. Risk factors for adverse drug events among nursing home residents. Arch Intern Med. 2001;161(13):1629–34.

9. Tinetti ME, Speechley M, Ginter SF. Risk factors for falls among elderly persons living in the community. N Engl J Med. 1988;319(26):1701–7.
10. Bloch F, et al. Psychotropic drugs and falls in the elderly people: updated literature review and meta-analysis. J Aging Health. 2011;23(2):329–46.
11. Shaw BH, Claydon VE. The relationship between orthostatic hypotension and falling in older adults. Clin Auton Res. 2014;24(1):3–13.
12. Zang G. Antihypertensive drugs and the risk of fall injuries: a systematic review and meta-analysis. J Int Med Res. 2013;41(5):1408–17.
13. Murad MH, et al. Clinical review: The effect of vitamin D on falls: a systematic review and meta-analysis. J Clin Endocrinol Metab. 2011;96(10):2997–3006.
14. Renneboog B, et al. Mild chronic hyponatremia is associated with falls, unsteadiness, and attention deficits. Am J Med. 2006;119(1):71 e1–8.
15. Boyd R, Stevens JA. Falls and fear of falling: burden, beliefs and behaviours. Age Ageing. 2009;38(4):423–8.
16. Lee J, Geller AI, Strasser DC. Analytical review: focus on fall screening assessments. PM R. 2013;5(7):609–21.
17. Barry E, et al. Is the timed up and go test a useful predictor of risk of falls in community dwelling older adults: a systematic review and meta-analysis. BMC Geriatr. 2014;14:14.
18. Moyer VA. Prevention of falls in community-dwelling older adults: U.S. Preventive Services Task Force recommendation statement. Ann Intern Med. 2012;157(3):197–204.
19. Robertson MC, Campbell AJ. Falls prevention and the role of home exercise programmes. J R Soc Promot Health. 2001;121(3):143.
20. El-Khoury F, et al. The effect of fall prevention exercise programmes on fall induced injuries in community dwelling older adults: systematic review and meta-analysis of randomised controlled trials. BMJ. 2013;347:f6234.
21. Cumming RG, et al. Home visits by an occupational therapist for assessment and modification of environmental hazards: a randomized trial of falls prevention. J Am Geriatr Soc. 1999;47(12):1397–402.
22. McCullagh MC. Home modification. Am J Nurs. 2006;106(10):54–63. quiz 63–4.
23. Cumming RG, et al. Adherence to occupational therapist recommendations for home modifications for falls prevention. Am J Occup Ther. 2001;55(6):641–8.
24. Bettez M, Tu LM, et al. Update: guideline for adult urinary incontinence collaborative consensus document for the Canadian urological association. CAUJ. 2012;6(5):354–63.
25. DuBeau CE. Beyond the bladder: management of urinary incontinence in older women. Clin Obstet Gynecol. 2007;50:720–34.
26. Shamliyan T, Wyman J, Kane RL. Nonsurgical treatments for urinary incontinence in adult women: diagnosis and comparative effectiveness. AHRQ Publication No 11(12)-EHC074-EF. 2012. doi:10.5489/cuaj.1224832.
27. McDowell BJ, Engberg S, et al. Effectiveness of behavioral therapy to treat incontinence in homebound older adults. J Am Ger Soc. 1999;47(3):309–18.
28. Ranson RN, Saffrey MJ. Neurogenic mechanisms in bladder and bowel aging. Biogeron. [Internet] 2015 [cited 20 Feb 2015]. Available from PubMed: http://www.ncbi.nlm.nih.gov/pubmed/25666896
29. DuBeau CE, Kuchel GA, Johnson 2nd T, Palmer MH, Wagg A. Incontinence in the frail elderly: report from the 4th international consultation on incontinence. Neurol Urodyn. 2010;29:165–78.
30. Miller SM, Miller MS. Urological disorders in men: urinary incontinence and benign prostatic hyperplasia. J Pharm Pract. 2011;24(4):374–85.
31. Engberg S, Sereika SM, et al. Effectiveness of prompted voiding in treating urinary incontinence in cognitively impaired homebound older adults. J WOCN. 2002;29(5):252–65. doi:10.1067/mjw.2002.127207.
32. Holroyd-Leduc JM, Mehta KM, Covinsky KE. Urinary incontinence and its association with death, nursing home admission, and functional decline. J Am Geriatr Soc. 2004;52(5):712–8.
33. John G, Gerstel E, et al. Urinary incontinence as a marker of higher mortality in patients receiving home care services. BJU Int. 2014;113(1):113–9. doi:10.1111/bju.12359.

34. Bing MT, Uhlman MA, Kreder KJ. An update in the treatment of male urinary incontinence. Curr Opin Urol. 2013;23(6):540–4.
35. Jamison J, Maguire S, McCann J. Catheter policies for management of long term voiding problems in adults with neurogenic bladder disorders (review). Cochrane Library. [Internet] 2013 [cited 20 Feb 2015]. Available from PubMed: http://www.ncbi.nlm.nih.gov/pubmed/24249436
36. Patel DP, Elliott SP, Stoffel JT, Brant WO, Hotaling JM, Myers JB. Patient reported outcomes measures in neurogenic bladder and bowel: a systematic review of the current literature. Neurourol Urodyn. [Internet] 2014 Oct [cited 20 Feb 2015]. Available from PubMed: https://www.ncbi.nlm.nih.gov/pubmed/25327455
37. National Institute for Health and Care Excellence (NICE). Urinary Incontinence – The management of urinary incontinence in women – NICE clinical guideline 171. 2013.
38. Gratzke C, Bachman A, Descazeaud A, Drake MJ, Madersbacher S, Mamoulakis C, et al. EAU guidelines on the assessment of non-neurogenic male lower urinary tract symptoms including benign prostatic obstruction. Eur Urol. 2015 [cited 20 Feb 2015]. Available from: doi:10.1016/j.eururo.2014.12.038
39. Gormley EA, Lightner DJ, Burgio KL, Chair TC, Clemens JQ, Culkin DJ, et al. Diagnosis and treatment of overactive bladder (non-neurogenic) in adults: AUA/SUFU guidelines. 2014. Available at: http://www.auanet.org/common/pdf/education/clinical-guidance/Overactive-Bladder.pdf.
40. Mohr S, Siegenthaler M, Mueller M, Kuhn A. Bulking agents: analysis of 500 cases and review of the literature. Int Urogynecol J. 2013;24:241–7.
41. Burgio KL, Goode PS, et al. Predictors of outcome in the behavioral treatment of urinary incontinence in women. Obstet Gynecol. 2012;102(5):940–7. doi:10.1016/S0029-7844(03)00770-1.
42. Lauti M, Herbison P, Hay-Smith J, Ellis G, Wilson D. Anticholinergic drugs, bladder retraining and their combination for urge urinary incontinence: a pilot randomized trial. Int Urogynecol J. 2008;19:1533–43. doi:10.1007/s00192-008-0686-8.
43. Roe B. Ostaszkiewicz, et al. Systematic reviews of bladder training and voiding programmes in adults: a synopsis of findings from data analysis and outcomes using metastudy techniques. J Adv Nurs. 2007;57(1):15–31. doi:10.1111/j.1365-2648.2006.04097.x.
44. Persu C, Braschi E, Lavelle J. A review of prospective clinical trials for neurogenic bladder: pharmaceuticals. Cent Euro J Urol. 2014;67:264–9.
45. Samuelsson E, Odeberg J, Stenzelius K, Molander U, Hammarstrom M, Franzen K, et al. Effect of pharmacological treatment for urinary incontinence in the elderly and frail elderly: a systematic review. Getriatr Gerontol Int. 2015;15:521–34.
46. Gaddey H, Holder K. Unintentional weight loss in older adults. Am Fam Physician. 2014;89(9):718–22.
47. McMinn J, Steel C, Bowman A. Investigation and management of unintentional weight loss in older adults. BMJ. 2011;342:d1732.
48. Payette H, Coulombe C, Boutier V, Gray-Donald K. Nutrition risk factors for institutionalization in a free-living functionally dependent elderly population. J Clin Epidemiol. 2000;53(6):579–87.
49. Ritchie CS, Locher JL, Roth DL, et al. Unintentional weight loss predicts decline in activities of daily living function and life space mobility over 4 years among community-dwelling older adults. J Gerontol A Biol Sci Med Sci. 2008;63(1):67–75.
50. Wallace JI, Schwartz RS. Epidemiology of weight loss in humans with special reference to wasting in the elderly. Int J Cardiol. 2002;85(1):15–21.
51. Seltzer MH, Slocum BA, Cataldi-Betcher EL, Fileti C, Gerson N. Instant nutritional assessment: absolute weight loss and surgical mortality. JPEN J Parenter Enteral Nutr. 1982;6(3):218–21.
52. Ensrud KE, Ewing SK, Stone KL, et al. Intentional and unintentional weight loss increase bone loss and hip fracture risk in older women. J Am Geriatr Soc. 2003;51(12):1740–7.
53. Fine JT, Colditz GA, Coakley EH, Moseley G, Manson JE, Willett WC, et al. A prospective study of weight change and health-related quality of life in women. JAMA. 1999;282(22):2136–42.

54. Newman AB, Yanez D, Harris T, et al. Weight change in old age and its association with mortality. J Am Geriatr Soc. 2001;49(10):1309–18.
55. Evans WJ, et al. Cachexia: a new definition. Clin Nutr. 2008;27(6):793.
56. Schiffman SS. Taste and smell in disease (first of two parts). N Engl J Med. 1983;308(21): 1275–9.
57. Shay K, Ship JA. The importance of oral health in the older patient. J Am Geriatr Soc. 1995;43(12):1414–22.
58. Lankisch PG, Gerzmann M, Gerzmann JF, et al. Unintentional weight loss: diagnosis and prognosis. J Intern Med. 2001;249(1):41–6.
59. Marton KI, Sox Jr HC, Krupp JR. Involuntary weight loss: diagnostic and prognostic significance. Ann Intern Med. 1981;95(5):568–74.
60. Wallace JI, et al. Involuntary weight loss in elderly outpatients: recognition, etiologies, and treatment. Clin Geriatr Med. 1999;13(4):717–35.
61. Hernández JL, Riancho JA, Matorras P, et al. Clinical evaluation for cancer in patients with involuntary weight loss without specific symptoms. Am J Med. 2003;114(8):613–7.
62. Wilson MM, Thomas DR, Rubenstein LZ, Chibnall JT, Anderson S, Baxi A, Diebold MR, Morley JE. Appetite assessment: simple appetite questionnaire predicts weight loss in community-dwelling adults and nursing. Am J Clin Nutr. 2005;82(5):1074.
63. Ruiz Garcia V, López-Briz E, Carbonell Sanchis R, et al. Megestrol acetate for treatment of anorexia-cachexia syndrome. Cochrane Database Syst Rev. 2013;3, CD004310.
64. Rabinovitz M, Pitlik SD, Leifer M, et al. Unintentional weight loss. A retrospective analysis of 154 cases. Arch Intern Med. 1986;146(1):186–7.
65. Metalidis C, Knockaert DC, Bobbaers H, et al. Involuntary weight loss. Does a negative baseline evaluation provide adequate reassurance? Eur J Intern Med. 2008;19(5):345–9.
66. White H, Pieper C, Schmader K, Fillenbaum G. Weight change in Alzheimer's disease. J Am Geriatr Soc. 1996;44(3):265.
67. Huffman GB. Evaluating and treating unintentional weight loss in the elderly. Am Fam Physician. 2002;65(4):640–50.
68. Padala KP, Keller BK, Potter JF. Weight loss treatment in long-term care. J Nutr Elder. 2007;26(3–4):1–20.
69. Young KW, Binns MA, Greenwood CE. Meal delivery practices do not meet needs of Alzheimer patients with increased cognitive and behavioral difficulties in a long-term care facility. J Gerontol A Biol Sci Med Sci. 2001;56(10):M656–61.
70. Young KW, Greenwood CE. Shift in diurnal feeding patterns in nursing home residents with Alzheimer's disease. J Gerontol A Biol Sci Med Sci. 2001;56(11):M700–6.
71. Wilson MM, Purushothaman R, Morley JE. Effect of liquid dietary supplements on energy intake in the elderly. Am J Clin Nutr. 2002;75(5):944–7.
72. De Jong N, Chin APMJ, de Graaf C, van Staveren WA. Effect of dietary supplements and physical exercise on sensory perception, appetite, dietary intake and body weight in frail elderly subjects. Br J Nutr. 2000;83(6):605–13.
73. Gillick MR. Rethinking the role of tube feeding in patients with advanced dementia. N Engl J Med. 2000;342(3):206–10.
74. Mitchell SL, Kiely DK, Lipsitz LA. The risk factors and impact on survival of feeding tube placement in nursing home residents with sever cognitive impairment. Arch Intern Med. 1997;157:327–32.
75. Takala J, Ruokonen E, Webster NR, Nielsen MS, Zandstra DF, Vundelickx G, et al. Increased mortality associated with growth hormone treatment in critically ill adults. N Engl J Med. 1999;341(11):785–92, 97.
76. Fox CB, Treadway AK, Blaszczyk AT, et al. Megestrol acetate and mirtazapine for the treatment of unplanned weight loss in the elderly. Pharmacotherapy. 2009;29(4):383–97.
77. Beal JE, Olson R, Laubenstein L, Morales JO, Bellman P, Yangco B, Lefkowitz L, Plasse TF, Shepard KV. Dronabinol as a treatment for anorexia associated with weight loss in patients with AIDS. J Pain Symptom Manage. 1995;10(2):89.

Common Infections

Christian Escobar, Sonica Bhatia, and Ania Wajnberg

Abstract

Infections represent a significant cause of morbidity and mortality in the home-bound patient. These patients, particularly those who are elderly, are at an increased risk of infection due to their multiple comorbidities, poor nutritional status, general debility, and reduced immunity [1]. Pneumonia, urinary tract infections, and cellulitis are some of the most common acute infections that homebound patients face and clinicians are challenged to treat. This chapter will discuss the diagnosis, etiologies, and therapeutic options for this group of diseases. Each specific infection has its own methodology for diagnosis and treatment in the home, as delineated by various current clinical practice guidelines.

Keywords

Common infections • Pneumonia • Bacterial pneumonia • Community-acquired pneumonia • Aspiration • Aspiration pneumonia • Cellulitis • Soft tissue infection • Staph infection • Staphylococcus • Streptococcus • MRSA infection • MRSA cellulitis • Urinary tract infection • UTI • Complicated UTI • Uncomplicated UTI

C. Escobar, M.D. (✉)
Department of Medicine, The Mount Sinai Hospital,
1 Gustave L Levy Place, 1216, New York, NY, USA
e-mail: Christian.Escobar@mountsinai.org

S. Bhatia, M.D.
Department of Geriatrics and Palliative Medicine and Department of Medicine,
The Mount Sinai Hospital, 1 Gustave L Levy Place, 1216, New York, NY, USA
e-mail: Sonica.Bhatia@mountsinai.org

A. Wajnberg, M.D.
Department of Medicine and Department of Geriatrics and Palliative Medicine,
The Mount Sinai Hospital, 1 Gustave L Levy Place, 1216, New York, NY, USA
e-mail: Ania.Wajnberg@mountsinai.org

© Springer International Publishing Switzerland 2016
J.L. Hayashi, B. Leff (eds.), *Geriatric Home-Based Medical Care*,
DOI 10.1007/978-3-319-23365-9_9

9.1 Key Points

- Urinary tract infections can often be diagnosed based on history alone in cognitively intact individuals
- Asymptomatic bacteriuria should not be routinely treated
- Previously healthy individuals without a recent preceding hospitalization can be treated for community-acquired pneumonia with a macrolide or tetracycline
- Elderly patients or those with extensive comorbidities or severe disease should be treated for community-acquired pneumonia with a beta-lactam AND a macrolide or only with a fluoroquinolone with activity against respiratory microbes (such as levofloxacin or moxifloxacin)
- Sputum cultures are often unnecessary and warranted only in specific situations
- Nonpurulent cellulitis can be treated with empiric coverage for streptococcus
- If the patient with cellulitis has purulence or abscess, has severe infection, systemic signs or has failed prior empiric treatment, then treat for methicillin-resistant *Staphylococcus aureus* (MRSA) and possibly additionally for streptococcus

9.2 Introduction

Homebound individuals are at an increased risk of infection due to several factors; they commonly have a number of coexisting chronic diseases that both cause disease and reduce innate immunity [1]. They often suffer from malnutrition, namely low protein states that also lower the body's natural defenses against foreign organisms [1]. Infectious diseases account for one-third of all deaths in people aged 65 years and older; infection-related mortality is nine times higher in older compared with younger cohorts [2, 3]. The elderly often present with atypical signs and symptoms when infected, which pose diagnostic challenges, and they often suffer more complicated courses of illness. Polypharmacy, variability in renal function, and multiple comorbidities result in more severe diseases and challenges in therapeutic considerations [1].

9.3 Urinary Tract Infections

A urinary tract infection (UTI) is defined as significant bacteriuria in a person with urinary signs or symptoms and no alternate source of infection. UTIs are the most common type of infection in the elderly. Traditionally, UTIs are categorized as either uncomplicated or complicated [1].

Uncomplicated UTIs occur in patients with a functionally and structurally normal urinary tract system. Conversely, complicated UTIs occur in patients with functionally or structurally abnormal urinary tract systems. Examples of functional abnormalities in the urinary tract system include ureteric reflux, incomplete bladder emptying, and chronic kidney disease. Examples of structural abnormalities include a cystocele, urethral stricture, an indwelling catheter, and prostatic hypertrophy. All of these abnormalities increase in frequency with age. Most UTIs in functionally impaired older adults (i.e., homebound geriatric patients) are considered complicated because the majority of these patients have some functional or structural issue with their urinary tract [1, 4].

In young, otherwise healthy adults, the diagnosis and treatment of a UTI are straightforward. The diagnosis can often be made solely based on a patient's history of dysuria, urinary urgency, and frequency; further evaluation with a physical exam and a urinalysis and culture may be utilized merely to confirm the diagnosis. Empiric antibiotic therapy is commonly prescribed on the basis of self-reported symptoms [4].

With older homebound adults, however, medical providers face several challenges in diagnosing UTIs. Functionally impaired patients may have difficulty communicating their symptoms because of cognitive, sensory, or impairment in the ability to communicate. Patients commonly have a history of urinary incontinence at baseline, making it difficult to notice an acute change in urinary urgency or frequency. In addition, older adults may not mount a fever in response to a UTI [1, 4].

Asymptomatic bacteriuria (ASB), asymptomatic UTI, and bladder colonization are all equivalent terms that refer to a positive urine culture obtained from an appropriately collected urine specimen in a noncatheterized patient, but without urinary frequency, urgency, dysuria, or suprapubic pain. Risk factors for ASB include female gender, advancing age, and being institutionalized. Duration of diabetes is associated with an increased risk of ASB in women. Prevalence rates for ASB for women over the age of 80 years living in the community have been estimated to be as high as 20 % [1, 5]. The prevalence of ASB is higher amongst geriatric patients in long-term care facilities (25–50 % in women and 15–40 % in men) compared to ambulatory older patients. Homebound older patients often have comorbidities that result in impaired voiding or indwelling catheterization, which in turn are associated with an increased prevalence of ASB [1, 5, 6].

The Infectious Disease Society of America recommends against treating ASB with antimicrobials except in some very specific instances (i.e., pregnancy and prior to a urological procedure with a high likelihood of mucosal bleeding) [1, 5].

9.3.1 Etiology

In the vast majority of cases, the bacteria causing UTIs are gastrointestinal flora that have colonized the perineum and traveled up the urethra to the prostate, bladder and/or kidney. Thus, patients with chronic-indwelling catheters or those who perform clean intermittent catheterization for conditions such as neurogenic bladder are at an increased risk of both UTIs and ASB because of the increased risk of introduction of bacteria to the urethra in these patients. Even external catheters (i.e., condom catheters) increase the risk of bacteriuria by increasing the pathogenic bacteria in the perineum. Less frequently, patients can develop a UTI from hematogenous spread of a pathogen causing a bacteremia from a nonurinary source.

Older women are more likely to have vaginal colonization with uropathogens, perhaps because they have less estrogen, which increases the pH of their genitourinary mucosa and decreases colonization with protective lactobacilli. In terms of structural abnormalities, older women are more likely to develop a cystocele with increasing age. In geriatric men, both prostatic hypertrophy and urethral stricture increase in prevalence with advancing age and can result in urinary obstruction, allowing stagnation of urine. In both older men and women, there is an increased risk of bladder diverticulae compared to their younger counterparts. Functionally, the bladder residual volume increases in older adults with age. Many neurologic illnesses that afflict the homebound elderly, including Parkinson's disease, Alzheimer's disease, and strokes can impair bladder emptying and thus increase the risk of UTIs [1].

Chronic bacterial prostatitis, an indolent type of UTI seen in older men, can be challenging to treat because of the poor penetration of antibiotics into the prostate. As such, the prostate in men with chronic prostatitis or those with prostatic calculi can become a reservoir for bacteria, resulting in frequent relapses of cystitis, sometimes with long periods of time between infections [1].

9.3.2 Differential Diagnosis

The differential diagnosis for geriatric homebound patients who are suspected of having a UTI varies depending on the presenting signs and symptoms (See Table 9.1). The differential diagnosis for perineal discomfort includes bacterial and fungal vaginitis in women and chronic prostatitis in men. Urinary frequency can be seen in new-onset or poorly controlled diabetes mellitus. Gross hematuria is seen in patients with urological cancer, nephrolithiasis, nephritis, and trauma associated with placing an indwelling catheter. Pyelonephritis presents with the triad of fever, costovertebral pain, and tenderness. Malodorous urine can be seen in patients with UTIs, as well as those with volume depletion and those with urinary incontinence and

Table 9.1 Differential diagnosis of UTI

Alternative diagnosis	Comments
Asymptomatic bacteriuria	Consider in patients presenting with delirium who lack the ability to give a urinary ROS
Volume depletion	Consider in patients presenting with malodorous urine without other urinary signs or symptoms
Poor hygiene	Patients presenting with malodorous urine
Urothelial cancer	Patients presenting with painless hematuria
Bacterial or fungal vaginitis	Patients presenting with perineal discomfort in elderly women
Chronic prostatitis	Patients presenting with perineal discomfort in elderly men
Pyelonephritis	Technically a specific type of a complicated UTI, presenting with the triad of fever, costovertebral pain, and tenderness
Nephrolithiasis	Patients presenting with hematuria, pain

poor hygiene [1, 5, 6]. An increase in agitation or confusion without accompanying urinary signs or symptoms in a patient with dementia may represent progression of dementia versus a delirium. The differential for delirium is broad and includes medication, side effects, a UTI or other infection, or some other change in the patient's environment. Increasingly, the anecdotal teaching point of checking a urinalysis (U/A) and urine culture on all elderly patients with delirium is coming under fire. In a patient with delirium, it is appropriate to check a U/A and culture if there are signs and symptoms pointing toward a UTI. However, in the absence of clear signs or symptoms pointing to a UTI, clinicians run the risk of checking a U/A and culture, and finding asymptomatic bacteriuria and then being left trying to determine if this is a "real" UTI or not, and subsequently whether or not to prescribe antibiotics. We recommend thinking carefully before ordering a U/A and culture in a patient with delirium without clear urinary tract symptoms [7].

9.3.3 Investigations at Home

Investigations at home should begin with a thorough history and physical examination. In homebound patients who may have cognitive impairment with or without urinary incontinence, this history may need to be obtained from the caregiver to reliably determine whether a patient is experiencing urinary frequency or dysuria. For functionally impaired patients, it may be challenging to ascertain whether a patient is experiencing urinary urgency. New or increased incontinence should prompt consideration of further work-up as a possible symptom of a UTI [4–6]. Caregivers and patients can be asked about foul-smelling urine, with the caution to clinicians in interpreting the significance of this sign: not all malodorous urine is due to a UTI, and not all UTIs produce foul-smelling urine. Malodorous urine may be associated with bacteriuria, caused by the polyamine production of the bacteria. However, malodorous urine does not help the clinician to understand if the patient is experiencing a UTI or ASB or simply volume depletion or dehydration [1, 5, 6]. Caregivers and patients should also be asked about gross hematuria, fever, and suprapubic and costovertebral pain.

When a UTI in a homebound elder is on the differential diagnosis, the clinician should pay close attention to certain aspects of the physical exam, including level of consciousness, vital signs, and suprapubic and costovertebral tenderness.

Urine dipstick testing for nitrite and leukocyte esterase (LE) can be done at home with results available within minutes. Nitrite is used as a surrogate for bacteriuria, but has a low sensitivity. Indeed when nitrite is positive, the test does not distinguish between asymptomatic and symptomatic bacteriuria [4]. Leukocyte esterase) is used as a surrogate for pyuria. Pyuria indicates an inflammatory process in the genitourinary tract, which can include, but is not limited to a UTI. While a result of positive LE is not conclusive in making the diagnosis of a UTI, a negative LE has high specificity for excluding a UTI [1].

Urine can also be collected in the home and be analyzed in a lab for more extensive microscopic testing, with results within hours. A urine culture can be collected in the home and sent to the laboratory with results available within days. Ideally, the urine sample collected for a urine culture should be a straight catheterization or clean catch sample to avoid contamination with perineal flora. Urine cultures should be obtained for all male patients with symptomatic UTIs and all women with presumed kidney involvement or underlying functional or anatomical GU abnormalities. Expert opinion and guidelines suggest that community-dwelling women with a history of recurrent uncomplicated cystitis who present with typical urinary symptoms can be treated empirically without a culture. However, if these patients present with atypical symptoms, have recently been on antibiotics, or have had a rapid recurrence of urinary symptoms following treatment for a presumed cystitis, a urine culture should be obtained to help guide diagnosis and appropriate therapy [4, 8].

It should be noted that most homebound elderly patients likely have some functional or structural impairment in their urinary tract system and thus most UTIs in the homebound elderly would be classified as having a complicated UTI. As such, it is rare for a female homebound patient to have both an uncomplicated UTI and typical symptoms. In the vast majority of homebound elderly patients with a suspected UTI, a urine culture should be obtained. Whether to treat the patient empirically while waiting for culture results or to wait for culture results and then choose an antimicrobial is discussed below [4, 8].

Significant bacteriuria is defined as greater than or equal to 10^5 colony forming units (CFU)/mL for noncatheterized patients. A clean catch specimen can be challenging to obtain in homebound elderly patients because of the possible visual, cognitive, and dexterity impairment, as well as the possibility of incontinence, and in this situation, the gold standard is a sample collected by clean intermittent catheterization (CIC) [1]. Most home-based practices obtain a culture by this method when there is a high clinical suspicion of a UTI, when the culture results are likely to change management (i.e., a patient who has previously had an multidrug-resistant UTI) and after having evaluated the individual patient's goals of care to weigh the risks and benefits of obtaining a urine sample by CIC. The procedure itself can lead to bacteriuria, cause some discomfort, and increase agitation in cognitively impaired patients [1, 6]. The urine sample being collected for culture should be sent to the laboratory as soon as possible to obtain accurate CFU counts.

For patients who have external (condom) urinary catheters at baseline, we institute the following procedure to decrease the risk of contamination with perineal flora. (1) Clean the glans. (2) Apply a new external catheter including a new collecting bag. (3) Collect the urine sample immediately after voiding [4, 6]. There is insufficient evidence as to what constitutes "significant" bacteriuria for patients with condom catheters.

For patients who have an indwelling urethral or suprapubic or intermittent catheterization, signs and symptoms compatible with a catheter-associated UTI include acute onset fever, rigors, delirium, malaise with no other identified cause, costovertebral pain, new onset of hematuria, and pelvic discomfort. Patients who have had their catheters removed may experience urinary urgency, frequency, or dysuria [6]. Spinal cord injury patients may experience increased muscle spasticity, autonomic dysfunction, or malaise [6]. Significant bacteriuria is defined as greater than or equal to 10^3 colony-forming units (CFU)/mL for patients with chronic-indwelling urethral or suprapubic catheters. Further complicating the diagnosis of a UTI in patients with chronic-indwelling catheters are the high rates of ASB found in these patients: ASB was found in 100 % of patients with chronic-indwelling catheters in one study [5, 6]. In a chronically catheterized patient suspected of having a UTI, if the catheter has been in place for more than 2 weeks, the catheter should be replaced and the urine culture should be obtained from the newly placed catheter ideally prior to starting antibiotics [6].

A common and controversial situation in the homebound, functionally impaired, noncatheterized elderly occurs when a patient presents with a change in mental status. In an ideal situation, the clinician would be able to elicit urinary symptoms from the patient or caregiver and order further work-up, or conversely, obtain a negative urinary review of systems (ROS) and investigate other possible causes of delirium. What happens more frequently is that a family member or caregiver of a more severely cognitively impaired, noncatheterized patient notes increasing lethargy and it is impossible to obtain an accurate urinary ROS. The clinician obtains a urinalysis and finds significant bacteriuria. The clinician now has to decide whether the bacteriuria represents ASB or a UTI. While we caution healthcare providers in attributing delirium without urinary symptoms to a UTI, as ASB has a higher prevalence in the functionally impaired elderly, most practices that treat functionally impaired geriatric patients acknowledge the challenges of obtaining a history regarding urinary symptoms from a patient with advanced cognitive impairment or who has baseline chronic urinary symptoms [1, 5].

Repeatedly treating ASB with multiple courses of antibiotics leads to resistant UTIs and other infectious complications including *Clostridium difficile*. Other potential harms of antimicrobial treatment include acute kidney injury, noninfectious diarrhea, nausea, and cachexia [1, 5, 6].

9.3.4 Pharmacologic Therapy

When a patient is suspected of having a UTI, clinicians must decide whether to start antibiotics empirically or wait for urine culture results. We suggest that this decision should be based on a combination of factors including the severity of the patient's clinical presentation, whether or not the patient has a chronic-indwelling catheter and the clinician's index of suspicion for a UTI.

For all patients with moderate to severe symptoms (fever defined as >37.9 °C or 1.5 °C above baseline temperature, CVA tenderness, rigors, hypotension, tachycardia, suprapubic pain, or gross hematuria), empiric antibiotic therapy should be initiated while waiting for the results of the urine culture results [8]. For patients (regardless of catheter status) with milder symptoms and when the clinical suspicion of a UTI is lower, we suggest waiting for the culture results to return before starting antimicrobial therapy [8]

For noncatheterized patients, we generally favor empiric treatment with either nitrofurantoin monohydrate/macrocrystals (100 mg orally twice daily for 5 days) or trimethoprim–sulfamethoxazole (TMP–SMX) (160/800 mg orally twice daily for 3–7 days). For a patient with a sulfa allergy, TMP monotherapy can be used. Both nitrofurantoin and TMP–SMX are cost-effective. Nitrofurantoin should be avoided in patients with renal impairment or those suspected of having pyelonephritis.

There are increasing rates of TMP–SMX and fluoroquinolone resistance in the community, as well as multidrug-resistant vancomycin-resistant Enterococci and extended-spectrum beta-lactamase producing *Escherichia coli* and *Klebsiella pneumoniae*. The Infectious Diseases Society of America (IDSA) recommends using TMP–SMX as empiric treatment for a UTI only if local resistance patterns show a resistance rate of *E. coli* of less than 20 % and it has NOT been used for this patient to treat a UTI in the past 3 months [1, 4]. The use of fluoroquinolones as empiric treatment for UTIs is controversial. Some studies have shown fewer adverse effects with ciprofloxacin use, while other guidelines advise against empirically using fluoroquinolones because of the risk of increasing uropathogen resistance. Moxifloxacin should not be used to treat UTIs as it has poor urinary excretion. Levofloxacin can cause glucose abnormalities in diabetic patients. Amoxicillin can be effective as a targeted therapy for Gram-positive organisms, but it is NOT recommended as a first-line agent because of the high prevalence of Gram-negative bacteria resistance to this agent. Amoxicillin/clavulanic acid and cephalosporins can also be effective as targeted therapy, but are also NOT recommended as empiric therapy because of their broad-spectrum activity and expense [1, 4]. Given the decrease in glomerular filtration rate seen in older adults, the cautious clinician should be sure to renally dosed antibiotics (see Table 9.2). For patients on warfarin who require antibiotic therapy, we recommend one of the two strategies. The first option is to check an INR

Table 9.2 Antibiotic coverage of UTIs

Antibiotic	Comments
Nitrofurantoin mononhydrate/macrocrystals	Recommended empiric treatment for noncatheterized patients. Contraindicated for patients with renal impairment
Trimethoprim–sulfamethoxazole	Recommended empiric treatment for noncatheterized patients if local resistance patterns show resistance rate of E. coli of less than 20 % and it has NOT been used for this patient to treat a UTI in the past 3 months
Trimethoprim	Alternative to TMP-SX for patients with sulfa allergy
Ciprofloxacin	Controversial use as a first-line empiric agent. Fewer adverse reactions. Increasing uropathogen resistance to this agent
Levofloxacin	Controversial use as a first-line empiric agent. Fewer adverse reactions. Increasing uropathogen resistance to this agent. Glucose abnormalities in diabetic patients
Amoxicillin	NOT recommended as an empiric treatment. Can be used as a targeted therapy for Gram-positive organisms
Amoxicillin/clavulanic acid	NOT recommended as an empiric therapy. Broad-spectrum. Expensive. Can be used as targeted therapy
Other cephalosporins	NOT recommended as an empiric therapy. Broad-spectrum. Expensive. Can be used as targeted therapy

within 1 week of initiating antibiotic therapy, regardless of the class of antibiotics, and adjust the warfarin dose as needed. The second option is to preemptively decrease the dose of warfarin by 15–20 % when antibiotics are initiated. There is insufficient data for us to recommend one strategy over the other [9, 10].

There is some evidence that topical estrogen therapy (but NOT systemic estrogen therapy) can decrease the risk of recurrent UTIs in elderly women. Pain and fever can be treated with acetaminophen [1].

9.3.5   Nonpharmacological Therapy

Oral hydration is recommended for UTIs, as well as for the isolated symptom of foul-smelling urine. Avoidance of unnecessary urinary catheterization, appropriate perineal hygiene, and incontinence care are recommended. The evidence for the use of cranberry products for the prevention of UTIs in the homebound elderly is inconclusive [1, 5, 6].

9.4   Pneumonia

Pneumonia is one of the most common diseases diagnosed and treated in the United States. Pneumonia is defined as an acute infection of the pulmonary parenchyma and can be caused by various pathogens including bacteria, viruses, or fungi. Most homebound patients will acquire pneumonia in the community (community-acquired pneumonia, CAP), including aspiration pneumonia (pneumonia contracted through aspiration of bacteria from oral or pharyngeal contents). Hospital-acquired pneumonia (HAP) is pneumonia that develops while patients are in the hospital, and healthcare associated pneumonia (HCAP) develops while patients are in other facilities such as nursing homes or other chronic care facilities. For the purposes of this discussion, we will focus on CAP and aspiration, as most homebound patients will be diagnosed with these types of pneumonia.

9.4.1   Differential Diagnosis and Etiology

Incidence of pneumonia increases with chronic illness, debility, and advanced age, as all of these conditions interact to impact pulmonary defense mechanisms and increase the risk of CAP. Specifically, conditions that increase the risk of CAP commonly seen in the homebound population include the following:

- Alteration in normal level of consciousness, which predisposes to aspiration (i.e., dementia, stroke, seizures, medications, drug/alcohol abuse)
- Tobacco or alcohol use
- Hypoxemia from any reason including chronic illness such as chronic obstructive pulmonary disease (COPD), chronic heart failure, interstitial lung disease, and others.

- Malnutrition
- Immunosuppression
- ≥65 years of age
- Chronic obstructive pulmonary disease (COPD)
- Dysphagia due to esophageal lesions and motility problems
- Bronchial obstruction due to stenosis, tumor, or foreign body
- Medications including acid suppressive therapy, antipsychotic medications, and corticosteroids

9.4.1.1 Differential Diagnosis for Bacterial Pneumonia

- Viral pneumonia
- Asthma
- Chronic obstructive pulmonary disease
- Bronchitis
- Pulmonary embolism
- Aspiration pneumonitis/pneumonia
- Chronic heart failure
- Pleural effusion
- Fungal pneumonia

9.4.2   Investigations in the Home

Pneumonia can present in a variety of ways in the elderly, especially in the home-bound patients. Studies examining the diagnosis of pneumonia by history and physical exam using X-ray as a gold standard find no combination of signs and symptoms (i.e., cough, fever, tachycardia, or crackles) that reliably predicted diagnosis with acceptable sensitivity [11]. Symptoms usually present acutely with patients complaining of changes over a few days. Common clinical complaints that should trigger evaluation for possible pneumonia include dyspnea, cough, fever, chest pain with pleuritic features, and increased sputum production, especially purulent sputum for bacterial pneumonia. Patients can also complain of not feeling "like myself," gastro-intestinal upset, and alteration in mental status.

Because many homebound patients suffer from neurological disease and/or dementia, aspiration pneumonia deserves special consideration. Any diseases that lead to reduced cognition or consciousness predispose to aspiration, as does dysphagia for any reason, esophageal disease, and the presence of a feeding tube. Prevention is key and will be discussed further below. Any patient with these risk factors diagnosed with pneumonia in the community should be suspected of having either CAP or aspiration pneumonia, regardless of whether an aspiration event was witnessed. Aspiration can be silent or occur during sleep and may develop into pneumonia even without a known inciting event. Of note, it is important to distinguish aspiration pneumonitis from a true aspiration pneumonia. Some aspiration events can result in a chemical pneumonitis with a pulmonary inflammatory response that presents as transient respiratory difficulty or distress but resolves quickly.

If pneumonitis is suspected, there is no role for antibiotics in treatment. However, it is important to suspect and recognize aspiration pneumonia as unlike in CAP, the organisms that cause aspiration pneumonia are more likely to be oral or upper airway flora including anaerobic bacteria, or much less commonly, Gram-negative bacilli or Staph aureus.

On physical exam, patients should be evaluated for fever, tachypnea, and tachycardia. In elderly patients, especially those with dementia, tachypnea may be the only sign, as fever is less likely. Counting the respiratory rate is an important component of the physical examination. If there is a consolidation, tactile fremitus will be increased and there will be dullness to percussion. On pulmonary auscultation, rales are the most common abnormal finding [12] but wheezes, crackles, or rhonchi may be audible in many patients, though not all. Pneumonia can be present with a normal lung exam. If the patient's history and physical exam do not clearly diagnose pneumonia, the gold standard in pneumonia diagnosis is plain chest radiograph. It is very helpful to partner with a radiology agency in the community that can obtain portable chest X-rays in patients' homes to help define pneumonia or other pulmonary pathology when history and physical are unclear.

Most clinicians who provide home-based medical care will be able to test basic laboratories in a timely fashion and the major abnormality to look for is leukocytosis with a leftward shift on differential. Other testing that may be helpful includes viral PCR, especially if influenza is suspected and may avoid unnecessary antibiotic use if diagnosed quickly.

Chest X-ray can show lobar consolidation or interstitial infiltrate which suggest different microbiological pathogens, but there are no pathognomonic chest X-ray findings for specific organisms. It is important to note that chest X ray can be falsely negative, especially in volume depleted patients and the clinical setting is by far the most important factor on which to base treatment decisions. One study found that approximately 11 % of negative chest X rays later had positive CT scan findings consistent with pneumonia [13].

Microbiological testing including sputum culture and blood culture can be done but are rarely helpful in the outpatient setting. Sputum culture may be considered if atypical microorganisms are suspected in a patient who is significantly immunocompromised, a cavitary lesion is noted on X ray, or is not responding to appropriate antibiotic therapy [14].

Though HAP/HCAP are not covered extensively here, it is important to remember that these etiologies must be considered in homebound patients recently discharged from a hospital, nursing home, or subacute rehabilitation facility to home and may require different, broader antibiotic coverage depending on local flora and antibiotic resistance patterns.

9.4.2.1 Prognosis and Risk Stratification

In general, significant morbidity and mortality from pneumonia are higher for chronically ill, frail, and/or elderly patients, many of whom fit criteria for homebound status. However, with timely diagnosis and treatment, even hospitalized patients (vs. homebound patients, most of whom will be treated in the home or

Table 9.3 CURB-65 in pneumonia

CURB 65 score	Mortality
One point for each: • Presence of confusion • Uremia (BUN >19) • Respiratory rate ≥30 • SBP <90 or DBP<60) • Age greater than 65	
0	<1 %
1	3 %
2	7 %
3	14 %
4	28 %
5	28 %

outpatient setting), had a mortality of <10 % [15]. There are multiple risk score calculators to help guide decisions like need for hospitalization, ICU, and treatment. The most commonly used two scores are the PSI and the CURB-65.

(a) **Pneumonia Severity Index (PSI):** PSI score is used to help determine need for hospitalization and ICU in patients with pneumonia. It is more comprehensive than the CURB-65 (see below) but difficult to implement in the home setting, as it requires multiple laboratory values including arterial pH level, blood urea nitrogen, sodium, and others. As the score increases, predicted 30-day mortality increases.

(b) **CURB-65:** This scale is more practical for use in the home setting as it is based largely on clinical criteria easily gathered during the history and physical exam, as well as one relatively routine laboratory test (BUN). The CURB-65 uses a 5-point system to predict mortality. (1) Presence of confusion, (2) uremia (BUN >19), (3) respiratory rate ≥30, (4) blood pressure (Systolic <90 or diastolic <60), and (5) age greater than 65. Each point on the scale from 0 to 5 confers a greater mortality rate: 0: 0.6 %, 1: 2.7 %, 2: 6.8 %, 3: 14 %, 4 and 5: 28 % [12, 16]. Patients with a score of 0–1 should be treated as an outpatient and those with score of 4–5 should be admitted, likely to the ICU. At the 2–3 range, patients must be closely monitored either in the home or hospitalized depending on their home support systems and goals of care (see Table 9.3).

9.4.3 Pharmacological Therapy

For previously healthy patients with no hospitalizations in the last 90 days, the IDSA/American Thoracic Society (ATS) "Consensus Guidelines on the Management of Community-Acquired Pneumonia in Adults" recommends empiric therapy for patients with CAP who are stable to be managed in the home setting with either a macrolide or doxycycline.

Table 9.4 Antibiotic Selections for Pneumonia

	First-line antibiotics
Community-acquired pneumonia	**Beta-lactam + macrolide** (e.g., azithromycin or clarithromycin) -or- **Beta-lactam + tetracycline** (e.g., doxycycline) -or- **Fluoroquinolone** (moxifloxacin or levofloxacin)
If anaerobic coverage required for true aspiration	**Clindamycin** -or- **Amoxicillin–clavulanate**

However, many homebound patients will not fall into this category as they are elderly, functionally impaired, or frail and many have multiple comorbidities including coronary artery disease, lung disease, liver or renal disease, diabetes, malignancy, or other comorbidities. For this group, a fluoroquinolone is the first-line recommended agent; a beta-lactam plus macrolide is an alternative to fluoro-quinolone in this situation. Specifically, an oral fluoroquinolone with respiratory coverage (levofloxacin 750 mg daily, moxifloxacin 400 mg daily, or gemifloxacin 320 mg daily) or a beta-lactam that can treat streptococcal pneumonia (amoxicillin 1 g three times daily, augmentin 2 g twice daily, or cefpodoxime 20 mg twice daily) AND macrolide (azithromycin 500 mg × 1 day, 250 mg × 4 days, clarithromycin 500 mg twice daily), or tetracycline such as doxycycline 100 mg twice daily. There is no evidence that treatment for over 7 days is better than 5–7 days, so recommendations are to treat for a 5- to 7-day course based on clinical response [17] (see Table 9.4).

9.4.3.1 Aspiration Pneumonia

Use of broad coverage for anaerobes in suspected aspiration pneumonia is controversial as some Thoracic Societies feel that the likelihood of true anaerobic infection without abscess is low. Most aspiration pneumonias should be treated as community-acquired pneumonias, as the most commonly aspirated organisms are nonresistant mouth flora. In patients presenting with severe symptoms, with obvious abscess on chest radiograph, oral abscesses or witnessed frank aspiration of gastric contents or those nonresolving with conventional treatment, especially with predisposing factors, many of whom are homebound (dementia and neurological disease) it is prudent to treat aggressively as the chance of a true anaerobic aspiration pneumonia is higher [14].

If one chooses to treat anaerobic aspiration pneumonia in the home setting, recommended first-line treatment includes clindamycin (450 orally 3 times daily) as first-line therapy in addition to usual CAP treatment. Alternative agents including amoxicillin–clavulanate (875 mg twice daily) or metronidazole (500 three times daily) *plus* amoxicillin (500 mg three times daily). Another option that is likely effective, but should not be used preferentially is fluoroquinolones as it will cover both CAP and aspiration. Duration is similar to recommendations above at 7 days.

9.4.3.2 Symptom Management

Patients treated for pneumonia at home may need oxygen for a brief course during their acute illness. Many durable medical equipment (DME) companies will supply home oxygen and it is useful to know how to order it with a local DME supplier before diagnosis. To order oxygen, hypoxia must be documented, so home-based medical care providers should carry a pulse oximeter and document the pulse oximeter results from the visit. In general under Medicare guidelines, oxygen will not be covered for pneumonia alone, but only if the patient has certain chronic conditions, such as COPD and CHF, exacerbated by pneumonia that now requires O_2 support as evidenced by documented hypoxia. Patients who are comfort-oriented at the end of life may be able to get home oxygen through a home hospice agency.

9.4.3.3 Prevention with Vaccinations

(a) Pneumococcal vaccine is recommended for every person aged 65 and older. For patients under 65, pneumococcal vaccine is recommended every 5 years if these patients have chronic illness including HIV, chronic renal disease, immunodeficiency, sickle cell disease, malignancy [18]. Many younger homebound patients may be immunocompromised due to chronic illness and may fall into this category [18]. Pneumococcal vaccine can be given to patients with pneumonia once they are on treatment with clinical improvement, or any time thereafter. There are now two types of vaccinations, each encompassing different serotypes, recommended for these patients. The two vaccines should not be coadministered and the 13-valent pneumococcal conjugate vaccine (PCV13) is preferentially given first and then the 23-valent pneumococcal polysaccharide vaccine (PPV23) 6–12 months after [18].

(b) Seasonal influenza vaccination is recommended for all adults yearly. Infection with influenza is associated with the development of pneumonia and higher rates of morbidity/mortality [19].

9.4.4 Nonpharmocologic Therapy

(a) Oxygen: As noted above, patients treated for pneumonia at home may need oxygen for a brief course during or after their acute illness.

(b) Positioning: During the acute illness, standing or sitting upright in a chair or elevating the head of the bed for patients who cannot get out of bed will promote lung expansion and improved air exchange. Aspiration precautions should always be followed, especially for homebound patients with cognitive impairment.

(c) Aspiration precautions: For patients at high risk for aspiration (see section above), all caregivers should be educated and instructed in preventive behavioral measures to avoid aspiration and aspiration pneumonia. These include good oral hygiene daily, keeping the head in a neutral position when swallowing, and keeping patients upright at 90° when feeding and for as long as possible after feeding. If a patient must be fed in bed, the head of the bed should be elevated to at least 30° for at least 1 h after eating/drinking. Caregivers should feed slowly and allow patients to complete their swallow before feeding continues. Many community nursing agencies will provide speech therapists who can evaluate patients' swallowing at home and make specific recommendations about food and liquid consistency to avoid aspiration, as well as provide education and modeling of the precaution behaviors outlined above.

9.5 Cellulitis

Cellulitis is an acute inflammation of the skin mainly involving the dermis and subcutaneous tissues, mostly caused by skin flora that are indigenous to healthy individuals. It is classically characterized by the four cardinal signs of inflammation: *rubor, calor, tumor* and *dolor*, or translated from the Latin: redness, warmth, swelling, and pain, respectively [20, 21]. It often presents in a localized area of the body, in a pattern that can be poorly demarcated on the skin. Erysipelas has many different connotations, but is commonly used to describe a superficial cellulitis with mostly lymphatic involvement [21]. This form of cellulitis is often indurated, with a sharp demarcated raised border. It can also show a dimpling of the skin as a result of localized edema (the "peau d'orange" effect).

9.5.1 Differential Diagnosis and Etiology

Most cellulitis is caused by naturally occurring colonized skin flora, most commonly streptococcus and secondarily most common, staphylococcus species. MRSA has emerged as a frequent cause of skin infections in the community. Patients are most at risk for MRSA if they were recently hospitalized, but there are strains of MRSA causing community-acquired cellulitis independent of recent institutionalization. Identification of possible MRSA infection affects management as described below. Severely immunocompromised individuals may become infected with organisms beyond the usual pathogens, including Gram-negative organisms such as *E. coli* and Pseudomonas and also with opportunistic organisms such as *Helicobacter cinaedi* and Cryptoccocus [21]. Diabetic patients' ulcers are also at risk of developing infections from Gram-negative organisms (Enterobacteriaceae spp., *Pseudomonas aeruginosa* and Acinetobacter spp.).

Risk factors for skin infections include any preceding acute or chronic process that results in localized damage to the superficial soft tissues of the body. This includes recent trauma, recent or concurrent dermatitis (either contact or ectopic), venous insufficiency, and chronic edema. The skin of older individuals is especially vulnerable to infection due to physiologic changes as a result of the aging process [1]. Any disruption to the lymphatics resulting in chronic or recurrent edema, such as those resulting after mastectomy or lymph node resection, can predispose to cellulitis. Animal or human bites cause cellulitis from trauma to the skin and transport of mouth flora to the resulting wound. Occasionally, osteomyelitis may evolve

Table 9.5 Differential Diagnosis of Cellulitis

Alternate diagnosis	Comments
Deep vein thrombosis	Determine pretest probability, consider ultrasound if medium/high
Changes of venous insufficiency/stasis dermatitis	Chronic changes, often darker red and hyper-pigmented changes, can get secondary infection especially if develops venous ulcers
Trauma without infection	Ecchymosis, history of trauma, possible hematoma present
Dermatitis (eczema or contact)	Often pruritic, can be chronic
Vasculitis	Systemic signs, lymphadenopathy in certain syndromes, presents diffusely
Insect bite	Local pruritis, very focal symptoms, can develop secondary cellulitis
Drug reaction	Less localized, more diffuse, often presents as hives, can be associated with symptoms of anaphylaxis
Other infections	
Fungal infection (Candida or Tinea)	Pruritic, scaly, often in intertriginous regions
Osteomyelitis	Acute or chronic, may present with systemic signs and sepsis
Septic bursitis	Localized swelling and redness, presents near a joint
Septic arthritis	Symptoms mostly localized at a joint with some involvement of surrounding skin. Often presents with joint effusion, joint tenderness, and decreased range of motion
Isolated skin abscess	Very focal or minimal to no erythema, purulent discharge present if abscess opened, otherwise fluctuant

outward to cause cellulitis of the overlying skin [21]. Finally, any immunocompromised state such as AIDS or neutropenia from leukemia, chemotherapy, organ transplant will be at increased risk of skin infections, often with unusual organisms [21].

Alternate diagnoses for suspected cellulitis include any process that also causes some or all of the signs of inflammation on the skin, including venous stasis changes, deep vein thrombosis, trauma, vasculitis, as well as other infective processes. Additionally, cellulitis can coexist or be a result of these alternate diagnoses (See Table 9.5).

9.5.2 Investigations at Home

History and physical examination are the mainstay in the diagnosis of skin infections. Appearance of new erythema, swelling, history of pain, and tenderness on palpation are often enough to diagnose a skin infection [20–23]. Predisposing risk factors and acuity of symptoms increase the probability of correct diagnosis. However, chronic venous changes and chronic ulcers can make diagnosis on visualization difficult. Skin cultures are usually of little to no diagnostic value as it will yield normal skin flora that represents normal colonization [23]. Abscesses and purulent drainage, however, should be cultured according to Centers for Disease Control (CDC) and IDSA guidelines as the results may change management, especially if infections fail to clear with empiric treatment [22, 23]. Start of empiric coverage does not have to wait for return of cultures. Blood cultures similarly are of little yield as most skin infections represent local processes [24].

Suspected cellulitis in the lower extremities and sometimes in the upper extremities often present similar to deep vein thrombosis. At those times, the clinician should consider assessing the probability of deep venous thrombosis (DVT) based on risk factors. The most studied clinical prediction rule is the Wells score [25, 26]. Those with a medium or high pretest probability warrant further evaluation for DVT, such as lower extremity ultrasound dopplers (either in the home, if home ultrasonography is available or office-based referral if necessary and within patient's capability). D-dimer may be elevated in both DVT and cellulitis as it is an acute phase reactant. A negative D-dimer may exclude DVT and rule in a cellulitis [26].

9.5.3 Pharmacologic Treatment

The CDC and the IDSA have issued updated guidelines for the antibiotic management of soft tissue infections in response to the emergence of increased incidence of MRSA causing infection in the community. Initial treatment choice depends on whether or not there is purulence, whereby the skin may be fluctuant, have a yellowish or whitish center or be frankly draining pus. Attempting to aspirate with a needle can also be done to prove purulence if the exam is unclear. An abscess with little to no systemic signs can be incised and drained with curative results and often does not need antibiotics. Additionally, if antibiotics are needed, purulence is suggestive of MRSA infection, and appropriate coverage of MRSA is needed. If there is no purulence, then typical coverage of susceptible streptococcus and non-MRSA staph is appropriate. However, if the patient fails initial therapy, has severe systemic signs (fever, tachypnea, tachycardia, leukocytosis on labs), and/or is immunocompromised, then MRSA should be covered along with streptococcal species. MRSA is resistant to all beta-lactam agents (penicillins and cephalosporins), with the exception of one of the newest IV cephalosphorins, Ceftaroline.

Appropriate oral antibiotic choices for non-MRSA cellulitis include beta-lactams, mainly penicillins and cephalosporins or clindamycin for those who cannot tolerate beta-lactam-based antibiotics (see Table 9.6). Recommended treatment

Table 9.6 Antibiotic coverage for non-MRSA cellulitis

Antibiotics	
Antibiotic	Dosing
Penicillins Penicillin V Dicloxacillin	250–500 mg orally every 6 h 500 mg orally every 6 h
Cephalosporins e.g., cephalexin	500 mg orally 4 times daily
Clindamycin	300–450 mg orally 4 times daily

duration is usually 5 days, but may be extended if the patient is not showing signs of improvement [23].

Patients in whom MRSA is suspected are often treated with oral trimethoprim–sulfamethoxazole, a tetracycline or clindamycin. Rifampin is also an option, although rarely used and should not be used as a single agent. Linezolid is also an option but the CDC suggests an infectious disease input before initiating therapy as it has very severe side effects and significant cost associated. Trimethoprim–sulfamethoxazole and doxycycline have unknown or poor coverage for streptococcus and use of a second agent (such as a beta-lactam) may be recommended to cover both strep and MRSA, especially for initial empiric coverage. Isolated abscesses that require antibiotics can be treated with MRSA coverage alone. Clindamycin covers both streptococcus and MRSA adequately but has a significant risk of causing *C. difficile* colitis. Fluoroquinolones and macrolides are not effective against MRSA due to high rates of resistance (see Table 9.7).

Additionally, IDSA guidelines give the option of steroid use (prednisone 40 mg oral daily for 7 days) as an adjuvant treatment for significant symptomatic cellulitis. This, however, is based on weak to moderate evidence.

Administration of prophylactic antibiotics is appropriate for patients with recurrent cellulitis. These are patients who have 3–4 episodes of cellulitis per year despite failed attempts to control risk factors. Patients can be treated with oral penicillin (250–500 mg orally twice daily) or IM benzathine penicillin (600,000 units for patients who weigh ≤27 kg; 1.2 million units for patients who weigh >27 kg) every 2–4 weeks. Staphylococcal prophylaxis can be tried with Clindamycin 150 mg orally once daily for adults. This continues until risk factors are eliminated [23].

Table 9.7 Antibiotic Coverage of MRSA Cellulitis

Antibiotic	Dosing	Comments
Trimethoprim–sulfamethoxazole (TMP–SMX)	1–2 double strength tabs twice daily	Only covers MRSA, consider adding beta-lactam for Streptococcus coverage (see Table 9.6)
Doxycycline or Minocycline	100 mg twice daily 200 mg orally once then 100 mg twice daily	Only covers MRSA, consider adding beta-lactam for Streptococcus coverage (see Table 9.6)
Clindamycin	300–450 mg twice daily	Adequate Strep coverage, can use as monotherapy Has increased risk of *Clostridium difficile* colitis
Linezolid	600 mg orally twice daily	Associated with myelosuppression, neuropathy, and lactic acidosis. ID consult recommended
Rifampin	600 mg once daily or 300–450 mg every 12 h	Not routinely used but can be used as adjuvant therapy for persistent Staph infections and or to eradicate colonization; use only in combination with other agents for Staph coverage as resistance with single use is very high

9.5.4 Nonpharmacologic Management

Purulent cellulitis requires drainage when possible, which will often prove curative if there are not extensive symptoms or systemic signs, such as febrile illness. Simple incision and drainage on most areas of the skin can be accomplished in the home. Abscesses on the face and hands or complex nonhealing wounds often require specialist intervention, either in the office or in the emergency department.

As an adjuvant to pharmacological therapy, elevation of affected extremities and warm compresses can aid in symptomatic control, both anecdotally promote drainage and thus improve pain and swelling [21, 26].

Finally, nonhealing or worsening cellulitis despite appropriate diagnosis and appropriate oral antibiotics may warrant intravenous antibiotics and possibly an infectious disease consult. This complication and/or possible systemic signs with a change in hemodynamics may warrant a higher level of care such as referral to an ER or hospitalization if such care is within the advanced directives of the patients. Signs of deeper tissue infection, including necrotizing infection, also warrant systemic IV antibiotics and hospitalization.

9.6 Summary

Infections contribute to significant morbidity and mortality in the homebound population. This population has multiple risk factors that increase their risk of infection. Urinary tract infections can be diagnosed based on history in cognitively intact individuals. True urinary infection can be difficult to distinguish from colonization in a patient who is cognitively impaired at baseline. Previously healthy individuals without a recent preceding hospitalization can be treated for community-acquired pneumonia with a macrolide or tetracycline, while more at risk patients such as the elderly or those with extensive comorbidities or severe disease should be covered with a beta-lactam AND a macrolide or only with a respiratory fluoroquinolone. Sputum cultures are only relevant in truly immunocompromised patients with cavitary lesions or other patients suspected of having infection with an unusual organisms. Initial evaluation for treatment of cellulitis involves assessing for severity of disease and for purulence as it will determine the type of empiric antibiotics. Nonpurulent cellulitis can be treated with empiric coverage for streptococcus only, while dual coverage for MRSA and for streptococcus should be done if the patient has purulence or an abscess, has severe infection, systemic signs, or has failed prior empiric treatment

9.7 Further Reading

Hazzard's Geriatric Medicine and Gerontology 6th edition McGraw Hill. Jeffrey B Halter, Joseph G Ouslander, Mary E Tinetti, Stephanie Studenski, Kevin P High, Sanjay Asthana. Section J Infection In The Elderly, 2009

Mandell, Douglas, and Bennett's Principles and Practice of Infectious Diseases, 7th Edition Edited by Gerald L. Mandell, John E. Bennett, and Raphael Dolin Philadelphia, PA: Churchill Livingstone Elsevier, 2009

References

1. High KP. Infection in the elderly. In: Halter JB, Ouslander JG, Tinetti ME, Studenski S, High KP, Asthana S, editors. Hazzard's geriatric medicine and gerontology. 6th ed. New York: McGraw-Hill; 2009. Chapter 124.
2. Mouton CP, Bazaldua OV. Common infections in older adults. Am Fam Physician. 2001; 63:257–68.
3. Pinner RW, Teutsch SM, Simonsen L, Klug LA, Graber JM, Clark MJ, et al. Trends in infectious diseases mortality in the United States. JAMA. 1996;276:189–93.
4. Gupta K, Hooton T, Naber K, Wullt B, Colgan R, et al. International clinical practice guidelines for the treatment of acute uncomplicated cystitis and pyelonephritis in women: a 2010 update by the infectious diseases society of America and the European society for microbiology and infectious diseases. Clin Infect Dis [Internet]. 2011 [cited 22 Jan 2015]; 52:e103–20. Available from: http://cid.oxfordjournals.org/content/52/5/e103.full
5. Nicolle LE, Bradley S, Colgan R, Rice JC, Schaeffer A, Hooton TM. Infectious diseases society of America guidelines for the diagnosis and treatment of asymptomatic bacteriuria in adults. Clin Infect Dis [Internet]. 2005 [cited 22 Jan 2015]; 40:643–54. Available from: http://www.idsociety.org/uploadedFiles/IDSA/Guidelines-Patient_Care/PDF_Library/Asymptomatic%20Bacteriuria.pdf4
6. Hooton TM, Bradley SF, Cardenas DD, Colgan R, Geerlings SE, Rice JC et al. Diagnosis, prevention, and treatment of catheter-associated urinary tract infection in adults: 2009 international clinical practice guidelines from the infectious diseases society of America. Clin Infect Dis [Internet]. 2010 [cited 22 Jan 2015]; 50:625–63. Available from: http://www.idsociety.org/uploadedFiles/IDSA/Guidelines-Patient_Care/PDF_Library/Comp%20UTI.pdf
7. McKenzie R, Stewart MT, Bellantoni MF, Finucane TE. Bacteriuria in individuals who become delirious. Am J Med. 2014;127(4):255–7.
8. Nicolle LE. Urinary tract infections in older people. Rev Clin Gerontol. 2008;18(2):103–14.
9. Baillargeon J, Holmes HM, Lin Y, Raji MA, Sharma G, Kuo Y. Concurrent use of warfarin and antibiotics and the risk of bleeding in older adults. Am J Med. 2012;125(2):183–9.
10. Ahmed A, Stephens JC, Kaus CA, Fay WP. Impact of preemptive warfarin dose reduction on anticoagulation after initiation of trimethoprim-sulfamethoxazole or levofloxacin. J Thromb Thrombolysis. 2008;26(1):44–8.
11. Metlay JP, Fine MJ. Testing strategies in the initial management of patients with community-acquired pneumonia. Ann Intern Med. 2003;138(2):109.
12. Wipf JE, Lipsky BA, Hirschmann JV, Boyko EJ, Takasugi J, Peugeot RL, Davis CL. Diagnosing pneumonia by physical examination: relevant or relic? Arch Intern Med. 1999; 159(10):1082–7.
13. Maughan BC, Asselin N, Carey J, Sucov A, Valente J. False-negative chest radiographs in emergency department diagnosis of pneumonia. Thode Island Med J. 2014. Available at: http://www.rimed.org/rimedicaljournal/2014/08/2014-08-20-cont-maughan.pdf. Accessed 23 Jan 2015.
14. Mandell LA, Wunderink RG, Anzueto A, Bartlett JG, Campbell GD, et al. Infectious Diseases Society of America/American Thoracic Society consensus guidelines on the management of community-acquired pneumonia in adults. Clin Infect Dis. 2007;44(Supplement 2):S27–72.
15. CDC/National Center for Health Statistics. Fast facts: pneumonia. Centers for Disease Control and Prevention. 14 July 2014. Available at http://www.cdc.gov/nchs/fastats/pneumonia.htm. Accessed 23 Jan 2015.

16. Lim W, van der Eerden MM, Laing R, Boersma W, Karalus N, Town G, Lewis S, Macfarlane J. Defining community acquired pneumonia severity on presentation to hospital: an international derivation and validation study. Thorax. 2003;58(5):377–82.
17. Dimopoulos G, Matthaiou DK, Karageorgopoulos DE, Grammatikos AP, Athanassa Z, Falagas ME. Short- versus long-course antibacterial therapy for community-acquired pneumonia: a meta-analysis. Drugs. 2008;68(13):1841.
18. CDC/National Center for Immunization and Respiratory Diseases. Vaccines and immunizations: pneumococcal vaccination: who needs it? 18 Sept 2014. Available at http://www.cdc.gov/vaccines/vpd-vac/pneumo/vacc-in-short.htm. Accessed 23 Jan 2015.
19. DC/National Center for Immunization and Respiratory Diseases .Vaccines and immunizations: seasonal influenza (Flu) vaccination . 18 Sept 2014. Available at http://www.cdc.gov/vaccines/vpd-vac/flu/default.htm. Accessed 23 Jan 2015.
20. Stevens DL. Infections of the skin, muscles, and soft tissues. In: Longo DL, Fauci AS, Kasper DL, Hauser SL, Jameson J, Loscalzo J, editors. Harrison's principles of internal medicine, 18 ed. New York: McGraw-Hill; 2012 (Chapter 125). http://accessmedicine.mhmedical.com/content.aspx?bookid=331&Sectionid=40726869. Accessed 21 Jan 2015.
21. Swartz MN. Clinical Practice: Cellulitis. N Engl J Med. 2004;350:904–12.
22. Gorwitz RJ, Jernigan DB, Powers JH, Jernigan JA. Strategies for clinical management of MRSA in the community: summary of an experts' meeting convened by the Centers for Disease Control and Prevention. Mar 2006. Available at http://www.cdc.gov/mrsa/pdf/MRSA-Strategies-ExpMtgSummary2006.pdf. Accessed 23 Jan 2015.
23. Stevens et al. Practice guidelines for the diagnosis and management of skin and soft tissue infections: 2014 update by the Infectious Disease Society of America. IDSA Clinical Infectious Diseases. 18 June 2014.
24. Perl B, Gottehrer NP, Raveh D, Schlesinger Y, Rudensky B, Yinnon AM. Cost-effectiveness of blood cultures for adult patients with cellulitis. Clin Infect Dis. 1999;29(6):1483–8.
25. Geersing GJ, Zuithoff NP, Kearon C, Anderson DR, Ten Cate-Hoek AJ, Elf JL, et al. Exclusion of deep vein thrombosis using the Wells rule in clinically important subgroups: individual patient data meta-analysis. BMJ. 2014;348:g1340.
26. Bates SM, Jaeschke R, Stevens SM, et al. Diagnosis of DVT: antithrombotic therapy and prevention of thrombosis, 9th ed. American College of Chest Physicians evidence-based clinical practice guidelines. Chest. 2012;141(2_suppl):e351S–e418S.

Wound Care in Home-Based Settings

10

Yasmin S. Meah, Peter M. Gliatto, Fred C. Ko, and David Skovran

Abstract

Wounds in homebound adults are common; clinicians who care for such patients require a working knowledge of prevention, diagnosis, prognosis, and therapeutics in order to minimize morbidity and maximize healing and comfort. The most frequently encountered wounds are decubitus wounds, also known as pressure wounds. Lower extremity ulcers are also common and can be venous, arterial, or neuropathic in origin. Wounds caused by malignant neoplasms are less common but are substantial causes of psychological and physical morbidity. Home-based medical providers who care for patients with wounds require a conceptual framework for dressings tailored to various types of wounds, as well as knowledge of home-based approaches such as negative-pressure wound therapy. Accurate and thorough documentation of wounds and wound care, appropriate billing, and collaboration with multiple disciplines are essential skills for the home-based clinician.

Keywords

Wound care • Home-based medical care • Interdisciplinary care • Decubitus ulcers • Pressure ulcers • Lower extremity ulcers • Venous ulcers • Chronic

Y.S. Meah, M.D. (✉) • P.M. Gliatto, M.D.
Departments of Medicine, Medical Education, Geriatrics and Palliative Medicine,
Icahn School of Medicine at Mount Sinai, One Gustave L. Levy Place,
1216, New York, NY 10029, USA
e-mail: yasmin.meah@mssm.edu; peter.gliatto@mssm.edu

F.C. Ko, M.D.
Brookdale Department of Geriatrics and Palliative Medicine, Icahn School of Medicine
at Mount Sinai, One Gustave L. Levy Place, 1020, New York, NY 10029, USA
e-mail: fred.ko@mssm.edu

D. Skovran, B.S.N.-R.N., A.N.P.-B.C.
Department of Medicine, Icahn School of Medicine at Mount Sinai,
One Gustave L. Levy Place, 1216, New York, NY 10029, USA
e-mail: david.skovran@mssm.edu

© Springer International Publishing Switzerland 2016
J.L. Hayashi, B. Leff (eds.), *Geriatric Home-Based Medical Care*,
DOI 10.1007/978-3-319-23365-9_10

venous insufficiency (CVI) • Arterial ulcers • Neuropathic ulcers • Debridement • Wound dressings • Wound bed preparation (WBP) • Negative-pressure wound therapy (NPWT)

10.1   Introduction

Although there are few specific data about the prevalence of wounds in a home-bound population [1], wounds are common in populations with similar functional level and comorbidities, such as patients in nursing homes [2]. The home-based medical provider will commonly encounter wounds from a variety of pathologic processes and should have a basic working knowledge of how to care for them. Every provider who takes care of patients in the home setting should be familiar with the major categories of wounds—pressure, venous stasis, arterial, neuropathic and malignant—be able to direct the management of these conditions and have a working knowledge of general strategies to prevent wounds. The virtues of interdisciplinary collaboration and teaching cannot be overemphasized.

This chapter will describe the prevalence, pathophysiology, prevention, and treatment options for the basic wound types listed above. In addition, current documentation and billing codes, which are often perplexing to providers, will be highlighted. Importantly, strategies to improve effective collaboration with various disciplines, including certified home health agency (CHHA) nurses, home health aides, physical therapists, surgeons, and podiatrists will be elaborated.

10.2   The Value of Interprofessional Collaboration in the Home-Based Care of Patients with Wounds

Interprofessional collaboration, communication, and partnership are keys to wound prevention, palliation, and healing. Alliances between healthcare personnel are built through clear and routine communication, a combined understanding of risk factors unique to each patient and shared realistic goals of wound healing and pain control. Providers should work in direct collaboration with nurses; joint home visits are occasionally necessary for complex or poorly healing wounds. Nursing agencies bill in 60-day episodes of care, so there should be no concern that a joint visit by the physician and nurse should negatively impact billing. Nurses who are highly competent in wound care are critical to successful healing; the most effective nurses possess extensive knowledge of dressings, readily counsel caregivers, and report changes in wound state to the primary clinician. Wound care nurses who offer direct or telemedicine consultation can be helpful in improving wound care outcomes in such situations [3]. Physical therapists are also essential to the care team as they can advise on durable medical equipment and repositioning techniques for caregivers and providers that can significantly improve the course of these ulcers.

Perhaps, most crucial for successful wound treatment in the home are vigilant and dedicated caregivers who maintain skin integrity and adhere to directions on positioning, repositioning, moisture containment, and nutritional augmentation; they also know when to call providers for emerging wounds, nonadherent dressings, new pain, or foul smell. Techniques for preventing pressure ulcers are not often intuitive; providers need to dedicate specific and proactive attention to training and counseling caregivers with at-risk patients. Though ulcers, particularly pressure wounds, may not be entirely avoidable in homebound persons, integrated multidisciplinary teams who are knowledgeable and complementary can increase likelihood of healing and decrease infection or pain. In situations in which wound closure is not the goal, palliation is most effective when caregivers, nurses, and home-based medical clinicians work in concert with aggressive attention to symptoms of distress [4, 5].

10.3   The Evaluation and Care of Pressure Ulcers in the Home

Pressure ulcers are among the most common types of wounds in the home-based medical care setting. The description of these wounds as pressure wounds is somewhat misleading as a number of other physical forces including friction, moisture, and shear stress cause wounds which are largely, but not completely, preventable and treatable. Understanding the physical stresses and the patient's characteristics that lead to these wounds is elemental to implementing effective prevention and therapeutics.

10.3.1 Physics and Anatomy of Wound Development

Correctly characterizing wounds is an essential first step for identifying and justifying preventative strategies and therapies, communicating with fellow providers, documenting and billing, and determining the likelihood of complete healing and/or recurrence.

The staging of pressure ulcers is complex, and substantial controversy exists on the validity of accepted scales [6]. The most widely accepted classification system used in clinical practice is the International National Pressure Ulcer Advisory Panel (NPUAP)/European Pressure Ulcer Advisory Panel (EPUAP) staging system, which categorizes pressure ulcers as six stages: Stages I–IV, and an additional two stages titled Unstageable and Suspected Deep Tissue Injury [7, 8]. In recent iterations of the scale, stages have been co-classified as categories [7, 8]; arguably, categories are more accurate descriptors that counter the common misconception of stages as progressive.

Static prolonged pressure is the crucial force for the development of true pressure wounds. It is important to understand that pressure ulcer stages or categories merely represent the VISIBLE degree of tissue injury. The McClemont Cone of Pressure theory describes the anatomic pressure gradient that develops when bone is pressed upon tissue against a static surface [9]. This concept is crucial to understanding why seemingly more superficial pressure ulcers are most commonly the end result of a deep pressure wound. Pressure on tissues causes capillary occlusion, tissue ischemia and, ultimately, tissue necrosis [6]. Because muscle is closest to bone, it suffers the greatest area of injury; subcutaneous fat is affected in smaller proportion and the skin the least [10, 11]. In addition, muscle and subcutaneous fat suffer far more irreversible damage to sustained periods of pressure than the dermis and epidermis. Thus, "what you see" is often not "what you get"—a phrase we often express when referring to true pressure wounds of the skin—as the skin damage is just the "tip of the iceberg" when a wound is the result of pressure [6, 12] (Fig. 10.1).

The most susceptible areas are over bony prominences; the most susceptible persons are those with limited or dependent mobility or sensory impairment [13]. Although current hospital practice dictates turning the body every 2 h to offload pressure on high-risk body parts, in truth, there is no clear minimum amount of pressure or time necessary to induce cell damage, and the practice of turning the body every 2 h is more convention than evidence-based therapy and prevention [14].

Shear forces are potent factors in the development of advanced wounds in home-based settings. Shear forces cause stretching and disruption of subcutaneous tissues and capillaries, making them far more vulnerable to damage by pressure [15]. Typical shear stresses in homebound persons include those generated on the sacrum when a person is shifted upward in bed or glides downward gradually from a partially upright position of 30–45°, and on the hip when the person is turned to the side by dragging the body along the greater trochanter. Shear forces accelerate the rate of ulcer manifestation and progression by several orders of magnitude over pressure alone. Older persons with more fragile and inelastic integument due to loss of collagen anchoring proteins and slower rates of tissue repair are more susceptible to injury from shear forces [16]. Minimizing or eliminating shear strain is a crucial primary and secondary prevention strategy, as this force more than pressure alone has been implicated in rapid tissue breakdown and ulceration [10].

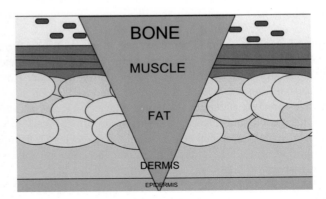

Fig. 10.1 McClemont Cone Effect: When a person is lying or sitting, muscle, fat, and skin are sandwiched between bone and the external surface. Prolonged compression of capillaries that supply these tissues causes ischemic compromise, particularly in tissues closest to bone. Pressure transmitted to these deeper layers of tissue can be up to five times that on the epidermis

10.3.2 Ulcer Stages and Categories

Stage/Category I ulcers emerge without frank denudation or ulceration of skin that is red and nonblanchable [8]. In persons with darker skin, these areas are hyperpigmented and the distinction as a pressure ulcer is often the relative warmth or tenderness to touch compared to the surrounding areas. Stage I pressure ulcers are complex wounds to categorize anatomically; though the skin is intact, the degree of damage to deeper tissues may be substantial. If the cause is friction, the damage to deeper tissues may be limited and thus the true thickness of tissue involvement is limited to the epidermis. The NPUAP and EPUAP caution against the classification of hyperemia exclusively due to friction a Stage I ulcer; however, many experts agree that distinguishing superficial hyperemia due to friction is difficult in clinical practice and perhaps underestimates the potent role that friction plays in the culmination of decubitus ulcers [8, 14]. Given the high likelihood of substantial deep tissue injury when pressure is the cause, Stage I ulcers should never be taken lightly; rather they should be seen not simply as at-risk skin involvement but serious deep tissue injury [6, 14, 17] (Fig. 10.2).

Stage/Category II ulcers are partial thickness wounds involving the epidermis and dermis [8]. They usually present as visible denudation of the epidermis and often have depth on the order of millimeters. They may also present as fluid-filled blisters. Although Stage II ulcers may be the result of pressure, they are more frequently the outcome of substantial friction over bony or nonbony areas. They may be promulgated by moisture from urine or feces, heavy exudate or sweat that separates the bonds between keratinocytes in the stratum corneum, a phenomenon called maceration [14, 18]. Most Stage II ulcers do not progress to Stage III or IV wounds [6, 17].

Stage/Category III ulcers are shear force or pressure injury wounds. They appear as full thickness skin loss involving damage or necrosis of subcutaneous fat that may VISIBLY extend down to, but not through, underlying fascia, with the

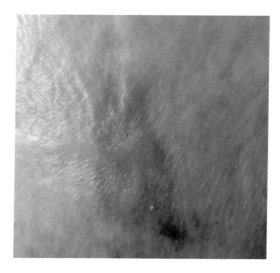

Fig. 10.2 Stage/category I pressure ulcer of the buttock

ulcer presenting to the naked eye as a deep crater [8, 14]. Classically, these are beefy red craters with depth. Depth, however, can vary based on the anatomic location. In areas in which there is little to no subcutaneous tissue, such as the ankle or scalp, a Stage III ulcer may be quite shallow; in contrast, in areas such as the buttock that have a substantial amount of fat, the depth can be substantial. Stage III ulcers may also extend underneath the dermal and subcutaneous layers of adjacent tissue, a phenomenon known as "undermining" or "tunneling." Deeper tissues such as muscle, tendon or bone, although likely affected, are not visible to the naked eye (Figs. 10.3 and 10.4).

Stage/Category IV ulcers are true pressure injury wounds. Like Stage III ulcers, they present with full thickness tissue loss; in contrast, however, deep tissue layers such as muscle, tendon, ligaments, or bone are visible. All other characteristics of Stage III ulcers apply to Stage IV ulcers including widely variable depth depending on the anatomic location and transgression to adjacent tissues through undermining and tunneling (Figs. 10.5 and 10.6).

Unstageable ulcers present as full thickness skin loss but the true depth of the ulcer is obstructed by necrotic tissue in the form of slough or eschar. Slough is characteristically yellow, tan, gray green, or brown and may be dense and adherent or soft and viscous. Eschar is tan, brown, or black and can also be dry and adherent or soft and pliable. It is important to recognize that though these necrotic elements may be located on the edge of Stage III and IV wound beds, wounds described as "unstageable" have such elements at critical points which obscure the fullest tissue depth of the wound. Until the slough or eschar is removed from the base of the wound bed, the actual depth of tissue involvement cannot be determined. This practice is generally contraindicated, however, when heel ulcers are the sites of injury. The development of eschar on the heel is considered protective, so dead tissue should not be removed if it is dry (Figs. 10.7 and 10.8).

Fig. 10.3 Stage/category III ulcer of hip

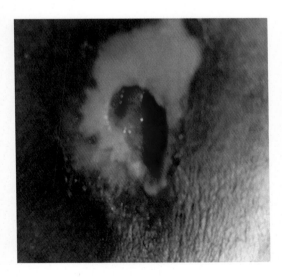

Fig. 10.4 Stage/category III ulcer with superficial slough and surrounding cellulitis

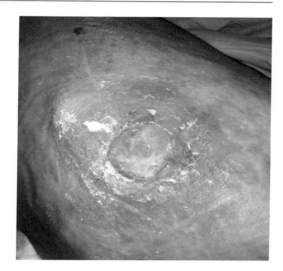

Fig. 10.5 Stage/category IV ulcer of sacrum with extensive necrosis

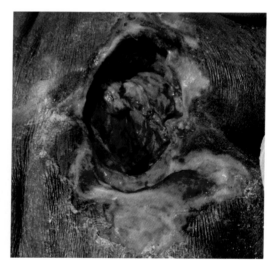

Suspected Deep Tissue Injury (DTI) characteristically presents as either a blood-filled blister or ecchymosis with purple or maroon colored intact skin in light-pigmented persons and brawny intact skin in darker-pigmented persons. Affected areas can feel edematous or boggy and are often warmer and tender compared to adjacent skin. DTI pressure ulcers are classically located over bony prominences with highest prevalence at the heel and lesser but substantial prevalence at the sacrum and buttocks [19] (Fig. 10.9).

Fig. 10.6 Stage/category
IV ulcer with dense slough
and maceration of the
periwound

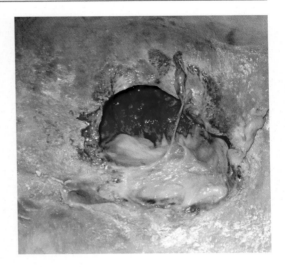

Fig. 10.7 Unstageable
heel ulcer with eschar

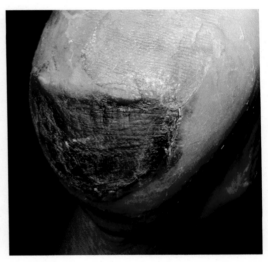

10.3.3 Effective Turning and Repositioning Techniques in the Home-Based Setting

High-risk skin areas in bedbound individuals should be inspected thoroughly at every home-based medical care visit. These include, in greatest incidence, the sacrum, ischium, heels and ankles, greater trochanters, and scapulae [20] and with lesser incidence the back, elbows, ear lobes, and scalp. Areas of vulnerability, however, can vary in persons with paralysis, kyphosis, and other anatomic abnormalities.

Proper repositioning is important for home-based medical care providers to understand; providers should instruct caregivers and interdisciplinary personnel on accepted methods for high-risk patients and for those with existing ulcers [21].

Fig. 10.8 Unstageable sacral ulcer with extensive peripheral eschar and slough

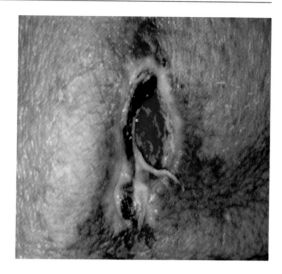

Fig. 10.9 Suspected deep tissue injury (sDTI) of the buttock

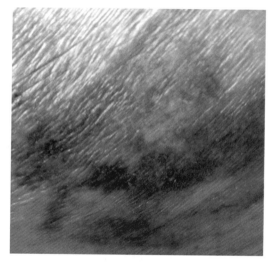

All providers should keep in mind, however, that optimal repositioning and repositioning schedules are controversial and little study has been devoted to the potential significance of small frequent weight shifts that may ultimately prove more practical and potent in home-based settings [22]. Regardless, we recommend the coupling of repositioning and frequent daily skin inspection as integral to preserving skin integrity in immobile patients with execution of the following repositioning and pressure-offloading techniques whenever possible. The following are suggested methods of positioning and repositioning to minimize friction, pressure, and shear force:

- Use bed linens as a shield and sling to turn and lift immobile persons in bed, rather than drag the body directly over surfaces.

- Allow partially mobile persons to move themselves when possible; use assistive devices such as a trapeze to assist patients in mobilizing themselves. Small movements at regular intervals are advised and caregivers may prompt for regular self-repositioning.
- When recumbent, place persons on their sides at a 30° tilt; avoid placing immobile persons directly on their sides to limit pressure on the greater trochanter and lateral malleolus of the ankle [23]. This is an awkward position for most people to maintain so the use of pillows is essential.
- Frequently turn and reposition lying patients every 2 h and seated patients every 15 min. The repositioning interval can be prolonged up to 4 h for recumbent positions and 1 h for seated persons when using pressure-reducing surfaces although this practice has not been validated [22].
- With the exception of eating and 30-min postprandial periods, do not leave immobile persons in an upright position more than 30° unless they are on a low air-loss mattress. Upright angles greater than 30° have been associated with higher sacral pressures when persons are on standard mattresses.
- Remain cautious about points of pressure and when possible keep bony prominences offloaded; for instance, never allow heels to remain static on a supine surface. Rather, elevate with pillows at placed just under the calves to keep heels off the bed surface. Pay attention to pressure points on bony surfaces when patients are placed in wheelchairs or transfer slings.
- Train and monitor caregivers regularly on effective repositioning and offloading. These techniques are not intuitive.

10.3.4 Ulcer Risk Scales and Utility in Clinical Practice

Several widely accepted scales are used in hospital based and nursing home settings to define the severity of internal and external risk factors that are most likely to lead to pressure ulcers. Though these scales have not been studied in home-based settings, their scoring breakdown is useful in determining and mitigating risk more holistically.

Decubitus ulcer risk scoring is a key component of the Outcome and ASsessment Information Set (OASIS) [24], which is used by Medicare-certified home health agencies (CHHAs) and must be conducted for each patient at defined intervals including on admission. The Braden Scale [25], a commonly used tool in the US, emphasizes risk as a mix of internal (patient specific) and external (environmental and physical) factors.

Because current evidence has shown that the use of risk assessment tools is not more effective than clinical judgment alone in preventing ulcers, home-based medical providers rarely use such time-intensive scales [26–28]. Nonetheless, it is important to think of these scales as a framework on which to determine risk and base prevention and therapy, as well as a common language for the interdisciplinary care team. We summarize the essentials here as a general inventory of risk factors. In addition, we have supplemented risk factors with practical considerations beyond what is captured in accepted scales.

10.3.4.1 Patient Characteristics Influencing Pressure Ulcer Development

- **Physiologic Age:** Advancing age with increased comorbid conditions that enhance the likelihood of incontinence, skin breakdown, and reduced capability of repair all contribute substantially to intrinsic risk.
- **Comorbid conditions:** Diseases such as cardiopulmonary disease, atherosclerotic disease, or diabetes, which impair tissue oxygenation increase the risk of tissue ischemia and thus pressure ulcer formation. Diseases such as dementia promulgate other risk factors such as immobility, sensory impairment, nutrition, and incontinence; dementia of all types poses the greatest risk for pressure ulcers.
- **Degree of immobility:** Poor or limited ability to make small adjustments in movement necessary to offset pressure-related ischemia is critical to the development of wounds. Highly immobile patients such as those with paraplegia, severe degenerative joint disease, or advanced dementia make them far more likely to experience high shear forces when mobilized and develop pressure wounds if not repositioned frequently, particularly if they are unable to make the small bodily adjustments that are critical to avoiding nocturnal ischemia in mobile persons.
- **Cognition:** Persons who suffer from impaired cognition or communication may lack the ability to move or direct their caregivers on turning and repositioning, particularly when in discomfort from prolonged periods of pressure. Furthermore, such persons may be incontinent and thus may be prone to urinary or fecal dermatitis.
- **Sensory impairment:** Those with impaired sensation such as those with spinal cord injuries, peripheral vascular disease, or scarred integument from previous deep tissue ulcers are unable to feel the painful stimuli from pressure-related ischemia and therefore unlikely to spontaneously move to relieve pressure.
- **Nutritional state:** A compromised nutritional state which often accompanies advancing age, frailty, and multiple comorbid conditions, particularly dementia, are clear risk factors for pressure ulcer formation. For one, as the patient loses weight, contact points of bony prominences are more pronounced and susceptible to pressure and friction injury. Additionally, the reduction in protein due to reduced intake or increased catabolism, as well as other nutrients such as vitamin C and zinc causes tissues to lose reparative capability [29]. Substantial controversy exists on whether nutritional supplementation with either protein or vitamin C and zinc actually improves outcomes. Typically, in persons with Stage III and IV ulcers, we advise a high protein diet (up to 1.5–2 g/ kg/day) with the addition of a daily multivitamin that contains vitamin C and zinc.

10.3.4.2 External Risk Factors for Pressure Ulcer Development

- **Friction and Shear forces:** Prolonged upright positioning and repositioning of the body without surface barriers such as a sheet can subject the body to both persistent and dynamic shear forces. Removing bed linens or diapers with the body pressed on the surface can cause significant friction and shear force injury. In terms of mitigating risk, the ability of caregivers and devices to relieve pressure adequately in immobile patients is highly associated with pressure ulcer formation and resolution. Pressure-relieving devices including foam or pillow offloaders and static and dynamic bed surfaces coupled with proper positioning and repositioning schedules can reduce risk.

- **Moisture:** Persistent moisture from urinary incontinence, fecal incontinence, sweat or heavily exuding wounds can cause maceration and dermatitis that can increase the likelihood of dynamic friction and shear forces to induce tissue injury. Wet skin is more prone to pressure ulceration than dry skin. Persistent moisture creates weakness in dermal bonds and localized edema; alkaline urine and fecal irritants, in particular, can weaken the stratum corneum making the skin far more prone to maceration and damage in the setting of friction and pressure. Fecal incontinence of soft stool or diarrhea is more potent than urinary incontinence in causing the perineal skin to inflame and, subsequently, to break down [14, 30]. Careful attention to hygiene is therefore important to emphasize with caregivers.

10.4   Direct Care of Pressure Wounds in the Home

The key to successful wound care is a comprehensive and collaborative approach; multiple interventions need to be implemented in order to maximize success and likelihood of wound closure and the prevention of wound recurrence. Collaboration with interdisciplinary personnel, consultants, and caregivers is essential to optimal wound healing. Adequate pain control with a low threshold for opiates when acetaminophen or nonsteroidal anti-inflammatory drugs are unsuccessful is also essential. Without adequate pain control, direct wound care is not simply difficult to perform but is counter to palliative care goals so intrinsic to good home-based medical care.

The comprehensive care of wounds can be separated into several direct and indirect tasks. Direct wound care is the most relevant to the home-based medical provider and perhaps the most daunting because of poor training and misconception of such care as germane only to surgeons or wound care nurses.

The following summary of wound care is most relevant to the care of decubitus wounds. Various principles, however, can be extrapolated to the care of venous stasis ulcers, arterial ulcers, neuropathic wounds, and diabetic foot ulcers. The care of each of these wounds is more nuanced than represented below and so the discussion of such wounds follows in more detailed format.

10.4.1 Pressure Wound Assessment

Accurate classification and measurements are important for effective communication with interdisciplinary providers, monitoring for progress, and identifying appropriate therapy. The therapy can be complex and involve an array of topical treatments, debridement modalities, support surfaces, and mechanical closure devices.

Classifying wounds not simply by stage but also by percentage slough, necrosis, characteristics of the surrounding tissue ("periwound"), and degree of tunneling and undermining is a critical skill for home-based providers.

Beyond staging, the following assessments should be performed for each wound:

1. Size of the wound in length, width, and depth. It is best to use paper tape to measure. The asymmetry of many wounds means that the length and width are often not simple. We, nonetheless, recommend the following approach:
   - Use the clockface as the reference for communication and documentation. Use the head and feet as reference points for 12 o'clock and 6 o'clock respectively.
   - Measure caudal–cranial width across the longest part of the wound.
   - Measure lateral width across the longest part of the wound.
   - Measure depth of the wound with a cotton swab or the finger gently placed to the base of the wound bed. Note the degree to which deeper tissues such as tendon and bone can be visualized.
   - Use the cotton swab to measure the depth of undermining and note the extent along the clock-face. In addition, use the cotton swab to measure the depth of tunneling. Be as descriptive as possible; for example, "Undermining from 2 o'clock to 6 o'clock with maximum depth of 3 cm at 4 o'clock and minimum of 0.5 cm at 2 and 6 o'clock."
2. Determine the percentage of slough and necrosis. Necrosis, or eschar, should be noted as wet or dry and adherent or friable.
3. Note the degree of exudate as mild, moderate, or heavy and the quality as serous, purulent, or bloody.
4. Document the quality and extent of the peripheral wound bed or periwound. The degree and extent of maceration, visible as bleached and edematous tissue, should be noted. In addition, any erythema or hyperpigmentation (especially in dark-skinned persons), bruising, tenderness, or crepitus should be noted. Finally, scar tissue, which is vulnerable to additional breakdown, should also be recorded.
5. Wounds should be classified as the most advanced stage by depth, and should not be reclassified as they heal. For example, as a Stage III pressure ulcer becomes more shallow, it should be described as a "healing Stage III ulcer," not reclassified as a Stage I or II ulcer.

10.4.1.1 Wound Bed Preparation: Cleansing, Initial and Maintenance Debridement, and Primary and Secondary Dressings

The general principles of direct wound care are summarized as follows:

1. Keep wounds with craters moist.
2. Keep wounds with intact skin covered with either a dressing or an absorptive emollient to prevent opening. Only intact skin with clear underlying pus or crepitus should be intentionally opened.

3. Fill dead space with packing materials tailored to the degree of exudate. Although evidence is limited, we often choose packing materials with antimicrobial activity in areas with a high-risk of infection [31].
4. Occlude all wounds with padding necessary to absorb excess exudate and adhesives that restrict entry of urine, stool, or sweat.
5. Keep the periwound dry with the use of barrier creams and/or skin preparations before applying adhesives.
6. Remove senescent or dead tissue with chemical, autolytic, or sharp debridement.

Wound Cleansing: Preservative-free normal saline should be used for most chronic wounds. In general, povidone–iodine solution, hydrogen peroxide, isopropyl alcohol and sodium hypochlorite (bleach that is commercially available as Dakin's Solution™) should be avoided given their high destruction of viable tissue and consequential delay in wound healing except in select circumstances. Povidone–iodine solution is used primarily to keep dry gangrene desiccated especially in heel ulcers whether pressure-related, neuropathic, or arterial. All arterial ulcers that are dry, in particular, should be kept dry with daily topical application of povidone–iodine solution by cotton swab or gauze [32]. Povidone–iodine use with wet wounds is limited to situations in which preparation of a sterile wound bed is necessary for sharp debridement. After the wound is debrided, the povidone–iodine solution is removed with saline. Dakin's Solution™ is advised as a time-limited application of ¼ strength solution to foul smelling wounds just long enough to control the smell. It is very caustic and painful, so in general it is to be avoided long-term and if pain should be significant, discontinued entirely. In palliative care settings, Dakin's Solution™ is rarely advised. On occasion, with extensive areas of dense senescent tissue (slough) or biofilm we will apply Dakin's full strength to the wound area once to remove the tissue or film. This is particularly useful for densely adherent slough with substantial surface involvement. Prior to application, adequate analgesia is usually necessary with subcutaneous or subsurface lidocaine 1–2 %.

Initial and Maintenance Debridement: Debridement, or the removal of visible and invisible nonviable tissue, is essential to reducing infection and promoting and speeding closure. Known as wound bed preparation (WBP), debridement is a two-phase process that may or may not follow sequentially. Initial debridement consists of the primary removal of visible nonviable tissue such as fibrin slough and necrotic eschar [33]. Maintenance debridement involves the ongoing periodic removal of cellular components such as nondividing or senescent fibroblasts and keratinocytes and proteins of the extracellular matrix that can impede an advancing tissue edge and the cellular turnover necessary for tissue healing [34]. Debridement should be a continual process until complete wound closure.

Mechanical debridement is perhaps the most nonspecific type of debridement with utility in limited settings. As the process can destroy both viable and nonviable tissues, it is most useful in wounds in which the slough or eschar is extensive or in areas of extensive bacterial biofilm [9]. We describe three methods of mechanical debridement below:

- Wet-to-Dry dressing debridement: As a practice, we do not employ this type of debridement in home-based settings. Saline-saturated gauze dressings are placed in a wound bed, long enough to allow the gauze to dry. The gauze is then pulled out, creating a type of mechanical debridement that is highly nonspecific for both viable and nonviable tissues [35]. As a wound care strategy, it is labor intensive, can promote a wound's bacterial burden, is painful, and is superseded by multiple other methods of effective debridement.
- Gauze debridement: Highly destructive and often painful, gauze debridement is performed with gauze moistened with saline to rub areas of slough, bacterial biofilm, or necrosis with force. It has limited use in home-based medical care except when slough, bacterial biofilm, or necrosis is semi-adherent and limited in area.
- High-pressure saline or water debridement: Saline or sterile water administered to a wound under high pressure removes bacterial biofilm and cellular debris; it has more limited usefulness with semi-adherent slough and eschar. For most deep ulcers, we perform high-pressure saline irrigation to reduce poorly visible biofilm and extracellular matrix that contain senescent fibroblasts and keratinocytes, as well as collagen which can ultimately form slough. In home-based wound care, we often create an impromptu yet highly effective device by attaching a 30–60 cc syringe to a 16, 18, or 20 gauge peripheral venous cannula (with the needle removed) or the tubing of a winged-infusion set (butterfly) and clipping the tubing to approximately 5–10 cm.

Autolytic debridement involves the use of dressings and formulations that promote the body's natural enzymes to continually remove cellular debris from the wound. In essence, all moist, occlusive dressings promote autolytic debridement, but as an exclusive means to care for the wound, autolytic debridement has limited use in treating shallow wounds.

Chemical debridement involves the application of agents that degrade or digest extracellular proteins sustaining necrotic or nonviable tissue in wound beds. This type of debridement is usually selective for senescent or dead tissue although penetration and effectiveness can be variable depending on the depth, density and moisture of the devitalized tissue. The application of nonspecific agents such as Dakin's Solution™, is less selective for devitalized tissue and though limited in effectiveness can be useful in certain wound care settings as described below.

Enzymatic debridement: Because collagen in healthy tissue is shielded by mucopolysaccharides, only exposed collagen in devitalized tissue is susceptible to degradation by metalloproteinases contained in such preparations as papain-urea and collagenase [36]. Papain-urea combinations were removed from the US market in 2009 because of allergic reactions associated with the papaya-derived papain component. Thus, home-based medical providers are left with only collagenase for the selective chemical debridement of wounds. For maximal success in using collagenase, dense slough, or eschar should be cross-hatched with a #10 blade to achieve penetration and uplifting of the collagen fibers which anchor the base of the eschar to the wound bed. In settings where sharp cross-hatching is not possible, however, application of collagenase can still promote substantial degradation of collagen [33].

Nonenzymatic debridement: Dakin's Solution™, or sodium hypochlorite (bleach), is a caustic chemical that can nonetheless achieve significant debridement of necrotic eschar or slough particularly if dense [37]. It is often used at ¼ strength to limit toxicity to surrounding tissue; the gauze saturated with Dakin's Solution™ must be changed every 12 h. On occasion, with wounds requiring more rapid debridement and in which sharp debridement is difficult to perform because of the location or high density of necrotic tissue, we use full strength Dakin's Solution™ as a one-time application. Before dabbing the area with Dakin's saturated gauze, we anesthetize the tissue with lidocaine to minimize the severe pain that can be associated with this application. In palliative care settings, the use of Dakin's Solution™ is generally not recommended because it induces significant pain.

Other chemical agents exist for this purpose such as honey [38] and cadexomer iodine [39]; the benefit of these preparations is that they often come in solid or semi-solid forms useful for packing or filling a wound and promoting a moist wound environment. They tend to be soothing rather than caustic to the wound bed. In addition, honey and cadexomer iodine preparations have antimicrobial properties that are particularly useful in wounds with a high burden of bacteria. Their superiority to collagenase in debriding devitalized tissue is not yet supported by the existing literature.

Sharp debridement of wounds is a useful skill for all home-based medical providers. Primary care clinicians should undergo appropriate training before executing this bedside skill. Some suggestions for resources include online training modules with videos, hands-on wound care courses with a sharp debridement skills laboratory or spending several clinical sessions working side-by-side with a clinician expert, such as a vascular surgeon, podiatrist or experienced primary care physician, or nurse with ample experience in debridement techniques. Some tips for successful bedside debridement are as follows:

1. Provide adequate analgesia locally and systemically. Before scalpel debridement, it is important to saturate the subsurface tissue with anesthetics such as lidocaine via local injection. In addition, it is advised to premedicate patients with opiates up to 30 min prior to debridement. Advising caregivers to administer analgesics prior to arrival helps to reduce provider-waiting time.
2. Use the right scalpel with a round rather than tapered edge such as a #15 blade or a dermal curette. The latter is more useful for less dense and less adherent yellow necrosis that usually affects fascia, muscle, or tendons.
3. Be able to physically and visibly distinguish between nonviable and vital tissue planes by lifting the edge of the necrotic tissue edge while advancing the scalpel.

Sharp debridement is indicated when chemical debridement has been unsuccessful, when more rapid tissue closure is desired or when preparing the wound bed for negative-pressure wound therapy (NPWT). Rates of wound closure can be accelerated on the order of days to weeks over chemical or autolytic debridement alone.

10.4.1.2 When Surgical Debridement and Closure are Necessary

Even in the home-based setting, it is occasionally necessary to consult a surgeon for operative debridement. In cases of extensive necrosis or infection or in the case of expansion of a wound despite aggressive home-based measures, surgical debridement and closure may be necessary, if such intervention is consistent with the patient's overall status and goals of care. In our practice, the majority of patients request in-home care alone, so external consultation is often difficult. On occasion, surgical consultants are able to make joint home visits to advise us on necessary next steps. For foot and ankle wounds, home-based podiatrists can also be important resources for more extensive debridement.

10.4.1.3 Bacterial Colonization, Critical Colonization, and Local Wound Infection

Reducing bacterial burden in the wound bed involves three main strategies including regular cleansing and irrigation, removing devitalized tissue, packing with antimicrobial dressings, and/or creating an acidic wound environment that inhibits bacterial proliferation [40]. Contamination and colonization of ulcers are common; several factors including bacterial burden, host immunity, and degree of devitalized tissue can cause colonization to progress to critical colonization (otherwise known as local wound infection marked by foul smell, local purulence or retarded wound healing but not generally requiring antibiotic therapy), invasive tissue infection with penetration of the surrounding healthy tissue (i.e., cellulitis or abscess) and, ultimately, systemic infection. The most common organisms invading devitalized tissue are *Staphylococcus aureus*, *Streptococcus pyogenes,* and *Pseudomonas aeruginosa* [41]; less common species include Proteus sp. and *Escherichia coli* [42].

In the event of surrounding tissue penetration or systemic infection, oral, intravenous, or intramuscular antibiotic therapy may be necessary and should be tailored to the most likely organisms in the affected area. For instance, sacral wounds may require enhanced coverage of Gram-negative species. Although not routinely recommended, if a wound bed is suspected to have a high bacterial burden given persistently foul smell, slow wound healing, persistent exudate on the order of days to weeks, or frank pus, sampling for culture can guide antibacterial therapy and uncover highly resistant species.

10.5 Common Primary Dressings, Secondary Dressings, and Adhesives in Home-Based Wound Care

In general, the choice of wound care dressings should be tailored to the appearance of the wound bed, the size and depth the degree of tunneling and undermining, the degree and quality of exudate, the degree and quality of devitalized tissue, and the appearance of the periwound. When ordering and documenting dressings, it is best to characterize layers as primary (i.e., directly on top of the wound), secondary (the layer directly adjacent to the primary layer), and tertiary (anchoring or adhesive) dressings.

The following tables summarize some of the common dressings and adhesives used in home-based settings with indications for each. This table is not meant to be restrictive or exhaustive, rather it should give the clinician a general repertoire and vocabulary for various dressing types. Home-based medical care providers should note that limitations in formulary are often be imposed by the nursing agency; some nursing agencies favor certain brands over others. Because the care of decubitus wounds is often similar to other wounds, we have used pressure ulcers as the standard indication and have noted when certain dressings are also indicated for other wounds (Tables 10.1 and 10.2).

Some guiding principles for wound dressings are as follows:

1. **Stage I and Suspected Deep Tissue Injury ulcers may be left uncovered or covered.** In areas subject to moisture or irritation from urine or feces, an emollient moisture barrier such as vitamin A and D cream or zinc oxide may be used. In addition, a thin adhesive barrier such as a transparent dressing or thin hydrocolloid is advised to limit friction. Adhesive barriers, however, are optional as the primary treatment when the skin is intact is to offload pressure.

2. **Stage II ulcers require different therapies based on the appearance and type.**
   - Blisters can be **left uncovered or covered** with an emollient such as vitamin A and D cream or zinc oxide or a primary dressing such as a thin transparent adhesive (Tegaderm™) or hydrocolloid. All barriers are optional but can facilitate the goal of reducing friction and limiting moisture.
   - Superficial ulcers should **always be covered and require filling** if there is substantial depth, i.e., more than 0.5 cm with dressings that are more hydrating if the exudate will barely moisten the primary dressing and more absorptive if the exudate is substantial and likely to saturate the primary dressing. Primary dressings such as hydrocolloids can be used for the majority of Stage II wounds with some degree of drainage. Hydrogels, which are hydrating and can come as a true gel or a solid matrix, keep the wound bed moist and cool. They are usually reserved for very shallow wounds without substantial devitalized tissue and with nominal exudate [14]. They may promote debridement of devitalized tissue albeit at a slower rate than the application of collagenase [33]. Packing with more absorptive dressings such as calcium alginate or carboxymethylcellulose (CMC)-based hydrofibers is necessary when the exudate is substantial and the depth is significant (i.e., greater than 0.5 cm). Occasionally, for highly exudative wounds, a foam dressing, secondary layers of gauze or woven abdominal pads are indicated. Barrier creams and skin preparations that promote waterproof seals between the skin and the adhesive dressing should be used to limit the maceration of the periwound.

3. **Stage III and IV ulcers are treated similarly.** The goal is to fill the crater bed with the right material to promote absorption while maintaining a moist, bacteria-free wound environment. We often use collagenase at the base of the wound if there is visible slough or eschar or hydrogel if there is a high degree of granulation tissue and mild drainage. Although hydrogel can be used in the wound base if there is dry

Table 10.1 Primary dressings in home-based wound care

Primary dressing	Primary forms	How it works	Optimal uses	Other indications and contraindications
Hydrogels	Manufactured as amorphous gel or gel sheets	Lubricates and softens tissue	Shallow wounds (depth less than 1 cm) with minimal exudate	Not recommended for moderately to heavily exudative wounds or venous stasis ulcers
		Promotes autolytic debridement	Deeper wounds (depth greater than 1 cm) with significant granulation tissue and without dense necrotic tissue or slough	Can be mixed with 2 % lidocaine gel or morphine liquid for additional analgesia
			Wounds with thin layers of necrosis or slough in preparation for sharp debridement	Ideal for palliative care settings as frequency of dressing changes can be up to 1 week; users are advised to refer to manufacturers insert of each product for details
			Painful wounds in which a cooling effect is desired	
Hydrocolloids	Manufactured as sheet, powders, and pastes, the latter with more absorptive capacity	Hydrophilic colloid particles bound to polyurethane which absorbs fluid from the wound and creates a gel-like covering	Well granulating wounds with mild exudate	Not recommended for use in deep wounds, infected wounds or venous stasis ulcers
		Over dry wounds acts as an impermeable barrier to moisture and a cushion against friction	Shallow wounds with thin necrosis or slough in preparation for sharp debridement	Often used as secondary dressing for Stage II or shallow Stage III ulcers
			Over bony prominences subject to repeated trauma from friction or shear stress such as the sacrum	Advised in palliative care settings as frequency of dressing changes can be up to a week

(continued)

Table 10.1 (continued)

Primary dressing	Primary forms	How it works	Optimal uses	Other indications and contraindications
Alginates	Manufactured as pads and ribbons. Pads can also be cut into ribbons	The absorption of wound fluid causes the seaweed-derived fibers to form a gel that promotes a moist wound environment	Given their high absorptive capacity, alginates are ideal for heavily exuding wounds	Not recommended for use in wounds with low drainage as the dressing can dry out the wound or impregnate into the wound causing difficulty in removing residual fibers
			Ideal for filling large craters, tunnels and undermining	Dressing frequency can be every other day
			Excellent primary dressing for venous stasis ulcers	For wounds with minor bleeding, alginates can induce hemostasis
			Can be used with antimicrobial gels in infected wound beds	
			When impregnated with silver, offers additional barrier to bacterial growth	
Hydrofibers (aka hydrocolloid fiber)	Manufactured as pads and ropes; many come impregnated with silver	Like an alginate, the absorption of wound fluid causes this synthetic carboxymethylcellulose (CMC) fiber to create a gel (similar to a hydrocolloid dressing) with enhanced absorption over alginates [43]	Same as alginates	Non-recommended uses are the same as alginates
				Benefit over alginates is that the frequency of wound care dressings can be several days longer [44]

Primary dressing	Primary forms	How it works	Optimal uses	Other indications and contraindications
Foams and hydropolymer derivatives	Manufactured as sheets (conformable or shaped to body part), sheets with peripheral adhesives or ropes; may be impregnated with silver or other antibacterial products that inhibit colonization	Foam dressings are composed of a polymer or urethane foam with craters that trap the exudate. The polyurethane coating enhances the creation of a moist wound environment thus promoting autolytic debridement or chemical debridement when coupled with an enzymatic ointment. Hydropolymers offer enhanced absorption with a backing layer that has breathability allowing for significant evaporation of wound exudate [45]. Differing antibacterial properties of impregnated and manufactured types are useful for limiting the bacterial burden of wounds in high-risk areas, wounds with foul odor or wounds that are chronically colonized	A primary dressing for any sized cavity with moderate to heavy exudate	Polyurethane foam dressings with high moisture-vapor transmission rates (MVTR) may allow for more days between dressing changes for highly exudative wounds
			A secondary dressing for heavily exudative wounds; may be placed on top of the primary dressing; the latter can include alginates or hydrofibers	Foams are not indicated as primary dressings for dry wounds or wounds with minimal exudate as they may stick to the wound bed and removal may cause trauma or pain
			A secondary dressing for non-exudative wounds to limit shear force during the healing process	
			Primary or secondary dressing for venous stasis ulcers	
			Primary or secondary dressing for friable or painful neuropathic foot wounds	

(continued)

Table 10.1 (continued)

Primary dressing	Primary forms	How it works	Optimal uses	Other indications and contraindications
Gauze	Dry gauze sheets or bandages, petroleum-impregnated gauze, iodine-impregnated gauze strips, elastic gauze bandage	Gauze sheets trap moisture through the lattice; layering multiple sheets maximizes absorption	Petroleum-impregnation offers a non-stick and less painful variation that can promote a moist wound bed with varying occlusive properties	Dry gauze is only used as a secondary dressing over dressings with more potential to keep wound beds moist
			Iodine-impregnated gauze strips offer wicking properties for small infected or moderately exudative wound spaces	With rare exception, dry gauze should not be applied as a primary dressing to any wound
			Elastic gauze bandages, when wrapped with tension, can compress venous stasis or bleeding wounds	Moist gauze as a wet-to-wet dressing is effective as a primary dressing for diabetic foot wounds
			As a secondary dressing, gauze can provide adequate offloading of pressure	Wet-to-dry gauze, in which moist gauze is allowed to dry before removal, is contraindicated in palliative care settings due to excess trauma and pain

Table 10.2 Secondary and tertiary dressings/adhesives

Dressing	Common uses and considerations in home-based wound care
Transparent film	Waterproof yet permeable to oxygen these are mostly used as secondary and tertiary adhesive dressings in home-based care. Used to anchor the primary dressing, transparent films provide occlusion so that moisture is trapped within the wound and maceration of the periwound is minimized. Adherence to the periwound is aided by the use of adhesive skin preparations. Transparent dressings can also be used as a primary dressing for shallow wounds, first-degree and second-degree burns, and blisters
Gauze	Dry gauze is used as an inexpensive common secondary dressing for heavily exudative wounds whether under a foam dressing or without; gauze bandages are also used to anchor primary and secondary dressings and to create substantial offloading particularly for foot wounds
Foam	Often used as a secondary dressing for heavily exudative wounds particularly sacral ulcers in which there is the added benefit of reducing friction and pressure, as well as venous stasis ulcers. For venous stasis wounds, we do not advise foam dressings with adhesive as the latter can denude the surrounding tissue during removal
Woven abdominal pads	Like foam, woven abdominal pads can offer substantial absorption, albeit at slightly less effective capacity but also at far less expense. Particularly for wounds requiring frequent wound changes and less bulk, woven abdominal pads are cost-effective alternatives to foam with higher absorptive strength than gauze
Paper tape	The closing ability of paper tape is adequate for wounds in which the edges are closely approximated and the area is free of moisture [46]. Its place in decubitus wound closure, however, is fairly limited to very small wounds (i.e., a centimeter or less in diameter and depth) as a secondary dressing. Paper tape offers the advantages of low cost and low allergenic potential. The primary disadvantage is that it poorly seals in areas with significant moisture or high shear stress. When placed exclusively over the dressing without contact with the skin, it can provide adequate adhesion
Cloth tape	Stretchable perforated cloth tape is a mainstay of home-based wound care. Unlike silk or rubber tape, stretchable cloth tape offers breathability, high adhesion particularly when coupled with adhesive skin preparations, and conformability to allow ease of movement. These qualities reduce moisture of the periwound, offer high occlusion to sweat, urine and feces and reduced blister-rates over traditional cloth tapes [47]. The cost of stretchable tape, however, is significantly greater than standard silk or rubber-based tape

eschar or dense slough, we advise its use solely to soften the eschar or slough in preparation for further sharp debridement within a week. Collagenase, though superior to hydrogel in this regard, is used similarly; cross-hatching with a #10 blade any dense areas of slough or eschar before application allows for increased penetration to the anchoring layers of the base; this step, however, is not absolutely necessary [48]. When drainage is moderate to severe, common dressings to fill such cavities include alginate, CMC-based hydrofibers, and foam dressings. Heavily exudative wounds often require significant layering with secondary dressings such as foam, excess gauze, or woven abdominal pads. The sacrum is particularly susceptible to substantial moisture from feces and urine; we invariably use several layers of secondary dressings for such wounds and a tight adhesive with conformability such as perforated cloth tape or a transparent adhesive dressing to maximize occlusion.

4. **Heel Wounds:** These wounds deserve special attention as the management of Stage III, IV and unstageable ulcers of this area differ considerably from the care of wounds elsewhere in the body. In general, heel wounds with eschar should be **kept dry** with daily painting of betadine [49]. Dry eschar is protective of the underlying tissue and if removed can lead to poor wound healing and limb loss. If the area is moist, use of the strategies for general Stage III and IV wounds can be applied.

10.6 Support Surfaces and Cushions in the Treatment of Pressure Wounds

As part of the armamentarium of pressure wound care, pressure-reducing and pressure-relieving support surfaces are integral. Although data are conflicting on ideal support surfaces for the prevention and healing of pressure wounds, there is consensus that higher-specification foam mattresses, as well as air, gel, and water-based surfaces and/or mattresses are superior to standard hospital bed mattresses [50, 51].

Pressure redistribution surfaces and cushions (wheelchair and heel, for instance) are classified as static or dynamic depending on whether or not they vary the pressure beneath the patient at timed intervals. The Centers for Medicaid and Medicare Services (CMS) has further classified bed surfaces into Group 1, 2, or 3 classifications based on their degree of pressure reduction or redistribution. In general, Group 1 surfaces provide the least amount of pressure reduction or redistribution and Group 3, the greatest [14, 52].

Static bed overlays or mattresses, also known as constant low-pressure devices, distribute weight over large contact areas thus reducing pressure to a single body prominence. These surfaces are largely considered preventive Group 1 support surfaces if composed of gels, foam, water, or air, therapeutic Group 2 if composed of a powered low air loss mechanism, or therapeutic Group 3 support surfaces if composed of fluidized air and particulates such as silicone beads [53]. Dynamic overlays, on the other hand, are largely considered therapeutic, Group 2 surfaces, though evidence also supports their use as preventative redistribution surfaces [14] Dynamic support surfaces such as alternating pressure cushions, mattress overlays or mattresses, contain air pockets that variably inflate and deflate to adjustable high- or low-pressure states. Kinetic or tilting beds allow for pressure redistribution through total body mobilization. The following table summarizes the qualifications for Group 1, 2 and 3 support surfaces as determined by CMS (Table 10.3).

Other foam and sheepskin pressure redistribution modalities are available which are particularly useful for bony prominences and other areas subject to high rates of shear stress even when a patient is on a bed support surface. For prevention and therapy of heel ulcers, in particular, sheepskin and foam boots are more effective

Table 10.3 Pressure- relieving support surfaces in home-based medical care

Pressure- relieving surface group	Group 1	Group 2	Group 3
Examples of support surfaces used in home care	• Gel mattress overlay • Alternating pressure pads • Static air or gel mattresses	• Powered alternating pressure mattress • Powered pressure-reducing low air loss mattress	Air-fluidized silicone bead beds
Criteria for coverage by US Medicare	All patients who are completely immobile qualify Partially mobile patients and patients with any stage pressure ulcer on the body quality of they have at least one of the following risk factors: • Incontinence (fecal, urinary, or both) • Poor nutritional state • Circulatory compromise • Sensory impairment	Patients must have either • Multiple Stage II pressure ulcers on the trunk or pelvis that have been under comprehensive treatment for the past 30 days. Treatment must have included the use of a group 1 support surface and clear documentation that the wounds have nonetheless worsened or not improved • Large or multiple Stage III or IV ulcers on the trunk or pelvis • Recent (i.e., within 60 days) of a skin graft or flap for a Stage III or IV pressure ulcer	Immobile patients with Stage III or Stage IV pressure ulcers who • Would require institutionalization if the device were not provided • Have previously failed therapy with a group 2 device
Conditions for discontinuation or downgrading to a lower group	–	Ulcer(s) healed Beyond 60 days of flap or graft skin closure	Ulcer(s) healed

(continued)

Table 10.3 (continued)

Pressure-relieving surface group	Group 1	Group 2	Group 3
Additional considerations	Advised for all bedbound individuals [14, 54]	Clinicians should be diligent about documenting the comprehensive care of the wound which should include modification of risk factors such as incontinence, nutritional state, and immobility by frequent and proper repositioning	Monthly, detailed documentation must be submitted to US Medicare to acquire and retain Group 3 support surfaces in the home
			Must adequately document that wound care is comprehensive and includes direct wound care management with qualified staff, limitation of incontinence associated moisture and nutritional support
			Must also document dedicated caregivers who assist with the comprehensive wound care plan and can respond quickly to a malfunctioning Group 3 bed which has lost power or is leaking air. Nonfunctioning Group 3 bed systems, which become rock-hard when air is lost or noncirculating, can cause expansion of a wound in hours

than mattress support surfaces alone in redistributing pressure to the calves, which are far less vulnerable to pressure and shear force related injury [51]. It is recommended that all immobile persons who are maintained on any group surface either wear sheepskin or foam boots or have their heels suspended in the air through the use of low-cost cushions or rolled towels placed under the calves [54].

10.7   The Care of Venous Ulcers and Chronic Venous Insufficiency in the Home

Chronic leg ulcers caused by chronic venous insufficiency (CVI) are the second most common wound-type treated in home-based medical care settings. CVI describes a condition that affects the venous system of the lower extremities. Varicose veins are the most common cause of CVI [55]. In studies of community-dwelling persons 60 and older, however, other comorbid vascular conditions such as peripheral arterial disease, diabetes mellitus, hypertension, and congestive heart failure have also shown potent links to venous ulceration [56]. Venous stasis skin changes can present as skin hyperpigmentation, eczema, or hard-thickened areas with unusual friability of the overlying skin when edematous. Thus, superficial trauma and pressure may accelerate venous ulcer development.

Risk factors for CVI include age (over the age of 30), family history, female sex, repeated venous thromboses, multiple pregnancies, and obesity. In the homebound population, the most common associations we see are in persons who are obese or remain in a seated position with dependent extremities for prolonged periods.

The initial management of CVI includes measures to reduce symptoms and prevent the progression of disease. This includes maintaining excellent skin care. The legs and feet should be cleaned daily with soap and water and a topical moisturizer should be applied such as petrolatum; lanolin-based products should be avoided given enhanced allergenic potential in areas of CVI. The moisturizer will help prevent dry skin, reduce fissuring and skin breakdown. Custom fitted or gradient compression stockings should also be applied and may be cost-effective in reducing the incidence and recurrence of venous ulcers [57]. This will provide graded external compression to the leg and oppose the hydrostatic forces of venous hypertension. The compression stockings should apply between 20 and 50 mmHg of tension. The pressure will result in improvement in pain, swelling, skin pigmentation, activity, and compliance [55].

Venous leg ulcerations occur between the knee and the ankle. They are classically but not exclusively located over the medial and lateral malleolus of the ankle. These wounds often begin as small shallow ulcerations with serous exudate that can rapidly expand over the course of days to weeks. The odor can be profound and cause significant distress [14, 32]. When ulcers erupt, the periwound is often very edematous, with substantial erythema, scaling, and weeping. The pain of such wounds is not usually severe unless there is an active infection; such discomfort must be distinguished from the frequently described "achiness" of CVI. Wounds, when infected, present with "burning" pain. Unlike decubitus ulcers, there is usually no eschar.

Fig. 10.10 Venous ulcer of the medial malleolus

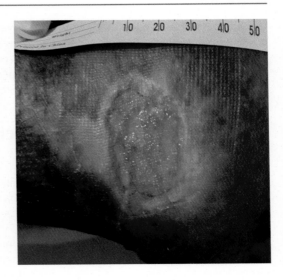

The wound bed often contains nearly homogenous granulation tissue; frequently they can also be shrouded with superficial fibrinous necrosis or slough [58] (Fig. 10.10).

Prior to developing a treatment plan for venous ulcers, it is critically important to differentiate the wound from an arterial ulcer, as the more substantial compressive therapies can be detrimental to persons with arterial compromise. Some symptoms that distinguish arterial ulcers are substantial pain of the extremity at rest with worse pain during elevation or activity. Arterial wounds usually have a pale, gray or yellow bed, nominal to no exudate and are often covered with eschar [56].

If a venous stasis ulcer is suspected and compression therapy is being considered, then the site should be evaluated for adequate blood flow via a palpable dorsalis pedis pulse or a bedside Doppler ultrasound. The resting ankle-brachial systolic pressure index (ABI) is a simple test that can be performed with a stethoscope and a sphygmomanometer at the bedside and is used to determine the quality of blood flow [59]. The person should be placed in the supine position for at least 10 min before performing the test; if the person smokes, the test should be performed no less than 2 h after the last cigarette. The systolic pressure is first taken over both brachial arteries with a sphygmomanometer; subsequently a systolic pressure is obtained at the dorsalis pedis and posterior tibialis arteries while an appropriately sized cuff is placed over the leg between the ankle malleoli and the calf. The higher systolic pressure of the two inferior arteries is divided by the higher systolic pressure of the arms to obtain the ABI. In cases in which the home-based medical provider has access to a portable Doppler probe, the measurements will be more accurate. An ABI between 0.91 and 1.3 is considered normal and the wound should be treated as a venous stasis ulcer. An ABI should not be completed on a person if they have excruciating pain in the lower legs or a suspected deep vein thrombosis [55]. In such cases, we advise referral to a mobile vascular laboratory or a home-based podiatrist for assessment of arterial flow by Doppler.

When a venous stasis ulcer develops, a compression dressing should be applied over a primary dressing. Cleansing prior to coverage should be performed with care to minimize trauma to the surrounding skin. We recommend gently patting the wound with saline or sterile water-doused gauze [60]. Additional dry gauze can be used to pat the wound dry. Primary dressings with high absorption are usually preferred such as alginates, CMC-based hydrofibers or foam. Hydrocolloids offer a soothing overlay but are less absorptive; they can be used over venous stasis ulcers with mild drainage. Finally, nonstick gauze or petrolatum-impregnated gauze may be used though their absorption capability is extremely low. They do offer the benefits of low cost and less painful removal.

Current evidence fails to show superiority of silver-impregnated dressings over standard dressings or of alginates or hydrofibers over hydrocolloids or nonadherent gauze dressings [61] in the care of venous stasis wounds.

Compression is the mainstay of effective venous stasis ulcer care. There are two main options for compression: an Unna boot and the four-layered bandage dressing. The Unna boot consists of a paste bandage that is impregnated with zinc oxide, glycerin, and gelatin. It is applied without tension in a circular fashion from the foot just distal to the metatarsals to below the knee. An elastic wrap or tubular support bandage is applied as a final layer and forms a cast after drying. The four-layered bandage involves the application of compressive elastic dressings at midstretch and with overlap to allow create an even distribution of tension across the limb. Excessive tension by the bandager is both unnecessary and potentially deleterious; thus clinicians should practice with the use of videos before applying [62, 63]. The first layer is an absorbent padding. It should be wrapped in a spiral fashion with a 50 % overlap. The second layer is a light-conforming wrap that is also wrapped in a spiral fashion with 50 % overlap. The third layer is a compression layer. It should be applied in a (Fig. 10.8) fashion with a 50 % overlap and 50 % stretch. This will apply about 17 mmHg pressure. The fourth layer is also compression. It is wrapped in a spiral fashion with 50 % overlap and 50 % stretch, which results in 20 mmHg pressure. Several studies comparing the Unna boot with the four-layer compression dressing have showed no differences in the effectiveness of healing venous stasis ulcers [64]. For ease of application and removal, we opt for the four-layer compression dressing in the home.

Regardless of type, compression is well supported as the standard for healing venous stasis ulcers over noncompressive dressings. Furthermore, evidence supports the greater effectiveness and faster healing times of a four-layer compression dressing over single component dressings, such as elastic gauze. For home-based persons for whom we cannot obtain an adequate arterial evaluation, we will use a two-layer compressive wrap composed of a primary absorptive layer and a single compressive layer; although the healing time is slower, it can be effective, nonetheless, particularly in persons who are recumbent [61].

Factors predicting a high likelihood of healing within 1 year of compression therapy include an ulcer width of less than 20 cm, eruption less than a year, significant reduction of lower extremity edema during the first 2 months of therapy and granulation tissue accounting for more than 10 % of the wound bed [65]. Conversely, risk factors that predict a lower likelihood of wound resolution within a year include larger wound sizes, wounds present for over a year, substantial necrotic slough within the wound bed, obesity, immobility, particularly at the ankle joint, and substantial lower extremity edema that persists beyond the early months of therapy. As venous stasis wounds are often difficult to heal and recurrent, such risk factors are useful in helping providers determine realistic chances of wound closure.

Other treatment strategies used in home-based medical care are largely targeted to prevention. These include pharmacologic therapy and exercise therapy to augment lower extremity mobility. In regards to pharmacologic therapy, four groups of drugs have been evaluated in the treatment of CVI including flavonoids, coumarins, and saponosides (horse chestnut extracts). However, these drugs are currently not approved for use in the United States. Horse chestnut seed extract has been found to be just as effective as compression stockings in reducing edema and pain but only in the short term [66]. Exercise therapy has also been used in the treatment of CVI. Home-based exercise programs which focus on lower extremity range of motion can theoretically improve the muscle pump action thus relieving symptoms. Studies in the home-based medical setting are lacking, however; in ambulatory patients, exercise has only been shown benefit when used in conjunction with medical or surgical treatment [67]. Although interventional management may be indicated, it is often not consistent with the goals of homebound persons with limited mobility or low desire for more invasive techniques and is not covered here.

10.8   Home-Based Care of Arterial Ulcers

10.8.1 Etiology, Risk Factors, and Signs and Symptoms of Arterial Ulcers

Peripheral arterial occlusive disease (PAOD) is common and associated with significant morbidities including arterial ulceration of the lower extremities. Thus, all patients presenting with lower extremity ulcers should considered for the concurrent presence of arterial insufficiency in order to identify and optimize management of arterial ulcers. Only those patients who will benefit from invasive management or whose therapeutics may change based on the presence or absence of arterial disease, however, should undergo further testing [68, 69].

Arterial ulcers develop secondary to PAOD in which arterial compromise causes reduced blood flow, thus leading to tissue ischemia, damage, and subsequent ulcer formation. The most common cause of arterial blood flow obstruction is atherosclerotic disease of the medium and large size arteries. Other causes and risk factors include diabetes, hypertension, hyperlipidemia, vasculitis, thromboangiitis, hypercoagulable states, anemia, obesity, advanced age, tobacco use, and traumatic injury to extremity [69]. Some of these risk factors are modifiable. Therefore, quality primary care in homebound patients that mitigates these chronic illnesses and adverse lifestyle choices (e.g., smoking cessation) is highly important in the prevention of arterial ulceration [70]. Moreover, providers should maintain a high index of suspicion for arterial ulcers in older patients with a history of vascular diseases [71].

Arterial ulcers frequently occur in areas of the lower extremities subjected to pressure or repetitive trauma [68]. Commonly affected areas include the metatarsal and phalangeal heads, web spaces between the toes, lateral malleolus, heels, tibia, and bony prominences of the foot frequently exposed to pressure from a shoe or brace (Fig. 10.11).

The ulcer often has well demarcated margins with a round, "punched out" appearance and minimal exudates. The wound base is usually pale pink, nongranulating, and may be necrotic or covered with an eschar. The ulcer depth ranges from shallow to deep depending on the anatomical location and the amount of underlying subcutaneous tissue. The skin surrounding the wound base may be thin, brittle, cyanotic, shiny in texture, hairless, and cool to touch. In addition, it may be pale on elevation and rubrous when dependent. Toenails distal to arterial ulcers may be thickened and opaque or absent. Arterial ulcers are particularly prone to infections; however, signs of infection may be subtle due to impaired blood flow. In patients with severe PAOD, gangrene of the extremities, missing limbs or digits and evidence of healed ulcers and scars from previous lower extremity surgery may be present [68, 70, 71].

Patients with PAOD may have diminished or absent peripheral pulses particularly in the dorsalis pedis and posterior tibial arteries. On physical examination, the presence of bruits in proximal lower extremity arteries indicates the presence of atherosclerosis. Patients with arterial ulcers have delayed capillary refill time (>3 s) and the return of color after raising an ischemic leg to 45° for 1 min [72]. A more accurate assessment of arterial blood flow in the extremities can be achieved by measuring the ankle brachial index (ABI) described above using a stethoscope or Doppler ultrasound. In home-based settings, the latter is often difficult to perform without the

Fig. 10.11 Arterial ulcer of the medial foot with necrotic eschar

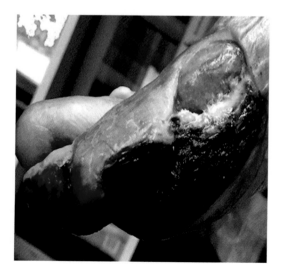

assistance of a home-based podiatrist unless a portable Doppler ultrasound machine is handy. The ABI provides a ratio of ankle to brachial artery systolic blood pressure, which predicts the effectiveness of peripheral circulation and severity of PAOD. The screening value for PAOD is defined by a resting ABI of ≤ 0.90 [58]. More specifically, an ABI that ranges from 0.91 to 1.30 indicates an absence of significant arterial disease and wounds, if present, are healable. An ABI that ranges from 0.41 to 0.90 indicates mild to severe arterial insufficiency with varying degrees of wound healing potential. An ABI ≤ 0.40 indicates critical lower extremity ischemia and low probability of wound healing [73]. Thus, the availability of ABI data can help clinicians gage the potential for arterial ulcer healing in homebound patients.

Sensory perception changes and pain are symptoms frequently associated with PAOD. Diminished or absence of temperature perception and proprioception and increased tingling are common in extremities with arterial ulcers. Muscle pain, ranging from resting pain to intermittent claudication, occurs in extremities with arterial insufficiency and worsens with activity or leg elevation. The arterial ulcers themselves may also be painful with or without an associated wound infection [68, 70].

10.8.2 Arterial Wound Management

The restoration of peripheral blood flow by revascularization (e.g., angioplasty, reconstructive surgery) is the intervention that will most likely promote healing of arterial ulcers. Indications for revascularization include the presence of nonhealing ulceration, gangrene, and progression of disabling claudication [68, 70, 74]. Operative interventions for arterial ulcers, however, are often poor options for homebound persons due to lifespan, severe immobility, and patient or family desire for more conservative methods.

The optimization of modifiable risk factors for PAOD and arterial ulcers should be considered and individualized in homebound patients. Smoking cessation must be advocated [74]. Exercise, such as walking, improves collateral arterial blood flow and should be advised when possible. Modification of other vascular risk factors, such as diabetes, hypertension, hyperlipidemia, and obesity should be considered in the context of the patient's overall goals for care and life expectancy [68, 74].

Avoidance of constrictive garments and elevation of the head of bed (4–6 in. but no more than 30°) to maintain lower extremity position below the level of the heart may improve arterial flow and should be advised [70]. In addition, attentive foot care and strategies that protect lower extremities from further excessive heat, cold or trauma should be exercised. These include daily foot examination for skin breaks, blisters and changes in skin color; avoidance of walking when barefoot; and ensuring the use of appropriate footwear (e.g., well-fitted shoes) free of friction and pressure points [73]. Taken together, these primary care focused interventions can be beneficial in the prevention and maintenance of new and chronic arterial ulcers, respectively.

The management of arterial ulcers distinctly differs from the care of other types of wounds in the following ways: maintenance of a dry wound bed; avoiding the unroofing of eschar; and mitigating the high risks of wound infection, pain, and malodor. Like pressure ulcers, arterial ulcers benefit from substantial offloading of pressure and friction. In order to keep the wound bed dry, healable and nonhealable dry ulcers should be cleansed with povidone–iodine or chlorhexidine and then patted dry to remove any excess solution; a nonhealable moist ulcer can be cleansed with normal saline or water and then patted dry to remove moisture. Subsequently, a protective dry wound dressing such as gauze can be applied. In contrast, in treating a healable moist ulcer with slough, the goal of management is moist wound healing and the use of autolytic debridement is appropriate provided that arterial inflow is adequate to support healing. Consequently, an appropriate dressing such as a hydrocolloid that maintains a moist wound environment can be applied to optimize cell migration and matrix formation in order to accelerate wound healing [69, 71, 72].

In general, the removal of necrotic or devitalized tissue and eschar by debridement promotes cell turnover and leads to faster wound healing. However, in the setting of arterial insufficiency, debridement of ulcer and unroofing of eschar may worsen tissue ischemia and enlarge the wound. Thus, in arterial ulcers with dry gangrene or eschar, debridement should only be performed after arterial blood flow has been reestablished [69, 71]. Furthermore, wound cleansing with normal saline and water should be avoided to prevent softening and unroofing of eschar, which could be a sign of wet gangrene.

Arterial ulcers are particularly prone to infections due to impaired arterial circulation. The signs and symptoms of a wound-related infection may include the following: (a) increased bacterial burden as suggested by a nonhealing wound, new necrotic slough, friable, or hypergranulation tissue, the absence of granulation tissue, increased exudate, and malodor; (b) localized infection as indicated by new or worsening pain, increased periwound induration, erythema, or warmth, and increased wound size; and (c) systemic infection as determined by the presence of lethargy, fevers, delirium, and sepsis [75]. The restoration of the arterial blood flow via bypass or atherectomy, which is often considered palliative, is central to controlling wound-related infection [14]. In homebound patients who are not candidates for revascularization surgery, however, systemic antibiotic therapy remains the treatment of choice for infected arterial ulcers [69].

Peripheral arterial disease and arterial ulcers are painful. The pain can be constant due to severe arterial insufficiency or intermittent secondary to wound dressing changes. Thus, clinicians must be cognizant of the inciting triggers of pain in order to optimize pain control. Positioning the lower extremities below the level of the heart may alleviate limb pain due to arterial insufficiency. This can be accomplished by hanging the affected leg over the side of the bed in order to improve flow. If dressing changes prove to be exquisitely painful, analgesic administration 30–60 min prior to wound manipulation is indicated. Because systemic analgesia is superior to topical therapies in achieving pain control, the administration of scheduled opioid analgesic at sufficient doses is frequently required to achieve optimal pain management. Moreover, the use of nonadherent dressings such as nonstick gauze or foam can minimize disruption of arterial ulcers and are less likely to cause pain on removal.

Wound odor typically results from tissue necrosis or bacterial colonization. While wound odor is not directly harmful to the patient, it may be indicative of an arterial ulcer's bacteria burden and pose a psychological burden on the patient and caregivers. Effective strategies to reduce development of malodor include practicing good hygiene, increasing frequency of dressing changes, and timely changing of soiled bed linen. If an underlying wound infection is suspected to precipitate malodor, appropriate antibiotic therapy should be initiated. Daily to three times weekly application of topical metronidazole (1 % solution, 0.75 % or 0.8 % gel or topical powder from crushed metronidazole tablets) is commonly performed to treat malodor and is particularly effective in treating wounds with high anaerobic bacteria burden [76]. In addition, odor-controlling dressings that contain activated charcoal or cadexomer iodine which can remove excess drainage and inhibit bacterial growth may be helpful in reducing malodor [77].

10.9 Treatment of Neuropathic Ulcers and Diabetic Foot and Ankle Ulcers

Although neuropathic ulcers can arise in multiple conditions that affect the peripheral nerves, diabetes accounts for the large majority encountered in community-based settings. In our practice, diabetic ulcers are frequently encountered as part of a constellation of poorly controlled diabetes, debility, and arterial disease (Fig. 10.12).

In general, the care of these wounds is similar to the care of pressure ulcers and arterial ulcers [78]. Diabetic foot and ankle ulcers may often be associated with arterial insufficiency and ABIs are essential to determining if large versus small vessel disease is involved. The former may require revascularization to enhance the likelihood of wound closure. Small vessel disease, however, requires glucose control coupled with pressure offloading through the use of specialized boots if ambulatory or sheepskin or foam heel protectors if bedbound or immobile [79]. As discussed

Fig. 10.12 Diabetic ulcer of the distal aspect of a mallet toe

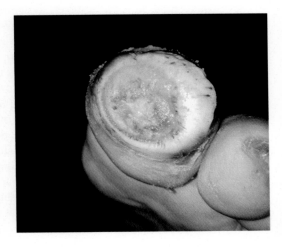

previously, heel ulcers which have dry eschar should be kept dry with topical betadine and exposure to air; a hydrocolloid dressing may be used to protect the area from friction when the person is ambulatory.

Direct care of diabetic neuropathic wounds of the foot often involves dressings that control a high bacterial burden. Cadexomer iodine preparations, which come as an ointment, gel, or paste, can be used to fill cavities, absorb excess exudate, enhance autolytic debridement, and reduce bacterial burden and have been shown to offer a lower cost alternative to more expensive antibiotic preparations and to twice-daily saline coated gauze dressings or moist-to-moist dressings [80, 81]. Though daily moist-to-moist dressings are an acceptable standard of care for diabetic neuropathic foot ulcers, it is labor-intensive and in home-based settings, not routinely possible [14].

Neuropathic wounds in persons without diabetes are treated with the same modalities used for pressure ulcers, as the etiologies are often quite similar. The absence of localized pain may be associated with substantial wound size and depth before noticed. Patient and caregiver vigilance in monitoring skin over bony or friction-prone surfaces is essential for prevention.

10.10   Home-Based Treatment of Malignant Wounds

Malignant wounds in the homebound are particularly challenging to manage because such wounds have a high morbidity and almost always occur when prognosis is grim and life expectancy is short. Malignant wounds occur when there is direct infiltration of tumor into the skin and subcutaneous tissues, leading to vessel erosion or occlusion and subsequent tissue death. The necrosis of superficial tissues in turn leads to sloughing, drainage, foul smell, and localized bacterial colonization. Such wounds can then become ulcerating or fungating [14]. Skin metastases can occur in as many as 1 in 10 patients with metastatic cancer [82].

The most common cancers associated with cutaneous spread leading to wounds are breast, head and neck, and skin cancers. Lung, colon, and kidney also have a high prevalence of fungating wounds [83]. Fungating wounds can be painful, itchy, malodorous, and/or have a large amount of drainage. Bleeding may be an issue, ranging from oozing to major hemorrhage if the tumor or ulcer erodes into a large vessel. The wounds pose a risk of infection [84].

Malignant wounds almost always occur in advanced cancer, which may limit treatment options directed to the cancer itself. Treatment of malignant wounds is often palliative rather than curative. The main symptoms to target are odor, drainage, pain, and bleeding.

One of the most distressing symptoms of malignant wounds is odor, resulting from the necrosis of tissue and products of anaerobic bacteria that colonize the wounds [85]. Topical metronidazole (cream preferred over gel which contains alcohol that may sting on application) [76, 77], medicinal honey, and oral chlorophyll [86] have been shown to reduce odors from malignant wounds. The drainage can be copious. Using absorptive dressings, like alginates, hydrofibers, hydrocolloids, or topical sucralfate cream are indispensable in the care of malignant wounds. Alginates and hydrofibers offer immediate hemostatic properties but their removal can be traumatic and lead to more bleeding; homecare providers are urged to use caution with such dressings and to consider saturating the dressing with saline just prior to removal. As with foul-smelling arterial wounds, silver or other antimicrobial-impregnated formulations can reduce odor [76, 77]. Using a nonstick initial layer to a dressing such as hydrogel wafers, petroleum-impregnated gauze, nonstick gauze, or foam dressings can help minimize pain and bleeding [83, 86]. A provider may need to balance the goal of managing drainage with minimizing the frequency of dressing changes, which can be painful and distressing. If the drainage is not manageable with highly absorptive dressings an ostomy bag may be used [14].

Malignant wounds have a tendency to bleed [86]. Erosion of the wound or tumor into a superficial vessel can also lead to frank hemorrhage. Minor oozing and spotting can be minimized with nonstick dressings and reduced frequency of dressing changes as mentioned above. Topical adrenergic agents like oxymetazoline (usually available as a nasal decongestant) can also be helpful. Topical or systemic tranexamic acid or systemic aminocaproic acid have also been effective in managing bleeding wounds Topical vasopressin and "Moh's paste," a chemical fixative containing zinc chloride, have also been used [83].

Pain from malignant wounds can be targeted with a number of local therapies, like topical lidocaine or morphine suspended in topical sucralfate or hydrogel, or with a systemic approach if warranted by the severity or persistence of the pain [14]. The quantities advised are approximately 1 mg of morphine to 1 g of hydrogel to achieve a 0.08–0.1 % mixture; a compounding pharmacy is often necessary to create this. The application of such agents can also be used to treat painful pressure and venous stasis wounds.

10.11   Indications for Negative-Pressure Wound Therapy

On occasion, providers may feel compelled to accelerate wound closure with the use of NPWT. NPWT involves the attachment of a semi-occlusive foam or gauze dressing to a vacuum device and a collection reservoir through plastic tubing. A solid seal that inhibits passage of air is critical to promoting a moist wound environment and preventing over-drying [87]. NPWT works through several theorized mechanisms:

- Macrodeformation, or the physical approximation of the wound surface
- Microdeformation, or the promotion of cellular proliferation at the wound surface
- Creation of a moist wound environment with low oxidative exposure
- Positive alterations in blood flow in the deeper wound bed despite reductions on the surface [88]

For poorly healing Stages III and IV ulcers, venous ulcers, and neuropathic wounds with minimal closure or expansion despite standard wound therapies over the course of 3 months, NPWT can greatly augment wound closure rates provided certain personnel are available [89]. One absolute requirement is the ready availability of caregivers, such as family, to care for the device when nonoperable or in need of adjustment. Home aides are usually prohibited from operating or adjusting the device. A second absolute requirement is nursing staff that are well-trained to operate the device and its attachments correctly. Familiarity with the device, possible adverse consequences and troubleshooting capabilities are essential. Though many companies offer help on demand, this is not a reliable means to provide the daily care necessary for effective NPWT. In our experience, the home-based medical provider's role is to ascertain the ability of caregivers to operate, troubleshoot, and call the providers when the device malfunctions or power is lost. Faulty equipment or dressing attachment can cause delays in wound healing and, more distressingly, can cause infection, pain or additional wounds to arise from maceration. Home-based medical providers should optimize the wound bed before application; this will mean adequate debridement to remove the majority of eschar or slough and treatment of underlying infection. Consultation with the NPWT on-staff nurse is essential before applying the device. Complications of these devices include bleeding and infection, the latter often due to retained dressings or infrequent dressing changes [90]. Because of the enhanced risk of hemorrhage, we never use these devices in patients on anticoagulant therapy or with evidence of a bleeding diathesis. Regular assessment of the wound with accurate and rigorous documentation is the responsibility of the primary provider for insurance coverage of the device; use up to 3 months without significant closure is a criterion for termination of the device. As this documentation and frequent follow-up can be labor intensive, many home-based medical providers are often reluctant to apply this nonstandard therapy.

10.12 Billing for the Assessment of Wounds and Wound Care

Careful and complete documentation is an important first step to accurate billing for wound care. Documentation should involve attention to intrinsic and extrinsic risk factors and discussions with caregivers and healthcare personnel on the mitigation of each. In addition to accurate documentation of the wound stage and size, wound bed preparation and methods of debridement must be clearly documented. In general, current procedural terminology (CPT) codes are used in home-based wound care ONLY if an active debridement modality such as mechanical, chemical, or sharp debridement is conducted on the day of the visit [91].

- Debridement of NONVIABLE tissues performed on the skin, epidermis, or dermis is reported with the active wound care management CPT codes 97597 and 97598. This code series can also be used when the tissues debrided are the superficial fibrin, exudates, or eschar at the base of deeper wounds when no specific tissue layer (i.e., fascia, muscle, or bone) is identified. This code series includes high-pressure irrigation of the wounds, application of chemical debriding agents, and sharp debridement. Anyone of these methods qualifies as an active wound management modality.

- In cases when debridement is of nonviable tissue is performed in preparation for NPWT and the goal is for closure of the wound by primary intention, CPT codes are of the 15002–15005 series.

Wounds cannot be billed by individual lesion; rather aggregate size of all of the wounds by square centimeter is what determines the appropriate CPT code and whether additional CPT codes are necessary. For instance, in the case of codes 97597 and 97598 for active wound care management, debridement of nonviable tissue for the first 20 cm^2 of aggregate wound size is billed with CPT code 97597; debridement of any additional square centimeters is billed with the addition of 97598 [92, 93].

10.13 Summary

Wound care and prevention are critically important skills for home-based practitioners to master. Pressure ulcers are ubiquitous in home care; their causes are multifactorial and not wholly avoidable. The care of such wounds, whether a superficial Stage I or deep Stage IV, is multidimensional and requires careful and regular attention, proper documentation, tailored dressings, comprehensive treatment regimens, and interdisciplinary partnership with shared goals of closure and palliation of pain and psychological distress. Venous stasis ulcers, arterial ulcers, neuropathic wounds, and malignant wounds are encountered less frequently but their management can be just as complex.

References

1. McDermott-Scales L, Cowman S, Gethin G. Prevalence of wounds in a community care setting in Ireland. J Wound Care. 2009;18(10):405–17.
2. Park-Lee E, Caffrey C. Pressure ulcers among nursing home residents: United States, 2004. NCHS Data Brief. 2009;14:1–8.
3. Vowden K, Vowden P. A pilot study on the potential of remote support to enhance wound care for nursing-home patients. J Wound Care. 2013;22(9):481–8.
4. Jaul E. Assessment and management of pressure ulcers in the elderly: current strategies. Drugs Aging. 2010;27(4):311–25.
5. Dam A, Datta N, Mohanty UR, Bandhopadhyay C. Managing pressures ulcers in a resource constrained situation: a holistic approach. Ind J Palliat Care. 2011;17(3):255–9.
6. Kottner J, Balzer K, Dassen T, Heinze S. Pressure ulcers: a critical review of definitions and classifications. Ostomy Wound Manage. 2009;55(9):22–9.
7. Black J, Baharestani M, Cuddigan J, Dorner B, Edsberg L, Langemo D, Posthauer ME, Ratliff C, Taler G. National pressure ulcer advisory panel national pressure ulcer advisory panel's updated pressure ulcer staging system. Dermatol Nurs. 2007;19(4):343–9.
8. Haesler E, editor. National Pressure Ulcer Advisory Panel, European Pressure Ulcer Advisory Panel and Pan Pacific Pressure Injury Alliance. Prevention and treatment of pressure ulcers: quick reference guide. [Internet] 2014. Available from: http://www.npuap.org/wp-content/uploads/2014/08/Updated-10-16-14-Quick-Reference-Guide-DIGITAL-NPUAP-EPUAP-PPPIA-16Oct2014.pdf
9. McClemont EJ. Pressure sores. No pressure - no sore. Nursing (Lond). 1984;2(21):suppl 1–3.

10. Bennett L, Kavner D, Lee BY. Shear vs. pressure as causative factors in skin blood flow occlusion. Arch Phys Med Rehabil. 1969;60:309–14.
11. Bouten CV, Oomens CW, Baaijens FP, Bader DL. The etiology of pressure ulcers: skin deep or muscle bound? Arch Phys Med Rehabil. 2003;84(4):616–9.
12. Bauer JD, Mancoll JS, Phillips LG. Grabb and Smith's plastic surgery. 6th ed. Philadelphia: Lippincott-Raven; 2007. p. 722–9. Chapter 74, Pressure Sores.
13. Cushing CA, Phillips LG. Evidence-based medicine: pressure sores. Plast Reconstr Surg. 2013;132(6):1720–32.
14. Alvarez OM, Kalinski C, Nusbaum J, Hernandez L, Pappous E, Kyrriannis C, Parker R, Chrzanowski G, Comfort C. Incorporating wound healing strategies to improve palliation (symptom management) in patients with chronic wounds. J Palliat Med. 2007;10(5):1161–89.
15. Gefen A, Farid KJ, Shaywitz I. A review of deep tissue injury development, detection, and prevention: shear savvy. Ostomy Wound Manage. 2013;59(2):26–35.
16. Ganceviciene R, Liakou AI, Theodoridis A, Makrantonaki E, Zouboulis CC. Skin anti-aging strategies. Dermatoendocrinol. 2012;4(3):308–19.
17. Berlowitz DR, Brienza DM. Are all pressure ulcers the result of deep tissue injury? A review of the literature. Ostomy Wound Manage. 2007;25:101–8.
18. Alvarez OM. Pressure ulcers: critical considerations in prevention and management. Clin Mater. 1991;8(3–4):209–22.
19. VanGilder C, MacFarlane GD, Harrison P, Lachenbruch C, Meyer S. The demographics of suspected deep tissue injury in the United States: an analysis of the International Pressure Ulcer Prevalence Survey 2006–2009. Adv Skin Wound Care. 2010;23(6):254–61.
20. Barczak CA, Barnett RI, Childs EJ, Bosley LM. Fourth national pressure ulcer prevalence survey. Adv Wound Care. 1997;10(4):18–26.
21. Seiler WO. Decubitus ulcers: treatment through five therapeutic principles. Geriatrics. 1965;40:30–44.
22. Krapfl LA, Gray M. Does regular repositioning prevent pressure ulcers? J Wound Ostomy Continence Nurs. 2008;35(6):571–7.
23. Moore Z, Cowman S. Using the 30° tilt to reduce pressure ulcers. Nurs Times. 2012; 108(4):22–4.
24. Centers for Medicaid and Medicare Services. Home health quality initiative [Internet]. 2015. Available from: http://www.cms.gov/Medicare/Quality-Initiatives-Patient-Assessment-Instruments/HomeHealthQualityInits/index.html
25. Braden B, Bergstrom N. Braden scale [Internet]. 1988. Available from: http://www.braden-scale.com/images/bradenscale.pdf
26. Anthony D, Papanikolaou P, Parboteeah S, Saleh M. Do risk assessment scales for pressure ulcers work? J Tissue Viability. 2010;19(4):132–6.
27. Kottner J, Balzer K. Do pressure ulcer risk assessment scales improve clinical practice? J Multidiscip Healthc. 2010;3:103–11.
28. Pancorbo-Hidalgo PL, Garcia-Fernandez FP, Lopez-Medina IM, Alvarez-Nieto CJ. Risk assessment scales for pressure ulcer prevention: a systematic review. J Adv Nurs. 2006; 54(1):94–110.
29. Dorner B, Posthauer ME, Thomas D. The role of nutrition in pressure ulcer prevention and treatment: National Pressure Ulcer Advisory Panel White Paper [Internet]. 2009. Available from: http://www.npuap.org/wp-content/uploads/2012/03/Nutrition-White-Paper-Website-Version.pdf
30. Beeckman D, Van Lancker A, Van Hecke A, Verhaeghe S. A systematic review and meta-analysis of incontinence-associated dermatitis, incontinence, and moisture as risk factors for pressure ulcer development. Res Nurs Health. 2014;37(3):204–18.
31. Dumville JC, Walter CJ, Sharp CA, Page T. Dressings for the prevention of surgical site infection. Cochrane Database Syst Rev. 2011;7, CD003091. doi:10.1002/14651858.CD003091.pub2.
32. Gist S, Tio-Matos I, Falzgraf S, Cameron S, Beebe M. Wound care in the geriatric client. Clin Interv Aging. 2009;4:269–87.
33. Milne CT, Ciccarelli A, Lasay M. A comparison of collagenase to hydrogel dressings in maintenance debridement and wound closure. Wounds. 2012;24(11):317–22.

34. Panuncialman J, Falanga V. The science of wound bed preparation. Clin Plast Surg. 2007;34(4):621–32.
35. Moore J, Jensen P. Assessing the role and impact of enzymatic debridement. Podiatry Today. 2004;17(7):54–61.
36. Shi L, Carson D. Collagenase Santyl ointment: a selective agent for wound debridement. J Wound Ostomy Continence Nurs. 2009;37(6 Suppl):S12–6.
37. Levine JM. Dakin's solution: past, present, and future. Adv Skin Wound Care. 2013;26: 410–4.
38. Nisbet HO, Nisbet C, Yarim M, Guler A, Ozak A. Effects of three types of honey on cutaneous wound healing. Wounds. 2010;22(11):275–83.
39. Schwartz JA, Lantis 2nd JC, Gendics C, Fuller AM, Payne W, Ochs D. A prospective, non comparative, multicenter study to investigate the effect of cadexomer iodine on bioburden load and other wound characteristics in diabetic foot ulcers. Int Wound J. 2013;10(2):193–9.
40. Basterzi Y, Ersoz G, Sarac G, Sari A, Demrikan F. In-vitro comparison of antimicrobial efficacy of various wound dressing materials. Wounds. 2010;22(7):165–70.
41. Ebright JR. Microbiology of chronic leg and pressure ulcers: clinical significance and implications for treatment. Nurs Clin North Am. 2005;40:207–16.
42. Bessa LJ, Fazii P, Di Giulio M, Cellini L. Bacterial isolates from infected wounds and their antibiotic susceptibility pattern: some remarks about wound infection. Int Wound J. 2015; 12(1):47–52.
43. Barnea Y, Weiss J, Gur E. A review of the applications of the hydrofiber dressing with silver (Aquacel Ag®) in wound care. Ther Clin Risk Manag. 2010;6:21–7.
44. Harding KG, Price P, Thomas S, Hofman D. Cost and dressing evaluation of hydrofiber and alginate dressings in the management of community-based patients with chronic leg ulceration. Wounds. 2001;13(6):229–36.
45. Carter K. Hydropolymer dressings in the management of wound exudate. Br J Community Nurs. 2003;8(9 Suppl):10–6.
46. Chao TC, Tsaez FY. Paper tape in the closure of abdominal wounds. Surg Gynecol Obstet. 1990;171(1):65–7.
47. Koval KJ, Egol KA, Polatsch DB, Baskies MA, Homman JP, Hiebert RNJ. Tape blisters following hip surgery. A prospective, randomized study of two types of tape. Bone Joint Surg Am. 2003;85(10):1884–7.
48. Smith and Nephew Inc. Measurement and application process for collagenase SANTYL® ointment [Internet] 2014. Available from: http://www.santyl.com/hcp/application
49. Shannon MM. A retrospective descriptive study of nursing home residents with heel Eschar or Blisters. Ostomy Wound Manage. 2013;59(1):20–7.
50. Legood R, McInnes E. Pressure ulcers: guideline development and economic modelling. J Adv Nurs. 2005;50(3):307–14.
51. McInnes E, Asmara JB, Bell-Syer S, Dumville J, Cullum N. Preventing pressure ulcers—are pressure-redistributing support surfaces effective? A Cochrane systematic review and meta-analysis. Int J Nurs Stud. 2012;49(3):345–59.
52. National Pressure Ulcer Advisory Panel Terms and Definitions Related to Support Surfaces [Internet] 29 Jan 2007. Available from: http://www.npuap.org/wp-content/uploads/2012/03/NPUAP_S3I_TD.pdf
53. Center for Medicaid and Medicare Services. Medicare policy regarding pressure reducing support surfaces – JA1014 [Internet] 24 Aug 2010. Available from: http://www.cms.gov/Medicare/Medicare-Contracting/ContractorLearningResources/downloads/JA1014.pdf
54. Junkin J, Gray M. Are pressure redistribution surfaces or heel protection devices effective for preventing heel pressure ulcers? J Wound Ostomy Continence Nurse. 2009;36(6):602–8.
55. Eberhardt RT, Raffetto JD. Chronic venous insufficiency. Circulation. 2014;130:333–46.
56. Greer N, Foman NA, MacDonald R, Dorrian J, Fitzgerald P, Rutks I, Wilt TJ. Advanced wound care therapies for nonhealing diabetic, venous, and arterial ulcers. Ann Int Med. 2013;159(8):532–42.

57. Samson RH, Showalter DP. Stockings and the prevention of recurrent venous ulcers. Dermatol Surg. 1996;22(4):373–6.
58. Lazarides MK, Giannoukas AD. The role of hemodynamic measurements in the management of venous and ischemic ulcers. Int J Low Extrem Wounds. 2007;6(4):254–61.
59. Aboyans V, Criqui MH, Abraham P, Allison MA, Creager MA, Diehm C, Fowkes FGR, Hiatt WR, Jönsson B, Lacroix P, Marin B, McDermott MM, Norgren L, Pande RL, Preux P-M, Stoffers HE, Treat-Jacobson D. Measurement and interpretation of the ankle-brachial index: a scientific statement from the American Heart Association. Circulation. 2012;126:1–20.
60. Kelechi T, Johnson JJ. Guideline for the management of wounds in patients with lower-extremity venous disease. J Wound Ostomy Continence Nurs. 2012;39(6):598–606.
61. O'Meara S, Cullum N, Nelson EA, Dumville JC. Compression for venous leg ulcers. Cochrane Database Syst Rev. 2012;11, CD000265.
62. Moffatt C. Four-layer bandaging: from concept to practice. Part 2: Application of the four-layer system. [Internet]. Mar 2005. Available from: http://www.worldwidewounds.com/2005/march/Moffatt/Four-Layer-Bandage-System-Part2.html#ref17
63. Introduction to Profore. [Internet] Date unknown. Available from: http://www.smith-nephew.com/professional/products/advanced-wound-management/profore
64. Polignano R, Bonadeo P, Gasbarro S, Allegra C. A randomised controlled study of four-layer compression versus Unna's Boot for venous ulcers. J Wound Care. 2004;13(1):21–4.
65. Milic DJ, Zivic SS, Bogdanovic DC, Karanovic ND, Golubovic ZV. Risk factors related to the failure of venous leg ulcers to heal with compression treatment. J Vasc Surg. 2009;49(5):1242–7.
66. Pittler MH, Ernst E. Horse chestnut seed extract for chronic venous insufficiency. Cochrane Database Syst Rev. 2012;11, CD003230.
67. Padberg Jr FT, Johnston MV, Sisto SA. Structured exercise improves calf muscle pump function in chronic venous insufficiency: a randomized trial. J Vasc Surg. 2004;39:79–87.
68. Hirsch AT, Criqui MH, Treat-Jacobson D, Regensteiner JG, Creager MA, Olin JW, Krook SH, Hunninghake DB, Comerota AJ, Walsh ME, McDermott MM, Hiatt WR. Peripheral arterial disease detection, awareness, and treatment in the primary care. JAMA. 2001;286(11):1317–24.
69. Hopf HW, Ueno C, Aslam R, Burnand K, Fife C, Grant L, Holloway A, Iafrati MD, Mani R, Misare B, Rosen N, Shapshak D, Benjamin Slade Jr J, West J, Barbul A. Guidelines for the treatment of arterial insufficiency ulcers. Wound Repair Regen. 2006;14(6):693–710.
70. Scottish Intercollegiate Guidelines Network. Diagnosis and management of peripheral arterial disease: A national clinical guideline [Internet]. 2006. Available from http://www.sign.ac.uk/pdf/sign89.pdf
71. Grey JE, Harding KG, Enoch S. Venous and arterial leg ulcers. BMJ. 2006;332(7537):347–50.
72. Sieggreen MY, Kline RA. Arterial insufficiency and ulceration - diagnosis and treatment options. Nurse Pract. 2004;29:46–52.
73. British Columbia Provincial Nursing Skin and Wound Committee Guideline: Assessment and Treatment of Lower Leg Ulcers (Arterial, Venous & Mixed) in Adults [Internet]. Aug 2014. Available from: https://www.clwk.ca/buddydrive/file/guideline-lower-limb-venous-arterial/
74. Hamburg NM, Balady GJ. Exercise rehabilitation in peripheral artery disease: functional impact and mechanisms of benefits. Circulation. 2011;123(1):87–97.
75. Wound infection in clinical practice. An international consensus. Int Wound J. 2008;5(Suppl 3):iii–11.
76. O'Brien C. Malignant wounds: managing odour. Can Fam Physician. 2012;58(3):272–4.
77. Fleck CA. Fighting odor in wounds. Adv Skin Wound Care. 2006;19(5):242–4.
78. Andrews KL, Houdek MT, Kiemele LJ. Wound management of chronic diabetic foot ulcers: from the basics to regenerative medicine. Prosthet Orthot Int. 2015;39(1):29–39.
79. Rai NK, Suryabhan, Ansari M, Kumar M, Shukla VK, Tripathi K. Effect of glycaemic control on apoptosis in diabetic wounds. J Wound Care. 2005;14(6):277–81.

80. Chow I, Lemos EV, Einarson TR. Management and prevention of diabetic foot ulcers and infections: a health economic review. Pharmacoeconomics. 2008;26(12):1019–35.
81. Apelqvist J, Ragnarson TG. Cavity foot ulcers in diabetic patients: a comparative study of cadexomer iodine ointment and standard treatment. An economic analysis alongside a clinical trial. Acta Derm Venereol. 1996;76(3):231–5.
82. Lookingbill DP, Spangler N, Helm KF. Cutaneous metastases in patients with metastatic carcinoma: a retrospective study of 4020 patients. J Am Acad Dermatol. 1993;29:228–36.
83. Recka K, Montagnini M, Vitale C. Management of bleeding associated with malignant wounds. J Palliat Med. 2012;15(8):952–4.
84. Probst S, Arber A, Faithfull S. Malignant fungating wounds: the meaning of living in an unbounded body. Eur J Oncol Nurs. 2013;17(1):38–45.
85. Fromantin I, Seyer D, Watson S, et al. Bacterial floras and biofilms of malignant wounds associated with breast cancers. J Clin Microbiol. 2013;51(10):3368–73.
86. Merz T, Klein C, Uebach B. Fungating wounds - multidimensional challenge in palliative care. Breast Care. 2011;6(1):21–4.
87. Orgill D, Bayer L. Update on negative pressure wound therapy. Plastic Recon Surg. 2011;127(Suppl 1S):105S–15.
88. Malmsjo M, Ingemansson R, Martin R, Huddleston E. Wound edge microvascular blood flow: effects of negative pressure wound therapy using gauze or polyurethane foam. Ann Plast Surg. 2009;63(6):676–81.
89. Orgill D, Bayer L. Negative pressure wound therapy: past, present and future. Int Wound J. 2013;10 Suppl 1:15–9.
90. Update on serious complications associated with negative pressure wound therapy systems: FDA Safety Communication. [Internet] 24 Feb 2011. Available from: http://www.fda.gov/MedicalDevices/Safety/AlertsandNotices/ucm244211.htm
91. Billing and Coding Guidelines: GSURG-051 Wound Care. [Internet]. 2011. Available from: http://downloads.cms.gov/medicare-coverage-database/lcd_attachments/28572_20/l28572_gsurg051_cbg_010111.pdf
92. Poggio A. A guide to coding for outpatient and in-hospital debridement. Podiatry Today. [Internet] 2011;24(8). Available from: http://www.podiatrytoday.com/guide-coding-outpatient-and-hospital-debridement
93. January 2015 Update of the Hospital Outpatient Prospective Payment System (OPPS). [Internet]. 22 Dec 2014. Available from: http://www.cms.gov/Outreach-and-Education/Medicare-Learning-Network-MLN/MLNMattersArticles/downloads/MM9014.pdf

Social and Ethical Issues in Home-Based Medical Care

11

Thomas E. Finucane

Abstract

Patients whose illness and frailty are severe enough to render them homebound are usually dependent on others for care. Individual autonomy is often restricted by financial and social limitations. The determination of capacity is extremely complex, and in many cases no "gold standard" can be used to make objective decisions about the presence or absence of capacity.

Lines of legal responsibility are often unclear or absent, making the designation of "neglect" difficult. Such relationships are often under a good deal of stress, and many have an extensive and disputed history. "Abuse" is essentially a criminal charge, a very serious allegation likely to disrupt relationships among patient, caregiver, and medical professional.

Decision-making about life-sustaining treatment can be complex, especially when a patient's capacity is in doubt or clearly lacking. Advance directives are imperfect tools that attempt to preserve the voice of a person who is no longer able to speak meaningfully about life-and-death choices. Their definitions, regulations, and nomenclature vary from jurisdiction to jurisdiction.

Home-based medical clinicians must routinely make sophisticated judgments about (1) whether the patient (and sometimes the surrogate) has decisional capacity, (2) whether current arrangements are illegal and could be improved by legal intervention, and (3) how best to honor the patient as a person when suffering and other burdens are rising and prognosis and other benefits are falling.

Keywords

Capacity • Competence • Abuse • Neglect • Living will • Health-care agent • Substitute decision-making

T.E. Finucane, M.D. (✉)
Johns Hopkins Bayview Medical Center,
5200 Eastern Avenue, Suite 2200, Baltimore, MD 21224, USA
e-mail: tfinucan@jhmi.edu

© Springer International Publishing Switzerland 2016
J.L. Hayashi, B. Leff (eds.), *Geriatric Home-Based Medical Care*,
DOI 10.1007/978-3-319-23365-9_11

237

11.1   Brief Summary

Ethical and social issues permeate the care of homebound patients who depend on others. Patients who can speak up for themselves often face very difficult choices. Patients who lack the capacity to speak for themselves may present even more complex decision-making problems. The determination of capacity generally cannot be done with simple or objective tests except in the most clear-cut cases. This determination is critical with respect to both the definition and management of potential elder abuse and to the use of advance directives.

11.2   Key Points

1. The determination of capacity requires an understanding of the task at hand.
2. This determination often requires judgment beyond the medicolegal.
3. Elder abuse is one extreme of a continuum of caregiver or companion behaviors that ranges from the heroic to the criminal.
4. In end-of-life decision-making, designated substitute decision-makers, sometimes called "health-care agents," are likely to be more useful than living wills in most jurisdictions.
5. Clinicians who make house calls are uniquely positioned to judge capacity, identify abuse, and help with advance care planning.

11.3   Introduction

In the poem "He Makes a House Call," Dr. John Stone wrote that "Health is whatever works, and for as long" [1]. He located this definition of health within the context of a house call and could well have been talking about a homebound patient with disabling conditions and the fabric of caregivers on whom such a dependent patient depends. Many homebound patients who are quite ill nonetheless lead full and authentic lives and are quite happy to do so. After making house calls for just over a year, a clinician once observed that as a result "I have radically redefined what I mean when I say that a patient is really sick."

Office visits and house calls differ in important ways that are relevant to the perspective of a home-based medical provider. First, in the more standard clinic-based encounter, a patient arrives at a clinician's place. The initiative for the visit has originated with the patient or companions, which may require a substantial commitment from both, and they frequently have an agenda. Clinicians are often, in a certain way, responding. In house calls, in contrast, the context and the contract are quite different; clinicians take the initiative to go to the patient. If the patient/companion initiative is not required, engagement with a home-based medical provider may be weaker. More often, when a patient recognizes the home-based medical provider's commitment to her health and the willingness to do what it takes to provide needed care, a high level of trust will develop and patient engagement is augmented. The difference between clinic visits and house calls in clinician-patient relationship can be seen indirectly. If a patient stops coming to the clinic, his clinician might or might not track him down. An unanswered knock on the front door of a homebound patient, in contrast, may create a distinctly different sense of obligation.

In addition, clinicians visiting a home may incidentally obtain additional dimensions of information almost completely unavailable in the clinic. The distinction between medical and social needs, always a challenging matter in care of vulnerable adults, may be far more direct and dramatic to a clinician in the living room. Meeting the medical and social needs of a homebound patient can present tragic challenges and trade-offs.

A third difference between clinic visits and house calls can be called the "locus of control." In the clinic, patients are usually outnumbered strangers in strange lands. The power dynamic strongly favors the health-care system. During a house call, patients are at home: "Here, you are in charge - of figs, beans, tomatoes, life" [1].

A lengthy array of ethical and social issues arise in the care (often long term) of a homebound patient who is often frail, dependent, chronically ill, cognitively impaired, impoverished or becoming so, or some combination of these characteristics. In this chapter, we will focus on two important issues: mistreatment of vulnerable adults and advance planning for life-threatening illness. Because the constructs of "vulnerable adult" and of "advance directives" both depend heavily on whether a patient has the capacity to make decisions, we begin with a discussion on capacity.

11.4   Autonomy, Capacity, and Respect for Persons

In general, referral to Adult Protective Services for review of relationships and living situation is reserved for vulnerable persons, who lack the physical or cognitive capacity to defend themselves in an abusive or neglectful situation. In general, advance directives take effect when the individual no longer has the capacity to make complex decisions about life-sustaining medical treatment but has previously left guidance about such decisions. In these models, "capacity" is considered as a binary value; patients either have it or lack it.

11.4.1 Decisional Capacity Is Not a Yes-Or-No Characteristic

In general, people are assumed to have the ability to speak for themselves; the possibility that they lack this ability is not routinely considered. Questions about capacity usually arise in patients with neurologic or psychiatric symptomatology. For practical purposes, it would be most useful to classify a patient as either having or lacking capacity. Several problems arise in this endeavor, however. First, cognitive capacity may wax and wane due to disease, medications, illness, and other patient-related factors. A common characteristic of Lewy body dementia and of severe infection is variability in sensorium. Second, decisions may change depending on circumstances. A competent, determined bedtime decision to get up at 6 a.m. and work in the garden may be replaced by an equally competent and determined decision at 6 a.m. to stay in bed. Third, judgments about capacity depend on the task at hand. Competence at playing bridge does not imply competence at playing shortstop. Similarly, a person may be capable of accepting the risk of a fall and consequent prolonged interval on the floor but not capable of deciding about major surgery or toxic chemotherapy. "Judgments of incompetence are therefore impossible to understand unless a task is assumed or specified" [2].

Fourth, and perhaps the most important, is the generally subjective nature of competency determinations. The essence of this problem was well summarized many years ago: "The search for a single test of competence is a search for the Holy Grail. Unless it is realized that there is no magical definition of competency to make decisions about treatment, the search for an acceptable test will never end … judgments (about competence) reflect social considerations and societal biases as much as they reflect matters of law and medicine" [3]. "Competence" is considered more to be a legal term and "capacity" to be a clinical term. The distinction is rarely useful when plain English is being spoken.

The general elements that suggest a patient has capacity are shown in Table 11.1, although this is necessarily a simplification. In addition, the ability to make a reasonable decision has been proposed as a criterion and discussed at length, without clear resolution. Here most clearly, decisions about what is "reasonable" may not be a matter for objective determination.

11.4.2 Threshold for Evaluation and Certification of Incapacity

Even when a person can satisfy these criteria, social considerations and societal biases will influence many determinations. The capacity to make decisions is most often sought when the outcomes are high stakes and the patient's wishes do not conform to the clinician's recommendations. Stated differently, patients may be perceived to be competent to say "yes" to a clinician but not competent to say "no."

In one view, great weight should be given to a marginally competent patient's stated preferences unless there is avoidable suffering or a clear risk of severe and avoidable harm; in these circumstances, coercive activity is more easily acceptable. Defining what level of risk is unacceptable may still remain a cause of argument.

In another view, a patient's dignity (and the social contract) may require action if the patient's situation surpasses some level of offensiveness even if no physical

Table 11.1 Suggested abilities to look for when determining capacity

Accurately understand the choices
Manipulate relevant information and weigh risks and benefits
Communicate a decision
Be consistent

harm results [4]. Extreme squalor, indifference to personal hygiene, and very odd social behaviors or relationships may provoke some clinicians to diagnose abuse or self-neglect and alert the authorities. Ignoring a cognitively impaired or mentally ill person who is being exploited or simply can no longer care for herself is unconscionable. But certifying that someone is incapacitated and then depriving her of her freedom simply to enforce a socially acceptable lifestyle is also wrong. Personal as well as societal biases will influence many determinations.

11.4.3 Practical Matters

The idea of capacity is closely linked to philosophical ideas about free will and personal responsibility; this is one reason the determination of capacity will remain controversial and difficult. The practical importance of this observation is that for any person who is conversational, the only valid way to judge capacity is to have a conversation with that person. Documentation of capacity is best done by a careful record of that conversation. Scores on popular cognitive tests have little additional value. The ability to describe the consequences of the proposed options and to explain why a particular option is being chosen is enough to satisfy most clinicians.

A sample note is given in Box 11.1. For patients whose communication abilities are limited, the determination of capacity will be more difficult. A plain English description of the patient's understanding of and reasoning about treatment options is generally the best way to document how the clinician judged the patient to have or lack decisional capacity about the specific management plan in question.

Box 11.1 Sample Informed Consent Discussion

Today Ms. Jones and I discussed her recent hospitalization, especially the fall, fracture, rhabdomyolysis, renal failure, and brief maintenance on dialysis. She describes this as the worst 4 weeks of her life and realizes that her life was in serious danger during that hospitalization. She insists, however, that she would rather go through the entire experience a second time, including the risk of death, than leave her home. She can name several important danger points, including the bathroom, the front steps, and especially the basement steps on the way back up with clean laundry. She feels she has made all home modifications that are reasonable and affordable and sees no other good options. Absolutely refuses to consider any alternative housing, including her daughter's home. Was interested in Shepherd's Pasture assisted living facility but is unwilling to spend that amount of money for room and board. She remains estranged from her husband and son, whom she does not wish us to contact. Her mini-mental state examination (MMSE) today is 21/30, stable. I believe she understands the risks of her decision to stay home and is willing to undertake them, especially given her lack of reasonable/acceptable alternatives.

Box 11.2 is taken from the court record of a man with severe traumatic brain injury suffered 4 years earlier. The proceeding is to determine whether his feeding tube should be replaced to prolong his life (which would arguably have violated his previously expressed wishes). His competence is at issue. Under life-and-death circumstances, experts could not decisively determine whether the patient had capacity. Questions about competence may range from the trivial to the unsolvable [5].

On this shaky platform are built the legal, ethical, and clinical frameworks for both elder mistreatment and advance directives.

Box 11.2 Excerpt from Trial Transcript Where Capacity Is at Issue [5]
"Dr. Kass acknowledged there was no way to verify whether Robert "really understood the questions or not," but "(t)he reason I asked those questions," Dr. Kass continued, "is because (Robert) was able to answer the previous questions mostly correctly. So I thought perhaps he could understand more questions." Dr. Kass believed Robert probably understood some but not all of the questions. Robert's speech pathologist, Lowana Brauer, testified generally that Robert used the augmented communications device primarily as therapy and not with enough consistency to justify leaving the device in his room for communication with other people. She did not, however, testify specifically about the interaction between Robert and Dr. Kass."

11.5   Elder Abuse and Self-Neglect

Tolstoy begins *Anna Karenina*, "All happyfamilies are alike. But every unhappy family is unhappy in its own way." Most care at home is provided with dedication and generosity and much of it in highly constrained circumstances. Some degree of caregiver impatience, burnout, and anger are probably common. Patient, caregiver, and circumstantial factors may increase the risk of decompensation. When the patient is somehow too vulnerable and the interactions are too cruel, a patient may be said to suffer "abuse." As with the concept of capacity, some cases are clear-cut and beyond dispute. In many situations, however, there is no bright line but rather a continuous gradation from niceness to criminal behavior occurring in the context of a family with its history and a cultural understanding that may differ from the clinician's.

In this section, we will consider homebound, vulnerable adults of any age. Because most such adults are elderly, the term "elder abuse" is commonly used.

The federal National Center on Elder Abuse notes that "Federal definitions of elder abuse first appeared in the 1987 Amendments to the Older Americans Act, however, these definitions are guidelines. Each state defines elder abuse according to its unique statutes and regulations, and definitions vary from state to state. Researchers also use varying definitions to describe and study the problem" [6]. Definitions are variable and generally unhelpful; focused on risk, harm, and safety;

Table 11.2 Common subtyping of abuse and neglect

Physical abuse
Social or mental abuse
Sexual abuse
Financial exploitation
Neglect
Self-neglect

Table 11.3 Some definitions related to elder abuse

World Health Organization [7]:
A single, or repeated act, or lack of appropriate action, occurring within any relationship where there is an expectation of trust which causes harm or distress to an older person
US Administration on Aging [8]:
Any knowing, intentional, or negligent act by a caregiver or any other person that causes harm or a serious risk of harm to a vulnerable adult
MedlinePlus [9]:
It is the mistreatment of an older person, usually by a caregiver. It can happen within the family. It can also happen in assisted living facilities or nursing homes
National Research Council [10]:
"Elder mistreatment" refers to (a) intentional actions that cause harm or create a serious risk of harm (whether or not harm is intended) to a vulnerable elder by a caregiver or other person who stands in a trust relationship to the elder or (b) failure by a caregiver to satisfy the elder's basic needs or to protect the elder from harm

and often discussed in the language of rights and victims. Table 11.2 shows a common schema for subtyping abuse and neglect.

Table 11.3 lists a variety of definitions [7–10]. Purported signs of abuse and neglect include pressure sores, weight loss, and medication nonadherence. The first two of these are common among chronically ill patients who are receiving absolutely good care. The third is highly prevalent in all care settings and patient groups. Here are three situations which might be classified differently according to the different definitions:

1. An elderly couple has a long tradition of bitter arguments. Hurtful remarks by each other are common and repetitive.
2. One partner asks for the tenth time in 2 h whether they've had lunch yet today. The other responds sharply with the intention of discouraging the further repetition of that question.
3. A bedfast patient with urinary frequency wears a diaper. The caregiver allows a certain interval of time to pass between diaper changes.

Each of these three interactions meets at least one of the definitions of elder abuse. How long a person may be left wet in a diaper, if there are no adverse medical consequences, before a finding of neglect should be made is a very complex question indeed.

Despite the lack of a serious definition, "elder abuse" is described as common, important, underdiagnosed, and underreported. A variety of laws have been passed, centers established, and guidelines promulgated—without consistent definition. Further, the US Preventive Services Task Force has concluded "that the current evidence is insufficient to assess the balance of benefits and harms" of screening vulnerable and elderly adults. Evidence is lacking, of poor quality, or conflicting and the balance of benefits and harms cannot be determined" [11]. Our failure to understand, diagnose, and prevent elder abuse is often attributed to a lack of research. An even more fundamental lack is a consensus definition on which to base the research. Homebound patients, often with high-level physical or mental disability or both, may require a great deal of long-term care in very difficult circumstances. In many cases, the caregiver is uncompensated and the patient is not a passive victim.

A state-by-state summary of relevant definitions, agencies, laws, and referral sources is available from the National Center on Elder Abuse of the federal Administration on Aging at http://www.ncea.aoa.gov/Stop_Abuse/Get_Help/State/index.aspx. Questions of referral to Adult Protective Services (APS) or consideration of guardianship are often more legal, tactical, medicolegal, and economic than they are medical, social, or ethical. Most states have mandatory reporting requirements for suspected abuse.

Because there are no data to suggest that referral to Adult Protective Services is more likely to help than to harm, clinicians in states with mandatory reporting of elder abuse are in an extremely difficult position. Taking on police or judicial functions is difficult for many physicians, who are primarily interested in finding the optimal situation, both medical and social, for their patients. In addition, the clinician's duty to protect her patient's confidentiality is in direct conflict with this duty to report, unless the patient requests that the information be conveyed. A general hesitation has been expressed previously with respect to intimate partner violence, a problem that overlaps substantially with elder abuse.

> Passionate entwined idiosyncrasies are often central to a marriage or other intimate partnership. These things are older than medicine. I think physicians should be very careful about medicalizing any one strand of such a profound and complex relationship. Some of this is none of our business. Preventing harm to patients is of course a central mission. But physicians should have good data [showing] that we can help before we break into a marriage, discover personal information from one of the partners, document this, and then make referrals to straighten the relationship out [12].

In addition to the social situation and historical clues, evidence of physical harm must be evaluated carefully. House calls will usually provide a much richer picture of the situation. Adjustments in the home environment may suggest themselves on-site. Possible alternative sources or sites of care may be realistically considered while in the home. Our practice is to ask something like "Are things OK on the home front?" in preference to the more widely touted "Do you feel safe at home?" For some elderly patients, this use of the word "safe" is taken as a question about grab bars in the bathroom and smoke alarms in the kitchen. Table 11.4 shows characteristics of patients and caregivers that have been associated with elder abuse.

Table 11.4 Characteristics of patient, caregiver, or both associated with risk of "elder abuse"

| High level of impairment and dependency with many care needs |
| Psychiatric illness and/or substance abuse |
| History of abusive relationships |
| Limited financial and/or social resources |
| Social isolation |

"Neglect," sometimes included as a form of elder abuse and sometimes considered separately, is also very difficult to define. Many caregivers, such as adult children, have no direct legal duty to the person for whom they care. If such caregivers, making the best of a bad situation, provide inadequate care by some test and are referred to APS, they may interpret the referral as a provocation and may then worsen the situation. If well done, in contrast, APS referral may work as a form of coaching, providing a new perspective and suggestions for improvement in a very cloistered situation.

However well-intentioned, referral of a patient to APS is generally equivalent to an accusation. This allegation of abuse or neglect is often being made against the person who is providing the bulk of the patient's care. This may lead to discontinuation of the clinician-patient and perhaps the caregiver-patient relationship, thus leading ultimately to harm. Ideally, such referrals would be made with the patient's permission and the consent of the caregiver. It would be seen as a step toward improving situations which are overwhelming to the caregiver. Involuntary referral is very similar to a slow-motion 911 call.

11.6   Advance Directives

For competent patients, decisions about potentially life-sustaining treatment can be very difficult. Three things are generally true about most patients: They do not wish to suffer, they do not wish to die, and they do not wish to talk openly about the trade-offs. Each of these wishes becomes more apparent to patients as death comes nearer. In a questionnaire study, subjects without cancer were more likely to decline noncurative, toxic chemotherapy for an advanced cancer than subjects who actually had advanced cancer [13]. Fair evidence shows that clinicians and caregivers may underestimate a patient's quality of life and desire to accept aggressive treatment.

In a separate study, the majority of patients with metastatic colon or lung cancer taking chemotherapy did not understand that this therapy was very unlikely to be curative. Patients who rated their physician most favorably had the highest rate of misunderstanding. "Physicians may be able to improve patients' understanding, but this may come at the cost of patients' satisfaction with them" [14].

Seeing patients at home, clinicians may be more able understand how a chronically ill patient is living and what the benefits and burdens of treatment might be.

Because of the relationship's nature, they may be able to improve a patient's understanding without undermining the relationship. A study done in a house call program, however, showed that homebound patients with poor prognosis remain reluctant to participate in advance care planning, except when death is near and certain [15].

The right of a competent patient to decline treatment, even if it would be life saving, is reasonably well established in most cases. A far more complex, and legally less well-defined, question arises when a patient can no longer decline, or accept, such treatment. In an attempt to preserve autonomy when capacity is no longer present, two legal instruments have been devised. These intend to allow a competent patient to leave advice about how medical decisions should be made if she were to become incapacitated. In a living will, the patient leaves specific guidance about certain medical treatments that may be considered in the uncertain future. With a health-care agent, the patient designates substitute decision-makers who are then authorized to make decisions on behalf of the patient.

The nomenclature can be confusing. (1) In some states, "advance directives" are synonymous with "living wills," and "health-care agents" are treated separately. In other states, "advance directive" is the umbrella term that includes both "living wills" and "health-care agents." We will use the latter schema. (2) A substitute decision-maker may be acting because the patient, previously competent, has designated her for this task. Some terms used by states to refer to the designated decision-maker include agent (e.g., Maryland), proxy (e.g., New York), surrogate (e.g., Florida), advocate (e.g., Michigan), health-care representative (e.g., Oregon), and (durable) power of attorney for health care (e.g., Delaware). (3) If no substitute decision-maker is designated, then a default decision-maker may be identified. Terms used to refer to this person are also quite variable and may overlap or directly contradict the terms used in other states.

To make matters worse, there is a great deal of variability among the states in the degree of authority that is granted to default substitutes compared to designated substitutes. In Virginia and Washington, DC, the default substitute has nearly as much authority as the designated substitute. Maryland tends to be much more restrictive in the authority of the default substitute. State-by-state advance directive forms are available online (http://www.caringinfo.org/i4a/pages/index.cfm?pageid=3289). Because of their wide variability, clinicians should know the relevant specifics if they are engaging patients in these discussions.

11.6.1 Living Wills

In general, the discussion of the living will is a complex matter for a patient. The patient must keep these two hypothetical circumstances in mind. The clinician asks him to imagine both that he has become sick enough that decisions about life-sustaining treatments are needed and that he has become unable to make those decisions. The patient then makes a binding, but revocable, decision about which treatments he would decline or accept. One way to phrase this to the patient, very carefully, is to ask if there are conditions where he would think himself better off dead than taking treatment to try to prolong life.

Many clinicians can recall patients who have left advance directives to limit treatment (e.g., "I never want to be intubated again") but then change their minds and do not reject treatment when it would avert death. The Wendland case referenced in Box 11.2 appears to describe exactly such a reversal [5].

A paper entitled "The End of History Illusion" raises further serious questions about the concept of advance directives. Based on measurements made on over 19,000 adults from age 18 to 68 years, the authors conclude that "Young people, middle-aged people, and older people all believed they had changed a lot in the past but would change relatively little in the future. People, it seems, regard the present as a watershed moment at which they have finally become the person they will be for the rest of their lives" [16]. If these subjects were reinterviewed 10 years later, they would presumably again report that they had changed greatly in the interim but would not change much in the future. Decisions about what would be worse than death might seem immutable at the time they are made and be highly inaccurate after some time has passed.

Perhaps because decisions like these may be so changeable, many states have strictly limited the situations in which living wills are valid. In several states, they refer only to treatment limitation in the event of terminal illness. In several, they are valid only if the patient is terminally ill or in a persistent vegetative state. Each state's designated categories should be carefully understood before completing a living will with a patient. In general, this document is far less useful for clinicians because of the very circumscribed circumstances that so limit its use in many jurisdictions.

11.6.2 Designated Substitute Decision-Maker

As noted above, the name for a substitute decision-maker who is designated by the patient varies greatly among jurisdictions (agent, representative, proxy, and surrogate, among others). Once again varying among jurisdictions, a substitute who has been designated is usually given a great deal of authority to make medical decisions on behalf of a patient who is no longer able to decide for herself. In Maryland, the health-care agent can make virtually any decision that the patient could make if she were still capable unless the signer has added restrictions to the document. An important exception is involuntary psychiatric treatment, which cannot be given on the basis of an agent's authorization. Other states place some restrictions on the authority of the agent to decline life-sustaining treatment. Finally, many states allow a patient to designate the substitute and grant decisional authority to that agent at the time the document is signed.

Designating a substitute decision-maker is generally a far simpler task cognitively than deciding about hypothetical treatment decisions during hypothetical future life-threatening illnesses in the context of a hypothetical incapacitating cognitive impairment, decisions which are often very difficult for a competent patient.

In addition, the discussion about designating an agent probably has less emotional impact than the discussion required to complete a living will (imagine you have both advanced cancer and Alzheimer disease). We suggest a discussion about health-care agents, built around this question. "You know that if we need to make any decisions about treatment, we'll ask you how you would like things to be done. But let's say that something happened to you. Let's say you hit your head on the windshield and we couldn't talk to you. Who is it that we should talk to about your care?"

The formalities for recording advance directives vary from state to state. Some but not all require notarization. In many states, lawyers are not required. Repositories in which to store advance directives are available online. There is little published experience about their utility. We advise patients to give copies of the documents to their physician, the person(s) named as agent, and one or two other close friends. An electronic solution to the problem of providing the document as needed should be forthcoming.

11.7 Conclusion

In an important essay, Broyard points out that "To most physicians my illness is a routine incident in their rounds, whilst for me it is the crisis of my life." In home-based medical care, the illness is neither routine nor an incident. The clinician has a far richer understanding of the patient's (and the caregiver's) situation. Decisions made in this context can more fully honor and respect the patient as a person [17].

References

1. Stone J. He makes a house call (Internet) 2014 (cited 15 Feb 2015) Available from: https://utmedhumanities.wordpress.com/2014/03/16/he-makes-a-house-call-john-stone/.   Accessed on 15 Feb 2015
2. Faden RR, Beauchamp TL. A history and theory of informed consent. New York: Oxford University Press; 1986. Chapter 8.
3. Roth LH, Meisel A, Lidz CW. Tests of competency to consent to treatment. Am J Psychiatry. 1977;134(3):279–84.
4. Foster C. Putting dignity to work. Lancet. 2012;379(9831):2044–5.
5. Conservatorship of Wendland (Internet). 2001. (cited 15 Feb 2015). Available from http://law.justia.com/cases/california/supreme-court/4th/26/519.html
6. State resources (Internet). (cited 15 Feb 2015). Available from http://www.ncea.aoa.gov/Stop_Abuse/Get_ Help/State/index.aspx
7. Elder abuse (Internet). (cited 15 Feb 2015). Available from http://www.who.int/ageing/projects/elder_abuse/en/
8. What is elder abuse? (Internet). 2015. (updated 12/31/2014; cited 15 Feb 2015). Available from http://www.aoa.gov/AoA_programs/Elder_Rights/EA_Prevention/whatIsEA.aspx
9. Elder abuse (Internet). 2014. (cited 15 Feb 2015). Available from http://www.nlm.nih.gov/medlineplus/elderabuse.html
10. Bonnie RJ, Wallace RB, editors. Elder mistreatment: abuse, neglect and exploitation in aging America (Internet). 2003. (cited 15 Feb 2015). Available from http://www.nap.edu/download.php?record_id=10406

11. Moyer VA. Screening for intimate partner violence and abuse of elderly and vulnerable adults: U.S. preventive services task force recommendation. Ann Intern Med. 2013;158(6):478–86.
12. Finucane TE. Intervening in abusive relationships. JAMA. 2003;289(17):2211–2.
13. Slevin ML, Stubbs L, Plant HJ, et al. Attitudes to chemotherapy: comparing views of patients with cancer with those of doctors, nurses, and general public. BMJ. 1990;300:1458–60.
14. Weeks JC, Catalano PJ, Cronin A, et al. Patients' expectations about effects of chemotherapy for advanced cancer. N Engl J Med. 2012;367(17):1616–25.
15. Carrese JA, Mullaney JL, Faden R, et al. Planning for death but not serious future illness: qualitative study of housebound elderly patients. BMJ. 2002;325(7356):125.
16. Quoidbach J, Gilbert DT, Wilson TD. The end of history illusion. Science. 2013; 339(6115):96–8.
17. Broyard A. Doctor talk to me. New York Times. 26 Aug 26 1990.

Further Reading

Broyard A. Doctor talk to me. New York Times. 26 Aug 26 1990.
Conservatorship of Wendland (Internet). 2001. (cited 15 Feb 2015). Available from http://law.justia.com/cases/california/supreme-court/4th/26/519.html
Finucane TE. How gravely ill becomes dying: a key to end-of-life care. JAMA. 1999;282(17):1670–2.
State Resources (Internet). (cited 15 Feb 2015). Available from http://www.ncea.aoa.gov/Stop_Abuse/Get_Help/State/index.aspx

Palliative Care

12

Christine S. Ritchie and Martha L. Twaddle

Abstract

Home-based palliative care is emerging as an important component of home-based medical care. Because a majority of homebound adults have serious illness and high symptom burden, every home-based medical provider should be well-versed in basic palliative care skills. This chapter describes communication strategies to clarify patient's goals of care, rationale and approaches to prognostication, and management of common symptoms experienced in the home (depression, pain, anorexia, and dyspnea). In addition, it covers the basic principles and framework of hospice care and tools to support advance care planning.

Keywords

Palliative care • Goals of care • Prognosis • Depression • Pain • Dyspnea • Hospice

12.1 Emerging Models of Home-Based Palliative Care

With an increasing recognition that many individuals with serious illness experience high illness burden and functional challenges for years and not just months, home-based palliative care is emerging as an important component of home-based medical care that presages and complements services provided by hospice.

C.S. Ritchie, M.D., M.S.P.H. (✉)
Division of Geriatrics, Department of Medicine, University of California San Francisco, 3333 California Street, Suite 380, San Francisco, CA 94143-1265, USA
e-mail: Christine.Ritchie@ucsf.edu

M.L. Twaddle, M.D.
Palliative Medicine, Northwestern University Feinberg School of Medicine, 211 E. Ontario, Suite 700, Chicago, IL 60611, USA
e-mail: martha.twaddle@northwestern.edu

© Springer International Publishing Switzerland 2016
J.L. Hayashi, B. Leff (eds.), *Geriatric Home-Based Medical Care*,
DOI 10.1007/978-3-319-23365-9_12

A number of home-based palliative care models are now filling the landscape of community-based care. The most common models fall into the following categories: home-based palliative care programs that are part of the continuum with hospital-based palliative care programs, home-based palliative care programs as a subset of home-based primary care programs, stand-alone consultative home-based palliative care programs, or palliative care programs provided by hospices and functioning outside of the traditional hospice benefit.

There is tremendous overlap between home-based primary care and home-based palliative care (Fig. 12.1). Practically speaking, because of the relative poor prognosis and high symptom burden of many patients seen in home-based primary care, all home-based primary care practices should be practicing *primary palliative care* (Table 12.1). However, for patients with particularly refractory pain or other symptoms; complex depression, anxiety, or grief; existential distress; or needs for assistance with conflict resolution around goals or methods of treatment, the provision of specialty palliative care in the home is appropriate.

Specialty palliative care involves healthcare professionals certified in hospice and palliative care. By definition, palliative care promotes an interprofessional approach that requires the active collaboration of medicine, nursing, and social work along with a combination of other disciplines such as mental health, pharmacy, and pastoral care when available [1, 2]. Specialist palliative care providers work in two ways: first, by providing direct care to patients and their families; and second, by providing consultative support to primary care or other specialty providers (as a consultant in the home or clinic) and enhancing and supporting their care of the patient and family. The critical competencies for home-based palliative care include the ability to manage complex and refractory symptoms, prognosticate, recognize the signs and symptoms of imminent death, address the associated care and support needs of patients and their families before and after the death, and support bereavement.

Palliative care does not lend itself well to fee-for-service payment models. The nature of the care provided is often time-intensive and involves team members who traditionally have no or limited direct insurance reimbursement mechanisms for their time and expertise (such as social work and chaplaincy). It is most effective (and has been best adopted) in integrated healthcare systems where care is value-driven. In this payment model, optimizing care in the home for individuals with serious illness can demonstrate improved patient and caregiver-centered outcomes while at the same time reduce the unnecessary suffering and added cost of care incurred in more expensive hospital or institutional settings. A randomized study of outpatient palliative care in lung cancer patients demonstrated better quality of life, improved survival of almost 3 months, and reduction of utilization across the entire course of illness [3]. A RCT of a home-based palliative care also demonstrated improved satisfaction, fewer hospital and emergency department visits, and lower costs [4].

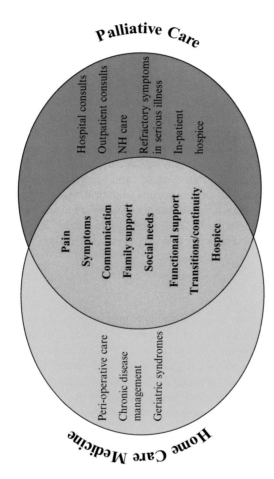

Fig. 12.1 Homecare medicine and palliative care: skills and settings

Table 12.1 Primary palliative care

Key components of primary palliative care
Pain/symptom assessment and management
Social/spiritual assessment
Understanding of illness/prognosis
Identification of patient-centered goals of care

12.2 Process of Care

12.2.1 Goals of Care and Treatment Preferences

Key elements of person-centered care include the elicitation of care goals and treatment preferences. This exploration naturally leads to the development of a care plan that aligns with patient and family values. Care goals are dynamic in nature and deeply contextualized by patients' personal definition of what constitutes meaning and significance, their cultural and social framework, their experience of illness, and the priority they place on certain health outcomes. Providers must become adept at eliciting and understanding patient's and caregiver's values and goals, recognizing that these goals will shift over time as their illnesses progress and/or what is important to them reprioritizes. A number of tools are available to elicit patient's and caregiver's values and goals. The questions in Table 12.2 offer examples of questions that can be used to better understand patients' values and goals.

12.2.2 Prognosis

Along with communication skills, the ability to prognosticate is one of the most important skills of those involved in the care of the very ill and one of the critical competencies in generalist and specialty level palliative care [5, 6]. Providing a time frame and when necessary, conveying a sense of urgency in light of limited life expectancy allows patients and families to make informed decisions as to how time their time will be spent and the opportunity to prioritize activities and treatment plans. The skill of prognostication requires knowledge of the typical trajectories of illness and insight as to the implications of physical signs and symptoms of illness as they manifest alongside and are impacted by the psychosocial and spiritual dynamics of the individual and their family. The provider must be familiar with the evidence from the literature, and have the ability to gather complete information in a patient assessment including exploring the psychosocial and spiritual aspects of the individual and family. The complex thinking and decision-making skills involved in prognostication also relies heavily on the wisdom honed from clinical experience. Most importantly, the ability to communicate prognosis to a patient and family is a critical skill—especially to know, because of culture, religion, or patient/family preferences what to convey, how, and to whom. Communication skills in delivering serious news require expert teaching, reinforcement through modeling and mentoring as well as intentional practice, ideally through the teaching technique of role play or using standardized patients. Increasingly, development of effective communication skills is a focus in the training of healthcare professionals. Table 12.3 provides a few considerations when engaging in conversations around prognosis.

Table 12.2 Useful questions to elicit patients' values and goals for care

What are the most important things in your life now?
What do you hope for?
What are your fears? Are there things about your current situation that worry you?
What do you understand about your condition and your overall health?
How much information about your condition do you find helpful? How much detail do you like or do you prefer to have me speak to your (daughter, son, husband, wife, friend) about these issues?
If you become sicker, how much are you willing to go through for the possibility of gaining more time?
How much does your family understand about what is important to you and your wishes for your treatment?

Table 12.3 Considerations when providing prognostic information

Find out what the patient/caregiver understands about the illness and their general sense about how things are going, e.g., "What is your understanding of your current health situation?"
Find out what kind of information the patient/caregiver desires, e.g., "How much do you want to know?" "Are you the kind of person that likes to hear numbers and facts or do you prefer more general information?"
Provide information while acknowledging limitations of prognostic estimations. For example, "Every person is different. What usually happens to someone in your situation is…"
Avoid specific numbers and use time ranges, e.g., "days to weeks," "weeks to months," etc.
Check for understanding
Acknowledge and support the expression of emotion

12.3 Physical Aspects of Care including Symptom and Safety Issues

12.3.1 Common Symptoms in the Home

Patients for whom home is the optimal setting for care delivery most often have advanced or complex illnesses coupled with significant functional impairment or disability. These individuals often experience a significant symptom burden as a result of their underlying diagnoses and comorbidities. Managing symptoms in the home setting presents unique challenges, particularly if symptoms are dynamic, tend to rapidly escalate or require intravenous medications for effective relief. In a study of 318 adults followed by a home-based medical care program, 43 % reported severe burden from one or more symptoms. The symptoms with the highest level of severity were depression, pain, appetite, and shortness of breath [7]. We briefly discuss management of these four most prevalent symptoms.

12.3.2 Depression

Depressive symptoms are prevalent in patients with advanced, life-threatening illnesses—up to 42 % experience depression at the end of life. Depression may be an indication of inadequately managed symptoms; therefore, addressing pain, dyspnea, and other symptoms as part of the overall treatment strategy is a key first step to addressing depressive symptoms.

Very few pharmacologic studies have been conducted that address depression in advanced illness; consequently, therapeutic recommendations do not differ greatly between palliative and nonpalliative patients. For patients with advanced illness, three factors influence choice of antidepressants (Table 12.4): (1) the time frame for treatment, (2) concurrent medical conditions, and (3) pharmacologic properties of the drug.

With respect to time frame for treatment, patients with a life expectancy of several months may benefit from a SSRI or tricyclic antidepressants (TCA) as long as the need for immediate onset of action is not present. The European Association for Palliative Care recommends mirtazapine, sertraline, and citalopram as reasonable considerations for first line therapy. For those who are weeks to a few short months from death, psychostimulants such as methylphenidate and modafinil offer more immediate onset within 24–48 h of initiation of therapy [9]. Concurrent medical conditions also guide therapy. For those with a history of seizure disorder, bupropion should be avoided. For those with chronic pain, antidepressants that also have a positive impact on pain (such as venlafaxine and duloxetine) should be considered. Relevant pharmacologic properties of antidepressants include availability of liquid formulation and side effects of the medication. Antidepressants that are available in liquid formulation (for when swallowing pills becomes more difficult) include fluoxetine, sertraline, paroxetine, citalopram, escitalopram, doxepin, and nortriptyline. Side effects such as orthostatic hypotension, dizziness, constipation,

Table 12.4 Considerations for pharmacologic treatment for depression in advanced illness

Antidepressant type	Timeframe for treatment	Concurrent medical conditions	Comments
Tricyclic antidepressants	≥2 weeks	Useful in setting of peripheral neuropathy	Greater risk for overdose Can prolong the QTc interval Can contribute to orthostatic hypotension
Selective serotonin reuptake inhibitor	4–6 weeks[a]		
Tetracyclic antidepressant e.g., mirtazapine	1–2 weeks	Reasonable in heart failure and diabetes May increase anticoagulant effect of warfarin	May increase appetite May reduce nausea Sedative effect may be beneficial for some Caution for serotonin syndrome in older adults
Psychostimulants	24–48 h		Caution in heart disease or cognitive disturbances (e.g., delirium)

[a]One-third of the overall effect of selective serotonin reuptake inhibitors (SSRIs) after 6 weeks of treatment is seen in the first week [8]

and prolonged corrected QT (QTc) interval tend to be most pronounced with TCA. Weight gain can be a potentially positive side effect of SSRI and mirtazapine. Sedation is also common with mirtazapine and trazodone and may be beneficial to patients with insomnia and depression, whereas agents with more activating properties (psychostimulants, SSRI) may be a side effect that is more beneficial to those with fatigue or psychomotor slowing [8, 10].

Nonpharmacologic therapy includes supportive psychotherapy and existential therapy. Supportive psychotherapy involves supporting adaptive coping mechanisms and minimizing emotional reactions such as shame and self-loathing that contribute to distress. Existential therapy often focuses on self-worth and self-determination in the context of increasing loss of control. Common forms of existential therapy include dignity therapy, therapeutic life review, and meaning-centered psychotherapy. Dignity therapy, a brief individualized psychotherapeutic intervention targeted at psychosocial and existential distress, has been shown to increase dignity, purpose and meaning and reduce depressive symptoms. [11] The questions commonly used in dignity therapy to elicit better understanding of patient/caregiver needs can be easily adapted to the home setting [12]. A useful overview question is "What do I need to know about you as a person to give you the best care possible?" Other related questions include many listed in Table 12.2 and questions to elicit other appropriate avenues for social and spiritual support: Who else should we get involved to help you through this difficult/challenging time?"

12.3.3 Pain

Pain is a common symptom experienced by individuals with serious or life-limiting illness, regardless of the underlying etiology. Pain is multidimensional in nature and can be exacerbated by depression, existential distress and psychosocial circumstances. Because of the complex nature of pain, careful assessment is needed to optimally characterize pain, determine, if possible, the cause of each type of pain being experienced and base management on the nature of the pain. Key elements of pain that ideally should be elucidated include character, location, frequency, relieving and aggravating factors of the pain, response to previous medication and treatment, and severity.

Pharmacologic pain management includes opioids, nonopioid analgesics (including acetaminophen), and nonsteroidal anti-inflammatory drugs (Table 12.5). Nonpharmacologic management may include guided imagery, transcutaneous electrical nerve stimulation (often facilitated through home physical therapy), therapeutic exercise, and treatments often considered alternative or complementary, such as acupuncture, massage, and other mind-body approaches.

12.3.4 Loss of Appetite

Appetite is affected by illness, drugs, dementia, and mood disorders. In a study of older adults from assisted living facilities or senior centers, decreased emotional

Table 12.5 Considerations for pharmacologic treatment of pain in advanced illness

Analgesic type	Concurrent medical conditions	Common adverse effects	Comments
Acetaminophen	Caution in liver disease and in advanced age	Can cause nausea Most side effects relate to impact on liver: itching, loss of appetite, dark urine, and clay-colored stools	Narrow dosing window Caution in accounting for the presence of acetaminophen in many OTC meds
Nonsteroidal anti-inflammatory agents	Caution in heart failure, kidney disease, hypertension, history of GI bleed	Gastrointestinal bleeding	Misoprostol or proton pump inhibitors reduce risk for GI bleeding
		Renal impairment and acute renal failure	
		Salt and water retention	
		Bronchial spasm/asthma	
		Cardiovascular risk	
Tramadol	Dose reductions necessary in older adults, renal impairment, and end-stage liver failure	Nausea and constipation common lightheadedness, dizziness, drowsiness, or headache	Lowers seizure threshold Risk for serotonin syndrome if provided concomitantly with serotonergic medications
Opioids	Avoid morphine in renal insufficiency	Sedation, nausea, and itching are common and often resolve Constipation rarely resolves with time and requires prophylactic bowel stimulants or osmotic agents	Start at low dose of short-acting opioid (e.g., morphine 5–10 mg) every 4 h; once total daily dose established from short-acting agents, long-acting agents can be considered Transdermal patch formulations should not be offered as first-line treatment until opioid dosing needs are known

well-being was most closely associated with poor appetite, highlighting the need to assess for and address depression [13]. Often, loss of appetite for patients with life-limiting illnesses such as metastatic cancer or end stage heart failure is a prognostic indication that the patient's condition is advanced. In these instances, helping caregivers be comfortable with the patient's reduced interest in eating and offering ways the caregiver can demonstrate love and affirmation other than through food is the most straightforward approach to manage loss of appetite.

For those who are not in the final stages of life, simple approaches to treat loss of appetite include removing dietary restrictions, supplementing intake by increasing the protein and calorie density of food, and considering nutritional supplements. Protein intake can be supplemented by adding milk powder, whey protein, dried peanut butter powder, egg whites, or tofu to food. Caloric density can be enhanced by adding olive or grape seed oil to sauces, fresh or cooked vegetables, and grains or pasta. Multiple small meals may be preferred over fewer large meals.

The value of nutritional supplements in frail older adults remains controversial but they appear most beneficial in older adults with evidence of undernutrition and are reasonable to consider as a time-limited trial. The three most common appetite stimulants used for anorexia include megestrol acetate, dronabinol, and mirtazapine. Megestrol acetate has been demonstrated to increase quality of life in patients with cancer and in nursing home residents. However, weight gain is not sustained and megestrol acetate can worsen heart failure, impair function of the corticoadrenal axis, and increase incidence of deep venous thrombosis so should be used cautiously [14]. Dronabinol has been shown to improve appetite in patients with AIDS and one small study has shown benefit in advanced dementia; however, it has significant CNS side effects and therefore has not been widely used in older adults [15]. As noted above, mirtazapine is more likely than other antidepressants to lead to weight gain and therefore is often considered in the setting of anorexia. Studies in nursing homes (not in the home), however, have not shown conclusive benefit [16].

Decisions regarding enteral nutrition at the end of life should be consistent with treatment goals and patient preference. With the exception of head and neck cancer and esophageal cancer, no studies have demonstrated improved survival in cancer or advanced dementia with enteral support. In advanced dementia, careful spoon feeding, allowing adequate time for feeding, avoiding distractions, and using verbal cueing are optimal.

12.3.5 Dyspnea

Dyspnea is common in the setting of advanced illness. Like with pain, characteristics of dyspnea and potential causes should be part of the initial and ongoing assessment. Common modalities that also can be effective include the use of a fan, breathing techniques, mindfulness and relaxation, anxiety management, and energy conservation. Breathing techniques that can reduce the sensation of dyspnea include pursed lip breathing, prolonged exhalation, and posture modification. In addition to mindfulness and relaxation, guided imagery and distraction strategies (e.g., music, TV, reading by self or caregiver) can be beneficial. Morphine and other opioids can mitigate against the sensation of breathlessness and often reduce dyspnea at much lower doses than are required to address pain.

12.3.6 Safe Prescribing in the Home

The practice of safe prescribing and administration differs in the home compared to the institutional setting. For example, in the home it is the patient themselves or a non-healthcare professional who is most often assessing the symptom burden in real time and dispensing the medication prescribed for relief. Education and the regular review of the safety issues involved in the storage and utilization of medications in the home is an important area of focus for visiting healthcare professionals. Each home visit ideally includes a review of the medications and a check as to where they are stored, how the safe disposal of used and unused, topical medications or needles are handled, and whether any family members, especially children, could be at risk because of the medications. Unfortunately, it is not unusual to have issues with the misuse of medications in the home setting, including diversion by the patient themselves or other people in the household or outsiders having access to the medications. These issues may range from misuse such as the patient taking medications for reasons other than for which it was prescribed (such as medicating anxiety with pain medication) to family members taking the medications or patient/family selling the prescribed medications. Home-based medical providers must assess the risk before prescribing, as well as pay careful attention to utilization and refill patterns. For patients receiving medications such as opioids or benzodiazepines, a medication "contract" with the patient is ideally a routine part of practice. This would include only one physician filling the medication at anticipated intervals with no refills/reissues after hours and on weekends and ideally one pharmacy dispensing. When misuse becomes evident, the medication, amount dispensed, or delivery route may need to be altered to enhance compliance and safety without sacrificing symptom control. Unfortunately, in cases where diversion is discovered, the patient/family must be notified that the physician or practitioner is no longer able to prescribe unless the issue can be securely corrected [17].

12.3.7 General Safety Issues in Advanced Illness

In addition to the safety issues related to the medication, general safety in the home is always of concern. For a detailed discussion of safety assessment in home-based medical care, please see Chap. 4. Given the correlation of functional impairment with advanced complex illness, the home-based medical provider should routinely assess for general patient safety with each visit. Issues may include the safe use of oxygen with patients who continue to smoke, the risk of falls with the presence of oxygen tubing, electrical cords, throw rugs, and uneven or poorly lit surfaces.

Safety in the bathroom includes assessing for the presence for or need for assistance devices such as handrails, bath benches, and perhaps an elevated toilet seat with sidebars. Reviewing how the patient navigates their home, how they exit and enter, and whether they are still driving despite advanced illness and impairment is vitally important. Here the interdisciplinary team of palliative care is particularly helpful as team members are available to help secure such resources as additional help in the home, assistance devices, food delivery, and transportation.

12.4 Psychosocial Aspects of Care in the Home

A number of psychosocial factors influence quality of life for patients with serious illness along with their caregivers. Environmental and social resources and constraints include the patient's home and the ability of the patient's home to accommodate his/ her physical needs, the patient's neighborhood, and built environment. Perceived or real discrimination, negative life events, high illness burden, and multiple comorbidities can be major sources of difficulty, while religious involvement and social support are often protective. Involving social work and pastoral care early can reduce both patient and caregiver distress.

12.5 Hospice Care

Over 1500 years ago, hospices emerged as places of "hospitality" for travelers on pilgrimage throughout the Middle East. These places of safety evolved into the early hospitals of Europe, most often operated and staffed by religious orders. Dame Cicely Saunders of Great Britain, trained as a nurse, social worker, and then as a physician, is recognized as the creator of the modern concept of hospice care. She pioneered the application of the scientific approach to the care of the dying, establishing many of the current best practices of palliative medicine, in particular, the control of pain via around-the-clock administration of analgesic therapy. Hospice entered the United States in 1974 under the guidance of Florence Wald, PhD, Dean of the Graduate School of Nursing at Yale University. Working in consultation with Dame Saunders, Dean Wald opened the Connecticut Hospice in New Haven 1974. This introduction of hospice care model into the United States was a significant shift from the British model as it emphasized care in the home, a model that is most common within the United States to this day [18].

12.5.1 Hospice as a Part of Healthcare

Hospice is the most organized and developed form of palliative care within the continuum and has been supported for over 30 years by defined insurance benefits, beginning with the United States Congress authorizing the medicare hospice benefit (MHB) in 1982. The MHB, through the *Conditions of Participation* [19] addresses the types of services provided within hospice care, the persons eligible to elect the benefit, and the payment system that supports the care. Hospice programs secure Medicare certification by demonstrating compliance with these federal regulations and may thus receive reimbursement for patient care from Medicare. Medicaid and commercial insurance programs generally mimic the MHB, with some variability in the levels of hospice care provided. In order to elect hospice care and receive reimbursement under the MHB, a patient must be deemed "terminally ill," or having a prognosis of 6 months or less if the illness(es) follow a typical course. This initial certification of the terminal illness is the responsibility of the hospice medical director (HMD) along with the patient's attending physician, if they have one.

12.5.2   The Medicare Hospice Benefit

The MHB is divided into benefit periods, initially two 90-day periods followed by an unlimited number of 60-day increments. Each benefit period requires the HMD to recertify and document in narrative form the patient's eligibility as to prognosis and goals of care. The MHB requires and covers four levels of care: routine home care (RHC), general inpatient (GIP), respite, and continuous care, which is also referred to as crisis care. More than 90 % of the hospice care delivered in the United States is provided in the patient's home via RHC, which increasingly includes the settings of long-term care and assisted living. The levels of care are described in Table 12.6.

12.5.3   Hospice Care Financing

The MHB is one of the original capitated reimbursement programs. The CMS determines the adjusted cap amount and works through Medicare Administrative Contractors (MACs) to distribute the funds for hospice services. Individual hospices submit their claims to their assigned MAC to receive reimbursement for care provided. Hospice is reimbursed through a flat per diem, which varies with the level of care. With the RHC per diem rate of roughly 150 dollars, the hospice program is responsible to provide the professional care of skilled nurses, social workers, chaplains, therapists, and the involvement of a physician as a HMD in an

Table 12.6 Levels of hospice care

General inpatient (GIP)	Provides support for short-term inpatient care to meet the needs of hospice patients for pain control or acute or chronic symptom management, which cannot be safely and effectively managed in other settings
Continuous (crisis) care	Continuous (nursing) home care is provided during brief periods of crisis as it is necessary to maintain the terminally ill patient at home
Respite care	Provides a short-term (5 days) facility stay for the patient so as to facilitate caregiver respite
Routine home care	Hospice care in the home setting (LTC, ALF, group home, or private residence)

interdisciplinary team structure. The per diem also covers all the medications, therapies, and procedures related to the hospice prognosis and any durable medical equipment necessary to care for the patient. The MHB also specifically calls for the involvement of volunteers to provide support to the patient and family.

Saunder's original hospice model and the current hospice financial model are based on the trajectory of illness in and anticipated prognosis of cancer patients. Despite significant advances in oncology treatment, the estimated survival for oncology patients with an Eastern Cooperative Oncology Group (ECOG) functional status of 3–4 who are no longer receiving disease-modifying treatments is still around 3–4 months [20]. As more patients with multiple significant comorbidities access hospice care at the end of life, the prognosis of complex illness is less predictable and the time spent in hospice care may vary widely. In 2013, approximately 34.5 % of hospice patients died or were discharged within 7 days of admission and 48.8 % within 14 days of admission. Approximately, 11.5 % of patients remain on hospice care for more than 180 days [21].

12.6 Challenges in Hospice Care

Although Medicare-certified hospice programs are regulated by the Conditions of Participation, there is variation in the care models they provide. Some have very active engagement of their physicians as specialists in palliative medicine; others have physician involvement limited to the administrative role of a medical director. Likewise, hospices vary as to the special modalities they provide for patients. Some will accept patients into their programs who are receiving oral chemotherapy, radiation therapy, or recurrent blood transfusions, others will not. Some require patients to have a "Do Not Resuscitate" status, others will not. "Open Access," a moniker that has fallen into disfavor, had been used in the past to connote programs that were more expansive in their admission criteria. Most importantly, patients, their families, and referring physician should ideally inquire as to the care model practiced by hospice programs and the role of the hospice physician in the plan of care.

12.6.1 The Physician Role in Hospice Care

The physician has distinct roles in hospice care. As a HMD, predominantly an administrative role, the physician is responsible for the written certification and recertification of the eligibility of the patient to access their hospice benefit. This responsibility is always provided in conjunction with input from the interdisciplinary team, but only a physician may serve as a HMD and certify or recertify eligibility. The HMD is also responsible for the medical plan of care, along with the patient's attending physician, if they have one. The HMD typically has responsibilities in areas such as quality improvement, pharmacy oversight, and ethics, as well as others. Only a physician of medicine or osteopathy may serve as a HMD.

The attending physician is a doctor of medicine or osteopathy and is identified by the individual, at the time he or she elects to receive hospice care, as having the most significant role in the determination and delivery of the individual's medical care. The HMD may serve as the attending physician (Attending of Record, AOR) when necessary and when requested by the patient at the time of election of the hospice benefit. A nurse practitioner may also serve at the AOR, although he/she may not serve as a HMD or provide certification of the terminal illness.

As of 2011, every hospice patient must have a face-to-face encounter to assess their ongoing eligibility prior to their third and all subsequent benefit periods with either a hospice nurse practitioner or hospice physician. These visits are administrative in nature and are covered as part of the RHC per diem. The purpose of these visits is not to certify eligibility, but to document the clinic status of the patient and provide the information to the interdisciplinary team and to the certifying HMD. If a medical issue is identified during a face-to-face visit, these may be separately documented and billed; however, a nurse practitioner may only bill and receive reimbursement under the HMB if he/she is the AOR.

Hospice patients frequently have complex medical conditions and benefit greatly from regular physician's follow-up in the home. These visits are coded and billed in the usual and customary fashion but may require the attachment of modifiers depending on which physician sees the patient and for what medical problem. The modifiers are as follows:

GV Modifier—used by the attending physician when seeing the hospice patient for issues related to their hospice diagnoses. In this case, the attending physician is not employed or under contract by the hospice.

GW Modifier—used by the AOR as well as the hospice physician when seeing the patient for issues unrelated to their hospice diagnosis.

Consulting physicians—clinicians who are not the AOR for a patient must be under contract with the hospice to bill and receive reimbursement for patient care. The patient and family elects who will be the AOR at the time that they elect to use their hospice benefit; this individual may or may not be the physician who referred them to hospice care. In home-based medical care, patients may be referred to hospice through their office-based oncologist or other specialist; this requirement will impact reimbursement for the home-based clinician so they must verify whether they are consulting or serving as the AOR. If consulting, they must submit their bills to the hospice and the hospice bills on their behalf and reimburse them as per the contractual arrangement [22].

12.7   Ethical and Legal Aspects of Care in the Home

Given the advanced state of illness providers typically confront when caring for people in home-based primary and palliative care, advanced care planning becomes a more pressing priority and immediate in its necessity. Despite sometimes living for years with functional limitations and chronic complex illness, these patients, like the greater population, are unlikely to have communicated actionable directives as to the intensity of healthcare interventions that they prefer. Meeting with people and their families in the home is an ideal location for these discussions as the patient is in a less vulnerable environment to explore goals of care and care preferences. In addition, the time spent in a home visit is typically longer than that in the ambulatory setting such that these conversations may have more time to evolve. Likewise, the setting more naturally lends itself to patient-centered discussions of meaning and value as there may be present many physical cues to initiate or bridge to these discussions—such as pictures of family members, mementos of life achievements, or evidence of hobbies and interests. Ideally, advance care planning is a series of conversations over time that starts with authentic interest in what matters most to the patient and to their family and how their priorities are impacted and informed by their health conditions.

The culmination of these discussions of "what matters most" is to create an actionable directive that can be honored by healthcare professionals. First and foremost, every patient needs to designate a decision-maker to speak for them in the event they are unable to communicate their preferences. This individual is often a family member but does not have to be. Ideally, the person identified as the surrogate decision-maker is an individual who can support and advocate for the preferences and directives of the patient. Surrogate decision-makers who are not aligned with the patient care preferences may experience significant stress in the role or seek to redirect interventions to care goals that are inconsistent with the patient's stated or implied preferences. The home-based medical care provider has a unique opportunity to counsel patients and families to identify a surrogate decision-maker who understands and supports the patient's goals of care and furthermore to support and educate the surrogate when they must assume the responsibility.

It is imperative that the home-based medical provider is knowledgeable as to the state laws that govern the identification and documentation of who serves as the surrogate decision-maker or healthcare power of attorney. Documentation of the care preferences of individuals can take several forms and may be identified by several different labels such as Living Wills, 5Wishes, Ethical Wills, etc. These care preference documents may be very helpful when they exist but are not actionable documents—meaning that emergency medical personnel called to the home cannot utilize a healthcare directive such as a Living Will to guide or in any way, modify, emergency interventions.

Increasingly, states are adopting documents based on the physician orders for life sustaining treatment (POLST) [23]. The POLST paradigm was initiated in Oregon by several medical ethicists in 1991 as a means to better honor the advance directives and end-of-life preferences of patients and families. POLST has been steadily adopted and adapted by other states throughout the USA by aligning with the local legal, medical, and cultural contexts and has been renamed in some settings as POST (physician order for scope of treatment), MOLST (medical orders for life sustaining treatment), and MOST (medical orders for scope of treatment). State law authorizes certain healthcare professionals to sign medical orders, and these individuals may also sign a POLST document.

POLST is not for everyone and is not an advance directive [24]. It does not replace the designation of the healthcare power of attorney. POLST is indicated for people with serious advanced illness and limited life expectancy who would benefit from having medical orders for treatment readily available to emergency personnel. People whose life expectancy is such that their primary care provider would not be surprised if they died in the next year will particularly benefit from the discussion and shared decision-making that is then reflected in the creation of a POLST document. In some states, the patient or family signs the completed POLST document to indicate agreement and consent to the treatment plan.

References

1. American Academy of Hospice and Palliative Medicine; Center to Advance Palliative Care; Hospice and Palliative Nurses Association; Last Acts Partnership, et al. National Consensus Project for Quality Palliative Care: Clinical Practice Guidelines for quality palliative care, executive summary. J Palliat Med. 2004;7(5):611–27.
2. Herman C. National consensus project updates palliative care guidelines. Aging Today Online. 2013 [posted on 26 Sept 2013 cited on 7 June 2015]. Available from: http://asaging.org/blog/national-consensus-project-updates-palliative-care-guidelines
3. Temel JS, Greer JA, Muzikansky A, Gallagher ER, Admane S, Jackson VA, et al. Early palliative care for patients with metastatic non-small-cell lung cancer. N Engl J Med. 2010;363(8): 733–42.
4. Brumley RD, Enguidanos S, Cherin DA. Effectiveness of a home-based palliative care program for end-of-life. J Palliat Med. 2003;6(5):715–24.
5. Glare PA, Sinclair CT. Palliative medicine review: prognostication. J Palliat Med. 2008;11(1): 84–103.
6. Matzo ML. Palliative care: prognostication and the chronically ill: methods you need to know as chronic disease progresses in older adults. Am J Nurs. 2004;104(9):40–9. quiz 50.
7. Wajnberg A, Ornstein K, Zhang M, Smith KL, Soriano T. Symptom burden in chronically ill homebound individuals. J Am Geriatr Soc. 2013;61(1):126–31.
8. Taylor MJ, Freemantle N, Geddes JR, Bhagwagar Z. Early onset of selective serotonin reuptake inhibitor antidepressant action: systematic review and meta-analysis. Arch Gen Psychiatry. 2006;63(11):1217–23.
9. Rozans M, Dreisbach A, Lertora JJ, Kahn MJ. Palliative uses of methylphenidate in patients with cancer: a review. J Clin Oncol. 2002;20(1):335–9.
10. Rayner L, Higginson IJ, Price A, Hotopf M. The management of depression in palliative care: European clinical guidelines. London: Department of Palliative Care, Policy & Rehabilitation. www.kcl.ac.uk/schools/medicine/depts/palliative/European Palliative Care Research Collaborative. www.epcrc.org; 2010.
11. Chochinov HM, Hack T, Hassard T, Kristjanson LJ, McClement S, Harlos M. Dignity therapy: a novel psychotherapeutic intervention for patients near the end of life. J Clin Oncol. 2005;23(24):5520–5.
12. dignityincare.ca/en/toolkit [Internet]. Dignity IN CARE; c2010 [cited 7 June 2015]. Available from: http://dignityincare.ca/en/toolkit.html
13. Engel JH, Siewerdt F, Jackson R, Akobundu U, Wait C, Sahyoun N. Hardiness, depression, and emotional well-being and their association with appetite in older adults. J Am Geriatr Soc. 2011;59(3):482–7.
14. Berenstein EG, Ortiz Z. Megestrol acetate for the treatment of anorexia-cachexia syndrome. Cochrane Database Syst Rev. 2005;2, CD004310.
15. Volicer L, Stelly M, Morris J, McLaughlin J, Volicer BJ. Effects of dronabinol on anorexia and disturbed behavior in patients with Alzheimer's disease. Int J Geriatr Psychiatry. 1997;12(9): 913–9.

16. Fox CB, Treadway AK, Blaszczyk AT, Sleeper RB. Megestrol acetate and mirtazapine for the treatment of unplanned weight loss in the elderly. Pharmacotherapy. 2009;29(4):383–97.
17. Inciardi JA, Surratt HL, Cicero TJ, Beard RA. Prescription opioid abuse and diversion in an urban community: the results of an ultrarapid assessment. Pain Med. 2009;10(3):537–48.
18. Twaddle ML, Kelley S. Hospice. In: Berger AM, editor. Principles and practice of palliative care and supportive oncology. 4th ed. Philadelphia: Wolters Kluwer Health/Lippincott Williams & Wilkins; 2012. Chapter 46.
19. Medicare benefit policy manual chapter 9 - Coverage of hospice services under hospital insurance (Rev 209, 05-08-15) [Internet] [cited 30 May 2015]. Available from: http://www.cms.gov/Regulations-and-Guidance/Guidance/Manuals/downloads/bp102c09.pdf
20. Oken MM, Creech RH, Tormey DC, Horton J, Davis TE, McFadden ET, et al. Toxicity and response criteria of the Eastern Cooperative Oncology Group. Am J Clin Oncol. 1982;5(6):649–55.
21. nhpco.org [Internet]. NHPCO's facts & figures: hospice care in America. 2014 [cited on 31 May 2015]. Available from: http://www.nhpco.org/sites/default/files/public/Statistics_Research/2014_Facts_Figures.pdf
22. Medicare Claims Processing Manual Chapter 11: Processing Hospice Claims (Rev 3118, 11-16-14) [Internet]. [cited 1 June 2015]. Available from: https://www.cms.gov/Regulations-and-Guidance/Guidance/Manuals/downloads/clm104c11.pdf
23. polst.org/about-the-national-polst-paradigm/history [Internet]. The National POLST paradigm; c2012-2015 [cited 7 June 2015]. Available from: http://www.polst.org/about-the-national-polst-paradigm/history/
24. polst.org/polst-what-it-is-and-what-it-is-not [Internet]. The National POLST paradigm; c2012-2015 [cited 7 June 2015]. Available from: http://www.polst.org/polst-what-it-is-and-what-it-is-not/

Caregiving

13

Claire Larson and Helen Kao

Abstract

As life span increases, many older adults in the United States are living longer with functional impairments. Informal caregivers are a significant part of the fabric of caregiving that enables older adults to avoid institutionalization. This chapter characterizes the growing population of caregivers, provides an overview of the economics of informal caregiving, discusses caregiver burden, describes different types of caregiving and settings of care, and concludes with clinical pearls for home-based medical clinicians to guide their interactions with caregivers.

Keywords

Caregiver burden • Caregiver education • House calls • Informal caregivers • Long term care • Residential care facilities

13.1 Who Are Caregivers?

Informal caregivers in the USA are a diverse but largely unrecognized and undervalued group. Traditionally, caregiving has been considered an expected family obligation. However, since the American family has changed over time, many older adults do not live with or near children or grandchildren. As family structures evolve, the USA faces an ever growing population of older adults who need caregiver support for functional deficits.

C. Larson, M.D. (✉) • H. Kao, M.D.
UCSF Division of Geriatrics, 3333 California St, #380, San Francisco, CA 94118, USA
e-mail: claire.k.larson@gmail.com; Helen.kao@ucsf.edu

© Springer International Publishing Switzerland 2016   269
J.L. Hayashi, B. Leff (eds.), *Geriatric Home-Based Medical Care*,
DOI 10.1007/978-3-319-23365-9_13

13.1.1 Overview of the Caregiver Population

A recent study found that a quarter of adults have served in a caregiving role [1]. Over half of the caregivers to older adults are themselves over the age of 50. Eighty-six percent of caregivers are relatives of the patient [2]. As life span increases, caregiving has changed from a short-term familial role to one that can last for years [3].

Patients may need a caregiver for a multitude of reasons. The most common conditions for which caregiving is implemented include old age (12 %), dementia (10 %), cancer (7 %), mental health disorder (7 %), heart disease (5 %), and stroke (5 %). Dementia often coexists with and complicates the care of other conditions.

The intensity and time commitment of caregiving are variable and fluctuate over time, in large part due to the variable needs of the care recipient. In 2009, the percentage of caregivers who provided assistance with at least one activity of daily living (ADL) was 58 %. Among the ADLs, caregivers assisted most frequently with transferring between bed and chair (40 %) and least with feeding (20 %). Furthermore, caregivers increasingly help with instrumental activities of daily living (IADLs): 83 % assist with transportation, 75 % with housework, 75 % with shopping, 65 % with meal preparation, and 64 % with finances [2].

As older adults live longer with disability, caregivers spend longer amounts of time in this role. Almost two-thirds of caregivers provide care for more than 1 year [2]. When a caregiver lives with the patient, the time dedicated to providing care equals a full-time job, on average 39.3 h/week [2].

13.1.2 The Economic Impact of Informal Caregiving

In 2009, 42.1 million caregivers were providing care at any given time, with an estimated economic value of $450 billion [4]. This figure is more than the 2009 annual expenditure of $361 billion for federal and state Medicaid contributions to health care and long-term care services [4].

The majority of informal caregivers receive no income or employment benefits for the care they provide. Additionally, these caregivers can accrue significant personal costs that impact their financial well-being and security. A 2014 survey of family caregivers for older adults found that 42 % of them spent >$5000/year on caregiving expenses [5]. One-third of caregivers use their savings to cover such expenses and another one-third reduce or stop saving for their own future [6].

Caregiving comes with significant financial impact and many family caregivers reduce hours or stop working outside the home to provide care. Almost three-quarters of caregivers maintain other jobs in addition to their caregiving responsibilities. Two-thirds of caregivers report their caregiving duties forced them to arrive late, leave early, or take time off from work [2]. Sixty percent of family caregivers reported that caregiving had a negative effect on their jobs [5].

If family caregivers can no longer provide care, then they must either hire in-home support or place their loved one outside the home. Some households supplement unpaid care with private paid help, though this can come at a significant cost [2].

13.2 Caregiver Burden and Assessment

13.2.1 Overview

Caregiving is associated with physical, psychological, and financial burdens. Caregiver burden is a major public health problem affecting the well-being of both caregivers and patients.

13.2.2 Incidence and Risk Factors for Caregiver Burden

Ninety-two percent of community dwelling residents requiring long-term care receive unpaid help, while 13 % receive paid help [7]. Unpaid family members provide the majority of long-term care and are at particularly high risk for burnout. Half of the caregivers report their level of burden as moderate or high [2].

Care needs, such as ADL and IADL assistance, are determined by numerous patient-related factors, including medical and psychiatric conditions. Caring for a patient with dementia is associated with a higher level of burden than caring for someone without dementia. Individuals with dementia often require supervisory care and are less likely to express gratitude to their caregiver [8]. Upward of 80 % of persons with dementia are cared for at home by family members [9]. As an individual's cognitive function declines, the caregiver's perceived burden increases [10]. Worsening dementia is associated with an increased need for caregiving and supervision, with a mean of 113 h/month for a patient with mild dementia, increasing to a mean of 298 h/month in a patient with severe dementia [11]. Increases in neuropsychiatric symptoms and behavioral disturbance, ADL and IADL impairment, and geriatric syndromes, such as falls and sleep disorders, also increase caregiver burden [10, 12].

Caregiver burden is not only influenced by patient characteristics, but also by caregiver characteristics (Table 13.1). Caregivers reporting the highest burden are more likely to live with the patient, have less education, and perceive that they had little choice in the caregiver role [13]. Caregiver characteristics associated with higher burden include being a spouse, of younger age, and having depressive symptoms [12]. Women may experience greater strain and burden related to caregiving

Table 13.1 Risk factors for caregiver burden

Patient characteristics	Caregiver characteristics
Dementia, especially with neuropsychiatric symptoms or behavioral disturbances [8] Increasing ADL/IADL dependence [10, 12] Presence of geriatric syndromes (e.g., falls, sleep disturbance) [10, 12]	Spouse and/or live with patient [12, 13] Lower education level [13] Perceive that little or no choice in caregiver role [13] Younger age [12] Depressive symptoms [12] Emotion-focused coping style [14]

than men [15]. Cultural differences among racial and ethnic groups may influence the perspective and expectations about caregiving, as well as the amount of extended family support.

13.2.3 Impact of Caregiver Burden

Caregiver burden can have adverse effects on patients, their caregivers, and society (Table 13.2). Caregivers suffering from burden are at a higher risk for committing elder abuse or neglect [18].

The mental health of caregivers is often affected with high rates of depression and anxiety. In one study of caregivers for individuals with dementia, a third of the caregivers met criteria for depression [16]. Caregivers are more likely to report that they are dissatisfied or very dissatisfied with their lives [1]. Caregivers have higher rates of emotional stress, less time for other friends and family, and often neglect self-care, such as healthy sleep, exercise, and diet [15]. Maladaptive coping strategies such as self-blame or wishful thinking have been linked with more anxiety and depression [14].

Caregivers report lower levels of physical and overall health. Twenty-three percent of adults who have been caregiving for over 5 years consider their personal health as fair or poor, compared to 13 % of the general adult population [2]. Seventeen percent of caregivers believe that their health has deteriorated as a result of providing care [13]. Elderly spouses who experienced caregiver burden had a mortality risk that was 63 % higher than that of controls [19].

While caregiving is associated with significant burdens, it can also have many benefits for the caregiver. Positive outcomes include enjoyment of role and personal

Table 13.2 Impact of caregiver burden

Impact of caregiver burden on:		
Patients	Caregivers	Economy
Individual may feel like a burden to his/her family and friends	Have high rates of depression and anxiety [16]	Informal caregivers receive no income or employment benefits
Individual may be subject to elder abuse or neglect by overwhelmed caregiver [17]	Have high rates of dissatisfaction with their lives [1]	Caregivers may use their own savings to cover caregiving expenses [5]
Individuals may spend down their savings to supplement informal caregiving with hired help [2]	Have less time for other family or friends [15]	Informal caregiving often has negative effect on one's formal job (e.g., forced caregiver to arrive late, leave early, or to take time off work) [2]
Individual may move out of private home to higher level of care due to burdens on family caregivers	Neglect self-care and rate personal health as poor or declining [13]	Informal caregivers provide care with estimated value of $450 billion annually [4]

fulfillment from helping a loved one. Caregivers at home are often family members or friends of the patient and caregiving allows them to have a continued rewarding relationship with their loved one.

13.2.4 Assessment of Caregiver Burden

Given the impact of caregiver burden, home-based medical care clinicians should assess caregiver's well-being. Multiple scales exist, but the most widely used is the 22-item Zarit Burden Interview (ZBI) (Table 13.3) [20]. This questionnaire was designed for research, rather than clinical use in daily practice. However, we include it in this chapter to describe the scope of issues to consider when assessing caregiver burden, with higher scores reflecting higher levels of burden. A 4-item screening version (Table 13.4) and 12-item short version of the questionnaire were developed and validated for easier screening of caregivers of community dwelling older adults with cognitive impairment [21].

Table 13.3 The Zarit Burden interview (choose the response that best describes how you feel)

	Never	Rarely	Sometimes	Quite frequently	Nearly always
1. Do you feel that your relative asks for more help than he/she needs?	0	1	2	3	4
2. Do you feel that because of the time you spend with your relative that you do not have enough time for yourself?	0	1	2	3	4
3. Do you feel stressed between caring for your relative and trying to meet other responsibilities for your family or work?	0	1	2	3	4
4. Do you feel embarrassed over your relative's behavior?	0	1	2	3	4
5. Do you feel angry when you are around your relative?	0	1	2	3	4
6. Do you feel that your relative currently affects our relationships with other family members of friends in a negative way?	0	1	2	3	4
7. Are you afraid what the future holds for your relative?	0	1	2	3	4
8. Do you feel your relative is dependent on you?	0	1	2	3	4
9. Do you feel strained when you are around your relative?	0	1	2	3	4

(continued)

Table 13.3 (continued)

	Never	Rarely	Sometimes	Quite frequently	Nearly always
10. Do you feel your health has suffered because of your involvement with your relative?	0	1	2	3	4
11. Do you feel that you do not have as much privacy as you would like because of your relative?	0	1	2	3	4
12. Do you feel that your social life has suffered because you are caring for your relative?	0	1	2	3	4
13. Do you feel uncomfortable about having friends over because of your relative?	0	1	2	3	4
14. Do you feel that your relative seems to expect you to take care of him/her as if you were the only one he/she could depend on?	0	1	2	3	4
15. Do you feel that you do not have enough money to take care of your relative in addition to the rest of your expenses?	0	1	2	3	4
16. Do you feel that you will be unable to take care of your relative much longer?	0	1	2	3	4
17. Do you feel you have lost control of your life since your relative's illness?	0	1	2	3	4
18. Do you wish you could leave the care of your relative to someone else?	0	1	2	3	4
19. Do you feel uncertain about what to do about your relative?	0	1	2	3	4
20. Do you feel you should be doing more for your relative?	0	1	2	3	4
21. Do you feel you could do a better job in caring for your relative?	0	1	2	3	4
22. Overall, how burdened do you feel in caring for your relative?	0	1	2	3	4

Reprinted from Zarit SH, Reever KE, Bach-Peterson J. Relatives of the impaired elderly: correlates of feelings of burden. Gerontologist. 1980;20 (6):649–55. Reference [20] by permission of Oxford University Press

Interpretation of Score:

0–21 little to no burden

21–40 mild to moderate burden

41–60 moderate to severe burden

61–88 severe burden

Table 13.4 Zarit Burden interview screening version

Do you feel...
That because of the time you spend with your relative that you do not have enough time for yourself?
Stressed between caring for your relative and trying to meet other responsibilities (work/family)?
Strained when you are around your relative?
Uncertain about what to do about your relative?

Answered as "Never" (0), "Rarely" (1), "Sometimes" (2), "Quite frequently" (3), or "Nearly Always" (4). A score of 8 or higher is suggestive of high burden, though an exact cutoff has not been established.

Reprinted from Bédard M, Molloy DW, Squire L, Dubois S, Lever JA, O'Donnell M. The Zarit Burden Interview: a new short version and screening version. Gerontologist. 2001;41(5):652–7. Reference [21] by permission of Oxford University Press

During the home visit, clinicians should ask questions to assess caregivers' mental health, coping, behavioral management, social support, and resources [22]. Examples of useful questions include the following.

- Are you feeling a lot of stress?
- Have you been feeling anxious or down?
- What do you do to relieve your stress?
- Does your relative/patient have behaviors that are difficult to manage or frustrating? How do you manage these?
- Does anyone help you with caregiving? Who and how often?
- Are you involved with any local support groups? If not, are you interested in learning about them?

After assessing caregiver burden, clinicians should provide education, support, and assist caregivers with identifying resources for support. These issues are addressed in the subsequent sections. The Family Caregiver Alliance National Center on Caregiving also has an online toolkit to help clinicians assess caregivers (https://caregiver.org/caregivers-count-too-toolkit). This resource provides a helpful overview of caregiving and resources, as well as a guide to conducting a caregiver assessment in Sect. 3.

13.2.5 Support for Caregivers

The primary support for most caregivers is their informal social networks and clinicians should inquire about friends or family that may be assisting them. Clinicians can provide education, as well as involve other skilled resources when needed. Finally, caregivers should be informed of local and national resources, including in-person and online support groups, counseling, education and skills trainings, and respite care [22].

Most support groups and organizations focus on sharing the caregiver's experience, as well as learning strategies and skills for caregiving. An intervention including counseling sessions and conversation groups resulted in a 6-month delay in nursing home placement [23]. Skilled therapy, such as cognitive behavioral therapy, is not as widely available, but has been shown to reduce depression in caregivers [24]. Interventions have been developed to address coping strategies, reduce anxiety, and increase satisfaction. A focus on problem solving and acceptance styles of coping is likely helpful for caregivers and can lead to a more positive caregiver experience [25].

Educational and supportive interventions have been shown to positively impact family and caregivers. Home visiting programs can help support caregivers and are most helpful in reducing burden among caregivers who live with patients [26]. Caregiver burden should be assessed and addressed, as this can improve quality of life for the caregiver and also ensure safety and sustainability of the caregiver–patient relationship. Additional resources are discussed at the end of this chapter.

13.2.6   Abuse and Neglect

While the majority of caregivers provide devoted, quality care, abuse and neglect of older, vulnerable adults remain prevalent. Elder abuse is intentional or neglectful act by a caregiver or trusted individual that harm a vulnerable older adult. One in 10 older adults experiences abuse or neglect by a caregiver each year and the incidence is expected to increase [18]. Elder abuse occurs most in home situations. Risk factors for elder abuse include shared living arrangements, cognitive impairment with disruptive behaviors, social isolation, caregiver's mental illness, and financial dependence on the older adult [17]. The US Preventive Services Task Force found insufficient evidence to assess the balance of benefits and harms of screening for abuse of older or vulnerable adults. However, clinicians in most states have professional and legal obligations to report and refer persons who are suspected of being victims of abuse [18]. Clinicians that perform home-based medical care are uniquely able to assess the dynamic of the caregiver and patient, as well as the safety of the home environment. Clinicians should be familiar with signs of and risk factors for elder abuse, so they can appropriately identify this underrecognized problem. Chapter 11, "Social and Ethical Issues In Home-Based Medical Care," addresses the complexities of assessment for abuse or neglect in these vulnerable patients.

Clinicians should ensure that they interview the patient alone without the caregiver present. Suggestions on how to interview the patient alone are described in detail in the section on Caregiver Education under "Interacting with Caregivers: Key Language and Techniques." The Elder Abuse Suspicion Index, available online, is a 6-item validated screen for use in primary care settings with cognitively intact patients [27]. The goal of the screen is to help identify possible cases of abuse to prompt providers to conduct more in-depth evaluation. Questions focus on neglect, emotional, financial, and physical abuse.

For patients with cognitive impairment, clinicians will need to rely on other possible red flags, such as:

- The caregiver often interrupts the patient to answer for him/her
- The patient has:
  - Bruising in unusual locations
  - Burns, hand slap, or bite marks
  - Evidence of dehydration or malnutrition
  - Poor eye contact or withdrawn behavior
  - An unusual delay in seeking medical attention for injuries
  - Frequently missed medications
  - Dirty clothing and poor hygiene

Any time elder abuse is suspected, the case must be reported to the local Adult Protective Services.

13.3 Levels of Care

Home-based medical care can be delivered in a variety of community settings: from private residences and small Board and Care homes to large assisted living facilities and entire "campuses" of a Continuing Care Retirement Community (Table 13.5). These settings provide varying levels of structural and programmed care that can enable an older adult to remain more independent, while also reducing burden on informal caregivers. Understanding the levels of care available to patients and caregivers in these settings, as well as the variable costs and availability of coverage through county programs or long-term care insurance, is useful for providers.

13.3.1 Private Home

The vast majority of older adults wish to live and die in their own home surrounded by loved ones. However, the presence of chronic diseases, injuries, or cumulative age related functional decline, often means that assistance is needed to remain at home. Options for caregiving in a private home include informal/unpaid and formal/paid caregiving, or a combination of both. In-home care can enable an adult to stay at home, but does not necessarily address social isolation and other needs.

13.3.2 Senior Centers and Adult Day Programs

Community-based Senior Centers and Adult Day Programs offer a wide array of centralized services and activities in a supervised and social environment. They provide much needed physical, cognitive, and social stimulation, such as exercise classes, group games, art or music sessions, and book clubs. Some provide

Table 13.5 Levels of care in the home or community (not including long-term care in skilled nursing facilities)

Level of care	Care available	Costs	Comments
Private home			
Senior Center/ Adult Day Program	• Centralized & supervised services/ activities • Socialization • Physical and cognitive stimulation (exercise, art, music, games, etc.) • Maintenance PT/OT • Transportation • Meals • Field trips	• National average ~$70/day • Private Pay • Medicaid HCBS • Veteran's Administration • Some state/local funding • Some long-term care insurance	• Range of services varies per site • Patient participation can enable family caregiver to maintain outside employment
Low-income government funded in-home caregiving	• I/ADL support • Supervisory care for dementia • Usually does not cover 24/7 care	• Income eligibility (often Medicaid thresholds or higher +/− share of cost)	• Must reside in county where care subsidy is provided • May enable family caregiver to get paid for their services
Paid In-Home Caregiving (agency)	• I/ADL support • Supervisory care • Can fit together shifts to provide 24/7 coverage • Usual "minimum" shift is 4 h at a time • Agency caregivers usually restricted from performing paramedical services	• $10–$40/h • Rate varies by geographic area and level of care needed • Long-term care insurance covers (and requires paid caregivers to be affiliated with an agency)	• Increasing legal protections for formal paid caregivers (maximum hours, mandated breaks, overtime etc.) • Agencies generally conduct basic background checks
Paid In-Home Caregiving (independent contractor)	• Same as agency caregiver but no restrictions on paramedical services • May enable more flexible scheduling	• Rate may be cheaper than for agency caregiver • May enable flexibility of offering live-in (room and board) arrangements in exchange for services • Long-term care insurance covers (but may require caregivers to be affiliated with an agency)	• Increasing legal protections for caregivers limit previously commonplace arrangements • Caregiver Agreement contracts recommended

(continued)

Table 13.5 (continued)

Level of care	Care available	Costs	Comments
Residential Care Facility for the Elderly (RCFE)	• Daily support with I/ADLs • Home like, community-based setting • Socialization • Similar activities to Senior Centers above • Inclusive of all meals • Transportation • Medication dispensation	• National average (2013) ~$3400/month Cost ranges greatly by location, size, level of care needs (e.g., $1000–$9000/month) • Private Pay • Some long-term care insurance covers/subsidizes	• Many individuals who, in past decades, would have been institutionalized in nursing facilities are able to reside in RCFEs if they have financial means
Continuing Care Retirement Communities (CCRC)	• Same as above • But resident can enter at fully independent stage • Care extends to and includes on-site skilled nursing and rehabilitation • "Tiered" approach to care	• Average $3000–$5000/month • Significant enrollment fee ($1000–$1 million) • Private Pay • Some long-term care insurance subsidizes	• Most expensive option • Enables resident to "age in place"
Respite Care	• Short-term time-limited care to relieve an informal caregiver • Can be provided in the home or through temporary placement of individual in a facility	• Private pay prorated for amount of time a formal caregiver is brought into the home or individual is placed in a facility • May be supported through some state programs or Medicaid waiver benefits • Some long-term care insurance covers	

transportation to and from home and may even offer scheduled group "field trips" to museums, parks, or other local cultural settings. The average cost for a full day of services is about $70. While many individuals pay out of pocket for these programs, public funding sources that support Adult Day participants include Medicaid Home- and Community-based Waiver Programs, the Veteran's Administration, and other state and local funding [28]. Some long-term care insurance will cover or subsidize participation in these programs. Senior Centers and Adult Day Programs can enable informal caregivers to maintain outside employment or provide family caregivers much needed daily respite from around-the-clock caregiving.

13.3.3   Residential Care Facilities for the Elderly

Residential care facilities for the elderly (RCFE) are settings that provide daily supportive services and often socialization and activities to older or disabled adults. RCFEs vary tremendously in size, services, and cost. Smaller, more intimate and home-like Board and Care homes, sometimes called group homes, are homes in residential neighborhoods that have been renovated to care for an average of 5–10 disabled adults. In contrast, an assisted living facility (ALF) is usually a large complex designed and built to house a higher number of residents, e.g., 100–200, in single or double-occupancy apartments. The increasingly higher level of care offered by some RCFEs has contributed to a notable shift in long-term care over the past few decades. Individuals with disabilities, who in the past would have required a nursing facility for long-term care, can now safely remain in the community at an RCFE if they have sufficient financial resources. RCFEs that have special dementia units or "hospice waivers," can sometimes even manage the complex and time-intensive care of a bedbound resident who requires hand-feeding. Family members can continue to play a valuable "informal" caregiving role in these settings, but with the comfort of knowing that the majority of their loved one's needs are attended to by formal staff.

RCFEs do not fall under the same strict regulatory requirements faced by skilled nursing facilities. Older adults choose an RCFE based on the type of setting, degree of care needs, "culture" of the facility, and cost they can afford.

All RCFEs provide meals and housekeeping and may provide medication management, transfer assistance, and help with ADLs. Most RCFEs provide some type of social or cultural activities. Board and Care homes with fewer resources may have visiting pet therapy, art, and birthday parties or holiday celebrations. In addition to these activities, ALFs may provide group exercise and art classes, film nights, bingo and card games, outings to shopping malls or cultural sites, and transportation to medical appointments. Some ALFs even provide on-site hair salons and nail care. Board and Care homes are generally more affordable than ALFs. The average cost of an RCFE in the US in 2013 was $3427 a month [29]. However, in some geographic regions costs can increase up to $7000–8000+/month, particularly if a resident has a higher level of care needs, which are often priced a la carte depending on the activity. Long-term care insurance may cover part or all of the fees depending on plan benefits and cost of the chosen facility.

13.3.4   Continuing Care Retirement Communities

Continuing care retirement communities (CCRC) integrate the services an older adult needs all in one community, as he or she transitions from independent living to assisted living to skilled nursing and hospice-level care. Often referred to as "tiered" approach to care, CCRCs are the most expensive of the long-term care options. They generally offer the same types of services and social activities as an ALF but with the additional security that an older adult can enroll while independent, transition into assisted care, and receive skilled nursing level support if needed in the same setting over time. An individual applies for and enrolls into a CCRC with an initial fee which can be anywhere from $100,000 to as much as $1 million. Monthly fees then range $3000–5000, but may increase if the resident has growing care needs [30]. As with RCFEs, long-term care insurance may cover part or all of the fees depending on plan benefits and cost of the chosen facility.

13.3.5 In-Home Caregiving

Informal or paid in-home caregivers can fulfill the needs of adults who require help with ADLs or IADLs in their own private residence or who may need to augment the services provided by an RCFE.

When paid formal caregivers are needed, patients or their families must choose a type of caregiver based on the cost they can afford, $10–40/h depending on geographic area and level of care needed [31]. The first option is hiring a caregiver through an agency. This is usually the most expensive hourly rate but provides several benefits to the employing adult. Agencies generally conduct background checks and ensure that the caregiver is a citizen or legal immigrant. Some agencies provide basic caregiver training and health insurance to employees and take the responsibility for finding a replacement for the client if a caregiver calls in sick. The second option is hiring an independent caregiver as a private contracted employee. The responsibility lies with the "employer" to conduct any background or reference checks, to train the caregiver for specific tasks, and to abide by federal and state laws regarding payment and taxes. If the caregiver calls in sick or resigns, the employing adult must scramble to find a replacement caregiver. The third type of caregiver is the "under-the-table" caregiver, which exists in every community, but is against the law and not advised. This arrangement can expose the caregiver to abuse, unfair working standards and hours, and low pay without benefits. The employing adult faces IRS taxes, penalties and interest if discovered. In this situation, the employing adult would also have to find a replacement if a caregiver decided to abruptly leave or became ill or injured [32].

Anyone hiring an independent caregiver is strongly advised to complete a formal Caregiver Agreement to define the responsibilities of both parties and detail the flow of payment. Caregiver Agreement templates are readily available for free online. Caregiver Agreements protect the caregiver and enable him/her to build employment history, establish credit, and have access to disability insurance, workers' compensation and public benefits. Agreements protect the employer from being taken advantage of especially when an adult is hiring a friend or relative [32]. Long-term care insurance can cover in-home paid caregivers, but may stipulate that the paid caregiver must be affiliated with an approved agency (i.e., not just a friend or independent contractor).

13.3.6 Respite Care

Respite care is short-term, time-limited care for an individual that can be provided in his or her own home, though more commonly is provided in a community program, an RCFE, or nursing facility. Respite services at home usually entail a formal caregiver coming to the home in place of the usual informal caregiver. Facility respite care entails moving the older adult to an RCFE or nursing facility for a short period of time. Respite care may be supported through special state programs or Medicaid, as well as through long-term care services and support programs, and long-term care insurance. Most long-term care insurance policies provide respite options. Medicare generally only covers limited respite care for patients enrolled in hospice services. For private pay, some respite programs offer sliding scale payment schedules and others prorate their monthly fee to the duration of time the individual is receiving respite services. Respite care provides a necessary break for informal caregivers to address their own personal needs, such as medical care, recovery from injury, travel to important family events, or simply to prevent burnout.

13.4 How to Assess the Level of Care Needed

Knowing when to hire caregivers or to move into a "higher level of care" and which level to move to is one of the hardest decisions older adults and their families must make. Home-based medical providers can play a vital role in evaluating and counseling patients and families when it is no longer safe to live at home. An individual's capacity to live at home can be evaluated through formal clinical assessments, as well as common-sense checklists available to the public via online web resources.

13.4.1 Kohlman Evaluation of Living Skills

Kohlman Evaluation of Living Skills (KELS) is an occupational therapy evaluation that has been shown to be an effective predictor of one's ability to live safely and independently in the community. Providers can request occupational therapy for KELS as part of a Medicare-approved Home Health care plan. The evaluation is more useful than simply assessing an adult's function with ADLs and IADLs [33, 34]. KELS evaluates an adult's living skills in areas of self-care, safety, health, money management, transportation, telephone, work, and leisure. KELS can be inaccurate for individuals with visual impairment or who grew up in another country with a different cultural background.

13.4.2 Functional Assessment

Any clinician practicing home-based medical care should be skilled in the thorough assessment of a patient's functional status. While it may not be as comprehensive as a formal comprehensive geriatric assessment or KELS, it can provide the clinician, the patient, and family with key information about the general areas of support someone needs to remain functionally and safely in his or her home.

As discussed in Chapter 4, the functional assessment includes ADLs: bathing, toileting, dressing, grooming, and transferring/mobility; and IADLs: food preparation, housekeeping, transportation, medication management, finances, and telephone use. Any impairment in these functional domains should warrant a discussion with the patient and family on how to assist the patient with identified deficits to enable the patient to remain at home. This could include nonpersonnel options such as monthly delivery of pre-filled pill packs, automatic bill-pay, home delivered meals, laundry service, and community transportation services. Alternatively, this could include personnel options ranging from family members taking over finances, medication management, and cooking to hired housekeepers, companions, or caregivers in the home.

13.4.3 Online Checklists

Several web-based resources provide free online "checklists" for families to have a systematic way in which they can assess a loved one's needs. These checklists are a valuable tool to aid in decision making regarding the safety and feasibility of an older adult remaining at home. The tools are easily accessible and educate caregivers how to identify practical and actionable issues.

Family Caregiver Alliance's website, www.caregiver.org, suggests families and caregivers consider not only ADL and IADL needs of the patient, but also three other domains: health care, emotional care, and supervision. If an individual does not have a preceding Advance Health Care Directive or Power of Attorney for Health, it is critical to establish one before she or he loses capacity. Emotional care is as important to patients' well-being as functional support. Isolation and loneliness have a significant impact on depression, wellness, and mortality. Caregivers must consider how to provide companionship, conversation, social engagement, and meaningful activities. Finally, for individuals with dementia, 24/7 supervisory care is essential if there is risk of wandering or home hazards, such as forgetting to turn off stoves or water faucets, even if the individual remains independent with his or her ADLs [35].

The web resource, www.caring.com, provides a useful guide to families and caregivers who want to know when the time has come to move a loved one to a more supportive environment such as an RCFE. The guide has an 11-category checklist of observable signs that suggest the individual needs more help:
https://www.caring.com/articles/moving-out-relative-question.

13.5 Caregiver Education

13.5.1 How to Interact with Caregivers in the Home

Home-based medical providers play a critical role in the education of patients and caregivers. There are several best practices to keep in mind in this educator role.

13.5.1.1 Setting the Stage

- The clinician should always address the patient first.
- Distinguish between the hands-on caregiver and the legal surrogate decision-maker, who may not always know how the patient is doing day to day.
- Be clear in communication when you are seeking collateral history from a caregiver and when you need to discuss decision making with the legal surrogate.
- If the patient has cognitive impairment or is severely hearing impaired such that direct interview is difficult, set the stage by first addressing the patient, and then by explaining that you will be asking his/her caregiver some questions as well.
- If needed, reserve time to speak to the caregiver in private away from the patient for sensitive history, e.g., the patient has paranoia, disinhibited sexual behaviors, violent aggression, depression, or other concerns.
- Always be explicit that the purpose of the visit is health care delivery and not a social visit.

13.5.1.2 Interacting with Caregivers: Key Language and Techniques

When greeting a patient who has a caregiver, even if the caregiver is the more reliable informant, always greet and acknowledge the patient. Let him/her know you will be asking the caregiver questions or ask him/her for permission to speak to the caregiver. For example:

- *Hi Mr. Smith (patient), I'm here to follow up on your leg pain. I'll be asking Ms. Jones (caregiver), some questions about how you're doing as well.*

You may ask the caregiver for time to meet with the patient alone, if needed. For example:

- *I like to have some time to meet with my patients privately just as I would in clinic. Do you mind going upstairs to another room while I speak with Mr. Smith? I'll call you back in when we're done.*

Home visits also provide an excellent opportunity to assess the caregivers' skills and knowledge with caregiving. Clinicians can provide in person education and feedback. For example:

- *Can you show me how you assist him in bed? How do your organize and give his medications? Can you assist me in rolling him to his side so I can examine his back?*

Listening and observation are critical to understand the caregivers' challenges and educational needs. Clinicians should:

- Validate the challenges of the caregiver role and give encouragement and "permission" for them to ask for help

- Encourage caregivers to take time for self-care
- Provide anticipatory guidance regarding disease progression

13.5.1.3 Addressing Barriers to Communication

- Ensure televisions and radios are turned off or muted during visits.
- Use the quietest room available with privacy, including closed door and windows with curtains that can be drawn.
- Use in-person contract interpreters, if financially possible for the practice, or telephone-interpreters for non-English speaking patients/caregivers. This avoids miscommunications that can occur when using family or informal caregivers to interpret.
- If caregivers only work certain hours, try to arrange home visits during the time that the caregiver is present for the most reliable in-person collateral history.
- If more than one caregiver rotates through the week, recommend that all caregivers make notes in a log to share key events and changes in condition, such as appetite, sleep patterns, urination and bowel movements, and falls, with each other and with the health care team.

13.5.1.4 Care Plan and Directions

Unless a portable printer is available, clinicians should be sure that key instructions for patients/caregivers/facility staff are clearly written down before leaving, especially if there is more than one caregiver but only one is present during the visit. RCFEs always require written or printed and signed orders for any care plan changes. Clinicians should provide caregivers with "levels of urgency" and red flag instructions for when to call the practice for phone advice and when, if within a patient's goals of care, calling 911 and emergency care are appropriate. When caregiver education is required and if home health nursing is not involved, clinicians can consider rotating days and times of visits in order to interface with other caregivers. This allows the clinician to obtain additional collateral and provide education and support to other caregivers. Family care plan meetings are often more easily arranged in the home than in clinic and hospital settings. Home-based medical providers can make use of this valuable forum to have meetings to establish goals of care or educate multiple caregivers or family members at once.

13.5.2 Educational Needs of Caregivers

The majority of informal caregivers receive no training on how to provide care. Eighty-one percent of caregivers feel inadequately trained for the tasks that they perform and have never received any formal education in caregiving [36]. They are expected to provide care for a complex adult with many needs with minimal to no instruction. Caregivers often feel overwhelmed and unsure about how to assist an adult, usually a spouse or parent, with ADLs or how to manage behaviors in dementia. Some caregivers simply learn through trial and error or from informal interaction with social contacts.

13.5.3 Educational Resources for Caregivers

Home-based medical clinicians are a valuable educational resource for the caregiver and can provide guidance regarding disease specific issues and behavioral management. They also can give insight, information, and anticipatory guidance about the patient's medical condition. During the medical encounter at home, clinicians can evaluate the caregiver–patient dynamic in the context of the home, assess home safety, provide counseling regarding behavioral management, and give suggestions based on their observations of the caregiver and patient at home.

Clinicians may involve other skilled professionals for education. Skilled home care is covered by most health insurances, including Medicare. Physical and occupational therapists assess the safety of the home environment and functional status of the patient. They may provide recommendations regarding environmental modifications, durable medical equipment needs, and mobility and exercise. In addition to addressing speech difficulties or dysphagia, many speech therapists perform cognitive rehabilitation and discuss ways to more effectively engage patients. Registered nursing may help with medication management, educating caregivers on how to assist with ADLs, and symptom monitoring. Pharmacists provide medication counseling and some provide prefilled medisets or blister packs. Finally, social workers (e.g., a Home Health social worker if a clinical practice social worker or community social worker is not available) can refer individuals to resources, such as respite care, transportation services, support groups, adult day programs, and higher levels of care, such as RCFEs. Development of an ADL impairment due to illness or physical or cognitive decline can qualify a patient for skilled home care. Home nurses, physical therapists, and occupational therapists can educate caregivers on how to assist a patient with ADLs.

In many communities, there are growing independent or franchise services which provide free or low-cost guidance to patients and families on choosing caregiver agencies or finding an appropriate RCFE. These range from national web resources to more personalized local services that conduct in-person patient evaluations and interviews. These services receive a placement fee from RCFEs for a successful match between a patient and facility. Clinicians may want to evaluate or meet with local franchise services to vet their commitment to patients and families and their track record for successful placements before recommending a particular local service.

Private pay services are also available, though perhaps not in all locations nationwide. Patients or families may pay for a private geriatric consultation, geriatric care manager (www.caremanager.org), or dementia behavioral specialist. Though not covered by Medicare, these consultants can help with care coordination and challenges with behavior management. Generally, the goal of these case managers is to minimize healthcare costs while optimizing function, independence, and communication.

13.6 Resources for the Caregiver

Access to education and support is essential for caregivers. Clinicians should provide education, but can also direct caregivers to national and local organizations for additional support and information. Importantly, clinicians should give caregivers "permission" to ask for help and validate the challenges of caregiving. Most caregivers receive the majority of support informally from families and social networks. Caregivers may benefit from increased social support, skills education regarding caregiving tasks, and assistance with coping. Many national organizations have online websites, with resources and educational materials for caregivers, as well as links to local chapters (discussed below).

13.6.1 National Organizations

National caregiver support organizations, such as the Alzheimer's Association and Family Caregiver Alliance, are an excellent resource for caregivers. These organizations, in addition to the others listed below, have websites that provide online educational materials about caregiving, dementia, and other chronic illnesses. In addition, national organizations can connect caregivers to local chapters and resources, such as respite care.

- Alzheimer's Association: http://www.alz.org
- National Family Caregiver Support Program: A national program funded by the Administration on Aging: http://www.aoa.gov
- Family Caregiver Alliance, National Center on Caregiving: www.caregiver.org
- AARP Caregiving Resource Center: www.aarp.org
- www.eldercare.gov

13.6.2 Support Groups

National organizations such as the Alzheimer's Association and National Family Caregiver Support program have local chapters and in-person and online support groups for caregivers. Support groups are also sometimes available through different health systems. Groups may be run by peers or professionals and provide a venue for caregivers to discuss shared experiences, learn skills and techniques about caregiving, develop more effective coping strategies, and foster camaraderie. These groups are effective at educating and increasing social networks and satisfaction with groups is usually high [15].

13.6.3 Counseling, Education, and Skills Training

Individual or group counseling led by a professional can be effective at addressing psychological concerns, such as anxiety or depression. Caregivers work with a practitioner to develop skills and techniques, such as through cognitive behavioral therapy, to address mental health issues and coping strategies [24]. Clinicians can provide trainings and education to increase caregiver knowledge [37].

As discussed previously, clinicians may refer patients to skilled home care services, including physical therapy, occupational therapy, speech therapy, registered nursing, and social work. These home care professionals can help to address a variety of caregiver needs.

13.6.4 Online Articles

Written for clinicians, these articles are available publicly online and include an overview about caring for caregivers. In addition, the articles include a handout for caregivers, as well as lists of additional online resources.

- Collins LG, Swartz K. Caregiver care. Am Fam Physician. 2011;83 (11): 1309–17.
- Parks SM, Novielli KD. A practical guide to caring for caregivers. Am Fam Physician. 2000;62 (12):2613–22.

References

1. National Alliance for Caregiving (NAC) in collaboration with AARP. Caregiving in the US. Funded by MetLife Foundation. Nov 2009.
2. Anderson LA, Edwards VJ, Pearson WS, Talley RC, McGuire LC, Andresen EM. Adult caregivers in the United States: characteristics and differences in well-being, by caregiver age and caregiving status. Prev Chronic Dis. 2013;10, E135.
3. Talley RC, Crews JE. Framing the public health of caregiving. Am J Public Health. 2007; 97(2):224–8.
4. Feinberg L, Reinhard SC, Houser A, Choula R. Valuing the invaluable: 2011 update, the growing contributions and cost of family caregiving. AARP Public Policy Institute; 2011.
5. Senior Care Cost Index 2014, based on family caregiver usage & attitudes survey [Internet]. 2014 [cited 2014 Dec 24]. Available from: http://www.caring.com/static/senior_care_cost_index_2014.pdf
6. National Alliance for Caregiving (NAC) and Evercare. Family caregivers: what they spend, what they sacrifice; The personal financial toll of caring for a loved one. Minnetonka, MN/ Bethesda: Evercare/NAC; 2007.
7. Kaye HS, Harrington C, LaPlante MP. Long-term care: who gets it, who provides it, who pays, and how much? Health Aff (Millwood). 2010;29(1):11–21.
8. Ory MG, Hoffman RR, Yee JL, Tennstedt S, Schulz R. Prevalence and impact of caregiving: a detailed comparison between dementia and nondementia caregivers. Gerontologist. 1999; 39(2):177–85.

9. Parks SM, Novielli KD. A practical guide to caring for caregivers. Am Fam Physician. 2000;62(12):2613–22.

10. Kamiya M, Sakurai T, Ogama N, Maki Y, Toba K. Factors associated with increased caregivers' burden in several cognitive stages of Alzheimer's disease. Geriatr Gerontol Int. 2014;14 Suppl 2:45–55.

11. Haro JM, Kahle-Wrobleski K, Bruno G, Belger M, Dell'Agnello G, Dodel R, et al. Analysis of burden in caregivers of people with Alzheimer's disease using self-report and supervision hours. J Nutr Health Aging. 2014;18(7):677–84.

12. Shankar KN, Hirschman KB, Hanlon AL, Naylor MD. Burden in caregivers of cognitively impaired elderly adults at time of hospitalization: a cross-sectional analysis. J Am Geriatr Soc. 2014;62(2):276–84.

13. Collins LG, Swartz K. Caregiver care. Am Fam Physician. 2011;83(11):1309–17.

14. Snyder CM, Fauth E, Wanzek J, Piercy KW, Norton MC, Corcoran C, et al. Dementia caregivers' coping strategies and their relationship to health and well-being: the Cache County Study. Aging Ment Health. 2014;19:390–9.

15. Connell CM, Janevic MR, Gallant MP. The costs of caring: impact of dementia on family caregivers. J Geriatr Psychiatry Neurol. 2001;14(4):179–87.

16. Covinsky KE, Newcomer R, Fox P, Wood J, Sands L, Dane K, et al. Patient and caregiver characteristics associated with depression in caregivers of patients with dementia. J Gen Intern Med. 2003;18(12):1006–14.

17. Lachs MS, Pillemer K. Elder abuse. Lancet. 2004;364(9441):1263–72.

18. Hoover RM, Polson M. Detecting elder abuse and neglect: assessment and intervention. Am Fam Physician. 2014;89(6):453–60.

19. Schulz R, Beach SR. Caregiving as a risk factor for mortality: the Caregiver Health Effects Study. JAMA. 1999;282(23):2215–9.

20. Zarit SH, Reever KE, Bach-Peterson J. Relatives of the impaired elderly: correlates of feelings of burden. Gerontologist. 1980;20(6):649–55.

21. Bédard M, Molloy DW, Squire L, Dubois S, Lever JA, O'Donnell M. The Zarit Burden Interview: a new short version and screening version. Gerontologist. 2001;41(5):652–7.

22. Bourgeois MS, Schulz R, Burgio L. Interventions for caregivers of patients with Alzheimer's disease: a review and analysis of content, process, and outcomes. Int J Aging Hum Dev. 1996;43(1):35–92.

23. Andrén S, Elmståhl S. Effective psychosocial intervention for family caregivers lengthens time elapsed before nursing home placement of individuals with dementia: a five-year follow-up study. Int Psychogeriatr. 2008;20(6):1177–92.

24. Chang BL. Cognitive-behavioral intervention for homebound caregivers of persons with dementia. Nurs Res. 1999;48(3):173–82.

25. Kneebone II, Martin PR. Coping and caregivers of people with dementia. Br J Health Psychol. 2003;8(Pt 1):1–17.

26. Melis RJ, van Eijken MI, van Achterberg T, et al. The effect on caregiver burden of a problem-based home visiting programme for frail older people. Age Ageing. 2009;38(5):542–7.

27. Yaffe MJ, Wolfson C, Lithwick M, Weiss D. Development and validation of a tool to improve physician identification of elder abuse: the Elder Abuse Suspicion Index (EASI). J Elder Abuse Negl. 2008;20(3):276–300.

28. The MetLife Mature Market Institute, National Adult Day Services Association (NADSA), The Ohio State University College of Social Work. The MetLife national study of adult day services: providing support to individuals and their family caregivers. New York: MetLife Mature Market Institute; 2010.

29. John Hancock National Study Finds Long-Term Care Costs Continue to Climb Across All Provider Options [Internet]. 2013 [updated 30 July 2013, cited 30 Nov 2014]. Available from: http://www.johnhancock.com/about/news_details.php?fn=jul3013-text&yr=2013

30. About Continuing Care Retirement Communities [Internet]. 2010 [updated 2010 Sept, cited 2014 Nov 30]. Available from: http://www.aarp.org/relationships/caregiving-resource-center/info-09 -2010/ho_continuing_care_retirement_communities.html

31. Matthews JL. How to pay for in-home care [Internet]. 2014 [cited 30 Nov 2014]. Available from: https://www.caring.com/articles/how-to-pay-for-in-home-care
32. Why You Should Use a Caregiver Agreement [Internet]. 2014 [updated 14 Feb 2014, cited 21 Dec 2014]. Available from: http://www.elderlawetn.com/02/caregiver-agreement/
33. Naik AD, Burnett J, Pickens-Pace S, Dyer CB. Impairment in instrumental activities of daily living and the geriatric syndrome of self-neglect. Gerontologist. 2008;48(3):388–93.
34. Burnett J, Dyer CB, Naik AD. Convergent validation of the Kohlman Evaluation of Living Skills as a screening tool of older adults' ability to live safely and independently in the community. Arch Phys Med Rehabil. 2009;90(11):1948–52.
35. Family Caregiver Alliance (FCA) and National Center on Caregiving. Caring for adults with cognitive and memory impairment [cited 13 Dec 2014]. Available from https://caregiver.org/caring-adults-cognitive-and-memory-impairment
36. The National Center on Caregiving at Family Caregiver Alliance. Caregiving: state of the art, future trends. Chicago: The American Society on Aging; 2007. March 6, 2007.
37. Coen RF, O'Boyle CA, Coakley D, Lawlor BA. Dementia carer education and patient behaviour disturbance. Int J Geriatr Psychiatry. 1999;14(4):302–6.

Index

A
Abuse. *See also* Elder abuse
  and neglect, 243, 276
  patient safety, 145–146
Accountable care organizations, 14, 17, 24
Activities of daily living (ADL), 62, 75, 82,
  270, 283, 286
AD. *See* Alzheimer's dementia (AD)
Adult day care centers, 44
Adult Protective Services (APS), 239, 244
Advance Beneficiary Notice (ABN), 24
Affordable Care Act (ACA), 18
Alzheimer's dementia (AD)
  epidemiology, 76
  pharmacologic treatment, 82–83
  prognosis, 88
  risk factors, 76
Amyotrophic lateral sclerosis (ALS), 119
  general management, 120
  referral to hospice, 122
  symptomatic treatments, 121
  symptom management, 121
Area agency on aging (AAA), 30
Arterial ulcer
  etiology and risk factors, 224–226
  of medial foot, 225
  signs and symptoms, 224–226
Arterial wound management, 226–228
Asymptomatic bacteriuria (ASB), 175
Autolytic debridement, 209
Autonomic dysfunction, 107

B
Bacterial colonization, 211
Behavioral and psychotic symptoms of
  dementia (BPSD)
  adult psychiatric care, 142–144
  management, 86–88

nonpharmacologic approach, 83
pharmacological treatment, 83, 84
Botulinum toxin (BoNT), 110
Bowel dysfunction, 118
BPSD. *See* Behavioral and psychotic
  symptoms of dementia (BPSD)

C
Caregiver
  abuse and neglect, 276–277
  assessment, 273–275
  burden
    impact of, 272–273
    incidence and risk factors, 271–272
  counseling, education, and skills training, 288
  economic impact, 270
  functional assessment, 282–283
  interaction
    addressing barriers to
      communication, 285
    care plan and directions, 285
    educational needs, 285–286
    educational resources, 286–287
    key language and techniques, 284
    stages, 284
  levels of care
    Continuing care retirement
      communities (CCRC), 280–281
    in-home caregiving, 278–279, 281
    private home, 277
    Residential care facilities for the elderly
      (RCFE), 280
    respite care, 281–282
    Senior Centers and Adult Day
      Programs, 277–279
  national organizations, 287
  online articles, 288
  online checklists, 283

Printed in the United States
By Bookmasters